BIRKHÄUSER

Birkhäuser Advances in Infectious Diseases

BAID

Series Editors

Advisory Board

Common Cold

Ronald Eccles
Olaf Weber

Editors

Birkhäuser
Basel · Boston · Berlin

Editors

Ronald Eccles
Common Cold Centre
Cardiff School of Biosciences
Cardiff University
Museum Avenue
Cardiff CF10 3AX
UK

Olaf Weber
Rheinische Friedrich-Wilhelms-Universität
Institute of Molecular Medicine
and Experimental Immunology
Sigmund-Freud-Straße 25
53105 Bonn
Germany

Library of Congress Control Number: 2009928444

Bibliographic information published by Die Deutsche Bibliothek
Die Deutsche Bibliothek lists this publication in the Deutsche Nationalbibliografie; detailed bibliographic data is available in the internet at http://dnb.ddb.de

ISBN 978-3-7643-9894-1 Birkhäuser Verlag, Basel - Boston - Berlin

Part of Springer Science+Business Media
Printed on acid-free paper produced from chlorine-free pulp. TFC ∞
Cover illustration: see p. 198; with friendly permission of Elizabeth Pappas
Printed in Germany
ISBN 978-3-7643-9894-1
9 8 7 6 5 4 3 2 1

e-ISBN 978-3-7643-9912-2
www. birkhauser.ch

Contents

List of contributors

Katherine E. Arden, Queensland Paediatric Infectious Diseases Laboratory, Sir Albert Sakzewski Virus Research Centre, Royal Children's Hospital, Brisbane, Australia and Clinical Medical Virology Centre, University of Queensland, Brisbane, Australia

Bruce Arroll, Department of General Practice and Primary Health Care, Tamaki Campus, University of Auckland, Private Bag 92019, Auckland 1142, New Zealand

Isabel Atzl, Berliner Medizinhistorisches Museum der Charité, Charitéplatz 1, 10117 Berlin, Germany; e-mail: isabel@atzl.info

Sheldon Cohen, Department of Psychology, Carnegie Mellon University, Pittsburgh, PA 15213, USA

Chris Del Mar, Dean, Faculty of Health Sciences and Medicine, Bond University, Gold Coast, QLD 4229, Australia; e-mail: cdelmar@bond.edu.au

William J. Doyle, Department of Otolaryngology, University of Pittsburgh, 3000 Mt Royal Blvd, Glenshaw PA 15116, USA; e-mail: docdoyle2@aol.com

Ronald Eccles, Common Cold Centre, Cardiff School of Biosciences, Cardiff University, Museum Avenue, Cardiff CF10 3AX, UK; e-mail: eccles@cardiff.ac.uk

Alex J. Elliot, Real-Time Syndromic Surveillance Team, Health Protection Agency, 6th Floor, 5 St Philips Place, Birmingham B3 2PW, UK; e-mail: alex.elliot@hpa.org.uk

Douglas M. Fleming, Royal College of General Practitioners Research and Surveillance Centre, Lordswood House, 54 Lordswood Road, Harborne, Birmingham B17 9DB, UK

Roland Helms, Berliner Medizinhistorisches Museum der Charité, Charitéplatz 1, 10117 Berlin, Germany; e-mail: rohebe@online.de

Harri Hemilä, Department of Public Health, University of Helsinki, Helsinki, FIN-00014, Finland; e-mail: harri.hemila@helsinki.fi

J. Owen Hendley, University of Virginia Department of Pediatrics, Charlottesville, VA 22908, USA

Tom Jefferson, Cochrane Acute Respiratory Infections Group, Via Adige 28a, Anguillara Sabazia, Roma, Italy, 00061; e-mail: jefferson.tom@gmail.com

Timothy W. Kenealy, Department of General Practice and Primary Health Care, Tamaki Campus, University of Auckland, Private Bag 92019, Auckland 1142, New Zealand; e-mail: t.kenealy@auckland.ac.nz,

Stephen B. Lambert, Queensland Paediatric Infectious Diseases Laboratory, Sir Albert Sakzewski Virus Research Centre, Royal Children's Hospital, Brisbane, Australia and Clinical Medical Virology Centre, University of Queensland, Brisbane, Australia; e-mail: sblambert@uq.edu.au

Ian M. Mackay, Queensland Paediatric Infectious Diseases Laboratory, Sir Albert Sakzewski Virus Research Centre, Royal Children's Hospital, Brisbane, Australia and Clinical Medical Virology Centre, University of Queensland, Brisbane, Australia

Florin Mihail, Am Ringofen 7, 42327 Wuppertal, Germany; e-mail: f.mihail@gmx.de

Sherif Beniameen Mossad, Department of Infectious Diseases, Section of Transplant Infectious Diseases, Medicine Institute, Cleveland Clinic, 9500 Euclid Avenue, S-32, Cleveland, OH 44195, USA; e-mail: mossads@ccf.org

Diane E. Pappas, Box 800386, University of Virginia Department of Pediatrics, Charlottesville, VA 22908, USA; e-mail: dep6b@virginia.edu

Mieke van Driel, Faculty of Health Sciences and Medicine, Bond University, Gold Coast, QLD 4229, Australia; e-mail: mvandrie@bond.edu.au

Olaf Weber, Rheinische Friedrich-Wilhelms-Universität, Institute of Molecular Medicine and Experimental Immunology, Sigmund-Freud-Straße 25, 53105 Bonn, Germany

Preface

The common cold is unlike any other human disease because of two factors: firstly, it is arguably the most common human disease and, secondly, it is one of the most complex diseases because of the number of viruses that cause the familiar syndrome of sneezing, sore throat, runny nose and nasal congestion. These two factors have made a 'cure' for the common cold one of the most difficult scientific and clinical endeavours (a topic often discussed in the popular media, where comparisons are made with the ease of putting a man on the moon). The present book brings together a wide range of experts from epidemiologists to virologists and pharmacologists to look at recent advances in our knowledge of the common cold. In some respects the book is unique, as it focuses on the common cold, a syndrome so familiar to the layperson but one that receives little attention from the scientist and clinician. The common cold can be viewed from many different aspects as illustrated in Figure 1.

The core knowledge for understanding the common cold must first come from virology and this is discussed in several chapters of the book. There have been major advances in this field because of the use of new methods of detecting viruses such as polymerase chain reaction techniques that have greatly aided our understanding of the epidemiology of viruses associated with common cold. The complexity of rhinovirus infection and epidemiol-

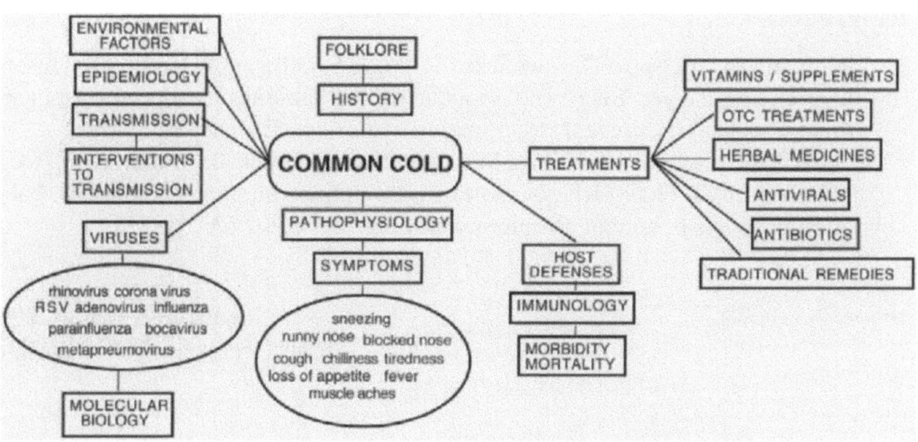

Figure 1. Areas of research and interest that contribute to our understanding of the common cold.

ogy, which is already a complex area because of the large number of rhinoviruses, is now further increased by the co-detection of viruses in any one subject and the fact that the evolution of rhinoviruses is complicated by genome recombination, which may lead to unique strains that may have distinct biological properties and clinical characteristics [1].

Recent research indicates that secondary bacterial infections associated with common cold viruses may be enhanced by rhinovirus infection [2] and this advance in our knowledge of the significance of common cold and morbidity is discussed in the book.

There is a great deal of information in this book on the treatment of common cold by a wide range of medicines, from over the counter medicines to a very wide range of alternative therapies. However, the large number of treatments for common cold in some respect indicates the relative lack of success in treating this common ailment; the large number of viruses involved in common cold makes it difficult to develop any vaccine or specific antiviral therapy.

As in the past, people today have accepted the common cold as something that inevitably happens. However, complications of what starts as a common upper respiratory tract infection frequently occur and pose a serious threat to those patients who are the most vulnerable, such as infants, the elderly or generally immunosuppressed people. In addition, there is a great economic impact of common cold because of the large number of consultations to general medical practice. Therefore, there is need to improve the current standards of treatment for the common cold.

The present book covers the different areas of research related to common cold and brings the reader not only an overview of the common cold but also focuses on recent advances in each area.

References

1 Palmenberg AC, Spiro D, Kuzmickas R, Wang S, Djikeng A, Rathe JA, Fraser-Liggett CM, Liggett SB (2009) Sequencing and analyses of all known human rhinovirus genomes reveal structure and evolution. *Science* 324: 55–59

2 Oliver BG, Lim S, Wark P, Laza-Stanca V, King N, Black JL, Burgess JK, Roth M, Johnston SL (2008) Rhinovirus exposure impairs immune responses to bacterial products in human alveolar macrophages. *Thorax* 63: 519–525

Cardiff and Bonn 2009
Ron Eccles and Olaf Weber

Common Cold
ed. by R. Eccles and O. Weber

A short history of the common cold

Isabel Atzl and Roland Helms

Berliner Medizinhistorisches Museum der Charité, Charitéplatz 1, 10117 Berlin, Germany

Abstract

A tickling in the nose, frequent sneezing, chills and a runny nose, followed by a scratchy throat, fatigue, a light headache and lots of thick mucus. Who does not know these symptoms of the classic common cold? For about 50 years, we have known the culprits to be rhinoviruses or other subgroups of the so-called picornaviruses, which lead to short-lived infections in the mucus membranes of the nose, throat and sometimes the bronchial tubes. If we look at the history of mankind and its illnesses, then the 50 years of certain knowledge about the cause of the cold make the discovery seem quite recent. This article offers insight into the history of medicine and examines the evidence – usually hidden – for the cold in various epochs and cultures. Between intuition and surprisingly exact descriptions from the past, sometimes with a blink of the eye, the focus is trained on the nose and the mucus accumulating there, in order to find out how the cold's appearance was construed. Therapeutic recommendations have ranged from black cumin to cauterizing irons to snuff. Sometimes the suggestions are completely foreign, yet at times they appear surprisingly modern, although ancient in origin.

Stone slabs and herbal arrows: Pre and early history

We know practically nothing about the medical ideas of Stone Age humans. How illness was understood, and how precisely it was treated, are things we can mostly only speculate about. Paleopathologists attempt, on the basis of changes in preserved bones, to draw conclusions about diseases that left traces between 5000 and 10000 years ago on the human skeleton. In this category are, for example, degenerative changes or the results of dietary deficiencies, such as rickets. Everything else is conjecture. Nothing certain is known about colds in the Stone Age.

Despite our lack of specific knowledge, we can be relatively sure that colds existed at that time. Once humans started living in large families and village-like communities, the ground was laid for the cold to spread, because where people live close together, colds thrive.

Many areas of life in the Stone Age were associated with the magical-mystical. The cycle of the seasons, success at hunting or the reason for an illness were attributed to a greater power that determined the lives of humans. Humans secured the favor and advocacy of this power through magical rites. Religious acts are therefore difficult to distinguish from medical ones and findings from this time period are not easy to interpret. It has been proven, however, that trepanation – the making of a hole or drilling in the skull – was performed on the living. Yet whether they intended to make an opening for the spirit of the disease to leave the body or they did it to relieve a person's headache has to remain speculation. It does not seem outside the realm of possibility that they also considered the head as the seat of a cold [1]. But whether they opened the head speedily on that account remains completely uncertain.

Since the earliest times, healing plants have been used to cure illnesses. The findings and observations from the corpse of the man from Hauslabjoch, better known as Ötzi, provide one source. Ötzi was carrying birch bracket, a polyporous bracket fungus, with him that possibly served as medicine [2]. Next to that – and here we find the magical mythical component – was a stone slab that has been interpreted as an amulet to ward off evil spirits. Tattoos on his skin pose a riddle. They can be seen as therapeutic manipulations, in which healing plants were impregnated in the skin. The marks on Ötzi's body are found, interestingly enough, at the meridian points that are commonly used today in acupuncture for the illnesses with which he has been diagnosed by western medicine [3].

But whether Ötzi had a cold or even knew of one, how he understood a cold or treated it lies in the realm of speculation.

Needles and burning: China

Acupuncture, moxibustion (the burning of healing plants on acupuncture points) and phytotherapy are the preferred practices in the therapeutic arsenal of Chinese doctors. They are applied when the flow of Qi, or life energy in the body, is blocked or when the opposing forces of Yin and Yang are out of balance.

Chinese healing approaches sickness and its therapy in a completely different way from western medicine [4]. The guiding idea postulates a close connection between humans and nature. The world is ordered according to a complex and dynamic system of opposites and dualities. The best known element of the medicine of dualities is the tenet of yin (the shady side of the hill) and yang (the sunny side of the hill). During the first millennium B.C., a system of diverse, dualistic categories developed and expanded to include many other phenomena of life, such as darkness – sunshine, female principle – male principle, cold – heat, wet – dry. Later, correspondences between certain natural phenomena and human organs were established.

The fixed pairs, water – kidneys, wood – liver, fire – heart, earth – spleen, metal – lungs, provided orientation for medical treatments for prevention and healing.

A well-developed pharmacy developed very early, whose creator is said to have been the mythical emperor Shen-nong (ca. 3000 B.C.). His pharmaceutical writings, called *Pen-ts'ao king* were probably collected into a book by unknown authors about the time of the birth of Christ. The work includes 347 products from the animal, vegetable and mineral kingdoms. Chinese pharmacy groups these in high, middle and low remedies. The higher medicines like ginseng root and magnolia fruit are never poisonous, should enhance life and delay getting older. The middle substances are sometimes poisonous and can provoke a reaction. They are meant to serve the principle of life and to remove deficiencies. Belonging to this group are, among others, parts of the plant *Ephedra sinica*. Specific diseases are treated with low remedies, frequently very effective, such as rhubarb root for constipation.

The essential work of traditional Chinese medicine is ascribed to another mythical emperor, Huang-ti (mid 3rd millennium B.C.) [5]. The *Nei-king*, originating between the 5th and 3rd centuries B.C., is divided into a part on fundamentals about anatomy, physiology, pathology and therapy as well as a section concerning acupuncture. Classical acupuncture is also based on the yin-yang system. The fleshy organs – the heart, lungs, spleen, liver and kidneys – are assigned to the principle of yin; correspondingly, the hollow organs – the stomach, gall bladder, intestines, urinary bladder and the 'three warmer', which is not clearly localized – are ascribed to yang. Special pulse and acupuncture points are accorded to each of these organs that together make up individual meridians or channels in the body. Each meridian has six different function points (stimulating, calming, regulating, strengthening, alarming, meridian crossing) that simultaneously serve in the diagnosis of the pulse and the therapeutic intervention of the physician. Treatment with needles has a calming effect on yang and burning herbs (moxibustion) a stimulating effect on yin.

Healthy people have a balance between light, dynamic yang energy and dark, quiet yin energy. External causes, such as the wrong diet, cold, wind or strong emotions can disturb this balance. For millennia, traditional Chinese medicine has believed that a cold is an illness of 'wind and cold' [6]. Wind and cold enter the body through the pores of the skin and penetrate deeper depending on the constitution of the individual and progress through various stages of development there. In vivid terms, it is said that the cold that has attacked the body's surface (chills at the beginning of a cold) becomes heat in the deeper layers of the body. If the body also protects itself by closing all the pores, then the cold can not leave the body. Fever results.

In addition to 'wind-cold' with symptoms like severe chills, low fever, neck pain, no sweating (dry skin), 'wind-heat' (few chills, more fever, noticeable sore throat, slightly moist skin, pulsing headache) as well as various influences of moisture and dryness can also be diagnosed. Chinese medicine therefore does not treat every cold the same way. It must also be established precisely in which stage of the cold a patient is. The physician must ask questions, examine the tongue and diagnose the pulse before deciding which kind of therapy is optimal for the patient. The goal of treatment is the 'opening' of the surface and the expulsion of the factors causing the illness. Acupuncture (primarily along the intestinal meridian), moxibustion or the administering of healing plants (foods that are spicy, heat and therefore sweat producing, such as garlic, ginger and herbal infusions) can all serve this aim.

Lead and honey: Egypt

From the 3rd to the 1st millennium B.C. the old empire of the Egyptians blossomed in the eastern part of the Mediterranean area. The Valley of the Kings and the pyramids are still witnesses today of the highly developed technology of this culture. Medicine and healing also flourished under the pharaohs. Physicians, serving the upper class and the public concerns for which they were commissioned, usually specialized in one part of the body and its diseases, so that the Greek historian Herodotus could report in the 5th century B.C.: "And the whole country is full of physicians, for some profess themselves to be physicians of the eyes, others of the head, others of the teeth, others of the affections of the stomach, and others of the more obscure aliments" [7].

The Egyptians' medicine was shaped by religion and magic. Thus certain gods, even more so than physicians, were responsible for individual parts of the body. Prayers, magic formulas and the use of amulets had great meaning. But empirical insights also found their way into therapeutic practice.

The Ebers papyrus and the Smith papyrus, both found in the 19th century and named after their discoverers, Georg Ebers (1837–1898) and Edwin Smith (1822–1906), belong to the most important Egyptian medical texts. The Smith papyrus provides information primarily about surgical measures, whereas the Ebers papyrus contains a description of numerous illnesses and suggestions for treatment with hundreds of incantations and formulas for remedies. The Ebers papyrus is considered the oldest medical book still in existence. Its 20-meter length points to its impressive coverage. Dating this document to deduce when these ideas emerged proves difficult. The writing was definitely used in the 16th century B.C. at the time of Pharaoh Amenophis I (ruled 1526–1506 B.C.), as evidenced by several calendar entries on the back. Yet the papyrus was probably written earlier and therefore reflects a much older medical tradition [8].

In addition to 20 different kinds of cough, the cold is also a topic in the Ebers papyrus. The formula for a spell that should drive the cold out of the body reads:

> "Flow out, fetid nose, flow out, son of fetid nose. Flow out, thou breakest bones, destroyest the skull, and makest ill the seven holes of the head" [9].

The milk of a woman who has borne a son or aromatic resin is proposed as therapeutic remedies. The spell must be said four times over these healing items. In order to drive the cold out of the body, it is recommended to spread a mixture of lead, incense and honey on the nose for 4 days. Irrigating the nose with date juice should also bring relief and force the cold out of nose and head.

Humors and medicine: Greco-Roman antiquity

References to the cold become more concrete during the course of Greco-Roman antiquity than was the case in earlier times and in other cultures. In this epoch, for the first time, comprehensive medical concepts are described in detail [10]. The Greek and Roman explanation for disease in the human body is derived primarily from so-called humoral pathology. This theory can be found in the Hippocratic corpus, a collection of medical texts that was generated around the Greek physician Hippocrates of Cos (5th/4th century B.C.), and in the works of the Roman physician Galen (129–199/216 A.D.), who based his insights on the Hippocratic corpus and then expanded this knowledge. The Galenic approach to the body and to illness accompanied western medicine well into the 19th century.

> "The human body contains blood, phlegma, black and yellow bile; Constitution, disease and health depend on them. Men are healthiest, when the mixture is balanced. Sickness occurs if one of the humors remains in great or minor quantity, when they separate from the rest or they are no more combined" [11].

This follows the precise formulation of Hippocrates' idea that the four humors are fundamental to health and sickness. In relation to the cold, mucus or 'phlegma' is the essential substance. Its seat in the body, according to Galen, is the brain:

> "Nature did not create an excreting organ for the phlegma, because it is cold and moist and a kind of half-digested nourishment. Therefore, the substance need not be carried out, it only needs to be changed. ... Perhaps it would be better to say mucin and not phlegma as people often do" [12].

Therefore, mucus in the nose is first and foremost a waste product, created when phlegma in the body is transformed, and not a direct sign for a serious imbalance of the humors.

Mucus is also associated with the season of winter. Hippocrates declared: "Phlegma increases in the human body in winter. It is closest to the nature of winter, because it is the coldest" [13]. The increased presence of mucus in the nose, noticeable several days after a cold begins, would have been interpreted by Galen, however, as a sure sign of sickness.

> "The white-colored substance (the phlegma) collects mostly … in those who have been chilled in some way" [14]. And Hippocrates wrote: "All diseases occur at all seasons of the year, but certain of them are more apt to occur and be exacerbated at certain seasons. – Of winter, pleurisy, pneumonia, coryza, hoarseness, cough, pains of the chest…" [15].

If we take a look at ancient pharmaceutical books, namely the *Materia medica* from Pedanius Dioscorides (1st century A.D.), we find medications that are useful against all kinds of symptoms of a cold: "mustard: … has the power to warm, to dilute, … and eaten to purge phlegm. … If pounded mustard is brought into the nose, it stimulates sneezing" [16]. Furthermore, Dioscorides describes radishes as anti-inflammatory for the throat and a cough, and onion juice mixed with honey – still used today – as helpful in discharging mucus. Sulfur was also considered effective: "It helps against cough and internal ulceration if it is eaten with eggs or applied by smoking. … It is useful against catarrh…" [17].

In addition to Hippocrates, Galen and Dioscorides, there were numerous ancient authors who documented their medical and therapeutic knowledge in writings. Among them, Pliny the Elder (23/24–79 A.D.) and Aulus Cornelius Celsus (1st century A.D.) are the most well known.

The religious aspect carried great weight in medical matters in antiquity. Alongside numerous gods that could be called upon in illness, the central god of healing, Asclepius, was considered accountable especially for cases of protracted sickness. The cold therefore hardly fell within his range of primary responsibility [18].

Medical knowledge and the religious component were passed down in the following centuries partially in the monasteries of the Christian west. The theoretical concept of humoral pathology, however, was transferred above all through the cultural area of the Near East to the rapidly developing Arabic medical world and returned *via* this channel back to Europe in the course of the 12th to the 15th centuries.

Sparks and cauterizing irons: Arabia

Medieval Arabic medicine fed in most cases on ancient authors. Hippocratic or Galenic works lived on through physicians and scholars and at the well-developed medical schools in the Byzantine Empire and in the neighboring Persian Empire of the Sassanids (Gundi-Schapur). The writings of antiquity they used existed in ancient Syrian, Persian or Hebrew translations or in the original Greek. Following Mohammed and his followers' conquests, many texts were translated quickly into Arabic and thus enriched the knowledge of Arabic physicians in Damascus, Bagdad or Cordoba.

Qusta ibn Luqa (ca. 830–ca. 920) of Baalbek considered how infectious diseases came into being: "Contagion is a spark that flies from a sick body to a healthy one, wherein the same illness develops as was in the sick body" [19]. Similar to Galen, he explained the typical development of an infection as the inhalation of "evil vapors", exuded from the body of the sick person, and the subsequent deterioration in the quality of the blood as well as the state of the organs. He did not mention the cold, however, as an infectious disease.

The cold is discussed in Arabic works dedicated primarily to pharmacy and dietetics. Mucolytic measures were advised according to the example of the ancients. A cold was thought to be caused by the cold in winter, but can be offset with appropriate clothing. A summer cold, however, declared the religious philosopher and physician Moses Maimonides (1135–1204) in Cairo, was caused by the seasonal heat that, "melted the hard excretions that are found in the brain and then they run down" [20]. Medicine to solidify the mucus needed to be used against this "acute catarrh", but a hat could also help hinder the liquefying effect of the sun's rays. Maimonides further advised in both cases to take preventive measures. One should avoid foods that "fill the head" such as milk and legumes, as well as alcohol that sedates the brain. Inhaling "aromatic scents of all kinds of spices" should also strengthen the brain's substance. His recommendations ranged from ground cloves to rose perfume [21].

If a cold had already materialized, the Arabic physician drew on the known *Materia medica*. The wealth of Greco-Roman medicinal knowledge had been taken over directly in the translations of Dioscorides and Galen and had been extended by several hundred new drugs. In connection with the cold, one can find, for example, in the *Additions to Dioscorides* by Ibn Gulgul (944–after 994) recommendations like banana for a dry cough, or ambra, a metabolic product from the sperm whale, for "illnesses coming from thick mucus" [22].

If "the brain has been attacked by cold and moisture", Arabic medicine advised the use of surgical measures.

The most well-known writer in the field of surgery is Abu l-Qasim az-Zahrawi (died 1013), born near Cordoba. The 30th book of his medical encyclopedia *Al-Tasrif*, dedicated to surgery, became the standard work for medieval Europe after its translation into Latin in the 12th century.

Abu l-Qasim believed cauterization to be an effective means for treating disease. This process involves destroying tissue with a cauterizing iron or a corrosive chemical. Ancient and medieval medicine used this radical method to burn out wounds, hemorrhoids, abscesses or growths, but also as pain therapy. The Syrian physician Ibn al-Quff (1233–1286) described in his manual for surgeons *Al-Umda fi sina at al-giraha* how one can fight the causes of a cold with the cauterizing iron when dietetic and purgative medicines no longer bring relief:

> "The method of application is as follows: the hair on the head is thoroughly shaven with a razor and the patient seats himself in front of the surgeon with crossed legs, hands on his thighs. Then the surgeon places the palm of his hand on the patient's nose with his fingers between his eyes. He finds the place where the extended middle finger ends on the head and takes his hand away. After this, he heats the olive-shaped cauterizing iron until it glows and cauterizes the aforementioned place and twists the cauterizing iron until the skull (bone) is visible. If the pain is great, he cauterizes a second time until the membrane of the bone (periosteum) appears, so that its substance becomes thin, the pores are opened and the matter can easily flow outward. Then he moistens a strip of cotton wool in water in which salt has been dissolved and places it on the wound for 3 days, changing it twice daily. Then he covers the wound with a strip of cotton wool that has been soaked in fat until the scab has disappeared. Finally, he treats the wound with salves that help form a scar" [23].

When the soul sneezes and the stars blow their nose: The Middle Ages

The warring conflicts during the 5th and 6th centuries in western Europe signified a deep cut in the transmission of medical knowledge. In the sequestered atmosphere of the monasteries, the ancient medical texts were preserved and copied. An active discussion about the meaning of illnesses in the Christian context began: Are they God-given and must therefore be borne, or is it permissible for humans to intervene in the process? Spiritual and physical salvation begins to be seen as intertwined [24].

Folk medicine existed parallel to the Christian interpretation. It was based on an extensive knowledge of herbs, but also drew on magic. Only very few magic formulas against diseases have survived, likewise, folk medicine can hardly be found in written sources. Drawing a connection between sneezing and the presence of the devil (who is tickling someone's nose) or a dark power belongs to this approach to the world. Written sources do not mention this idea until much later, but it appears to be completely plausible for the Middle Ages. Three sources from the early Middle Ages relevant to the history of the cold point to the foundation for the treatment of disease in the framework of monastic medicine. The first is the *Lorsch Pharmacopoeia* from the end of the 8th century that includes copies of numerous parts of ancient medical works as well as many recipes for medications [25]. The second is the 9th century ideal plan for the St. Gallen monastery, showing an herbal garden within the monastic walls, where medicinal herbs were planted [26]. This area was not far from the cells where sick monks were treated. Third, the 9th century poem *Hortulus* by the abbot Walahfried Strabo

(808/9–849) from Reichenau names the plants that were probably planted in his own monastery [27]. Among them are the time-honored salvia, radish and fennel that can be found in antiquity as well as in the pharmacopoeia of later centuries for use against a stuffy nose, cough and infectious illnesses in the nasal and throat area.

The most important woman among the representatives of monastic medicine was the abbess Hildegard von Bingen (1098–1179). Her *Book of Simple Medicine* (*Liber simplicium medicinae* or *Physica*) is a description of the effect of vegetable, animal and mineral healing substances. Hildegard's experiences stem primarily from the flora and fauna of her Rhineland home, especially evident in the plants of the abbey garden. For colds and coughs, she recommended tansy (*Tanacetum vulgare*) in soups, cake or with meat. Inhaling the powder of redstem filaree (*Erodium cicutarium*), Mount Atlas daisy (*Anacyclus pyrethrum*) and nutmeg should also bring relief [28].

Hildegard's theory of illness differed little from ancient humoral pathology. Above all, the *Book of Compound Medicine* (*Liber compositae medicinae* or *Causae et curae*) reflected the abbess's knowledge of Galen's theory of qualities. For her as well, a cold results from a collection of cold, moist substances in the brain that develop into a poison and that must be expelled. In this view, a person is just a reflection of the cosmos, because "the stars in the air also cleanse themselves in this way and the earth also rids itself of certain dirty, foul-smelling substances" [29]. Hildegard even saw in sneezing a self-cleansing mechanism of the body that can be vital: "When the blood in a person's vessels is not lively and quick, but rather lies there as if sleeping, and when his humors do not flow quickly, but sluggishly, the soul notices this of course and jars the whole body with sneezing and lets the person's blood and humors wake again and return to their correct condition. Namely, if water was not held in motion through storms and flooding, it would become putrid; and likewise, a person would also rot internally if he did not sneeze or would not clean his nose through blowing it" [30].

In order to reduce or purge these horrible humors, Hildegard recommended several recipes in her *Book of Compound Medicine*. For example fennel and dill should be heated, the steam inhaled and finally the remains eaten with bread. The smoke from heated pine wood also makes nasal mucus flow better. A lye solution can be made from the ashes, which can be used to wash the head [31].

In the 12th and 13th centuries, the popes ended medical activities at the monasteries through several conciliar decrees. Hildegard von Bingen thus became the last great representative of healing practice during the flowering of monastic medicine. Clerics were forbidden from practicing healing. This activity was transferred to the schools and universities that were slowly developing.

Already in the 10th century, long before the papal decrees, the medical school of Salerno represented the crucible of secular European medicine. Although many texts were translated later in Toledo at the translation school there, in the southern Italian town a variety of ancient Arabic sources were also being made available in Latin. Constantine Africanus (1018–1087) was the most famous teacher and translator in Salerno. Under the aegis of Norman and Hohenstaufen rulers in southern Italy, the first training and licensing regulations for physicians were prepared and implemented [32].

Between the 12th and 15th centuries further places for learning and investigation were created, for example, in Paris, Bologna, Oxford or Montpellier. During the 13th century they began calling themselves universities. They held a privileged status from the king, emperor or pope and were communities to teachers and students (universitas magistrorum et scolarium), bound legally by a set of statutes. The medical faculties of the schools in Paris, Bologna and Padua formed the crystallization points for the communication of medical knowledge. Instruction, however, was provided for a very long time in schematic ways according to the scholastic method [33]: Teachers conveyed the writings of the ancient authors, usually Galen, without critique and students seldom questioned what they were taught. Humoral pathology with its specific diagnostics (taking the pulse, examining the urine) and therapeutic measures (blood letting, purging, vomiting) thus remained the guiding theory of illness during the Middle Ages. The typical 'scholastic' physician who had studied at a university carried out a type of medicine that was, in extreme cases, far from the physical realities of his patients. He was, however, well read in the relevant literature that he applied to each case. The practical side of medicine, on the other hand, remained in the background.

A short digression: The Dreckapotheke (dirt pharmacy)

Medicine in the early Mesopotamian high culture (Assyria, Babylonia) frequently took supernatural influences into account when considering the origin of illnesses. The influence of the gods on human health could not just be the healing of afflictions, but must also indicate punishment by allowing demons causing illness to get the upper hand in a person's body. The goal of the doctor, therefore, was to carry out treatments that would irritate or expel the interloper, i.e., the source of illness, from the human body. In order to achieve this goal, he would prescribe bitter or nauseating substances, such as urine, feces, menstrual blood or rancid fat of human or animal origin. Egyptian and Greco-Roman medicine also resorted to these kinds of substances for treatment. Thus Galen said of feces: "You do not just need it as an additive in remedies that you apply externally, but also in ones you use internally" [34].

Urine and excrement also found use in fighting coughs. Pliny the Elder prescribed jaguar urine and hare feces to be used internally [35]. The late ancient author Sextus Placitus gave coughing children crow excrement to be used internally [36].

At the end of the 17th century, the medical work of Paullini's *Heilsame Dreck-Apotheke* (Healing Dirt Pharmacy) [37] recorded in more than 200 pages a list of diverse cases of illness where human and animal waste products could find use. Thus colds should be able to be healed by applying human feces and urine externally, as well as the excrement of sheep, cattle, goats, pigs, horses and doves. For the physician Christian Franz Paullini (1643–1712), feces, dirt and earth were all one. The human was earth and returned to earth:

> "God is and remains the old potter, and thus daily turns and forms all manner of things from feces on his wheel. How do we retain the complete health we have or regain our lost health? With remedies made from herbs, roots, animals and minerals. If you investigate all of their origin, however, you will find Dreck (trans: dirt, here: feces) and nothing more.... Whoever disrespects feces, disrespects his origin" [38].

Folk medicine also knew prescriptions from the Dreckapotheke. Slavic tradition, for example, recommended taking ground stork excrement in honey water for a sore throat; for a cold you inhaled it as fine dust [39].

Here as elsewhere the consumption of one's own urine is repeatedly advised, for example, against a cough:

> "First thing upon waking, pass some urine, then take some of the midstream in the palm of your hand and inhale it deeply into the nose. Continue this several mornings. It will clear your head" [40].

A look at the best seller list proves that the Dreckapotheke is still considered effective today: One of the most successful reference works in 1993 was a book with the title *Ein ganz besonderer Saft – Urin* (A Very Special Liquid – Urine) [41].

Herbal books and good advice: The Early Modern period

In the 15th and 16th centuries changes were introduced that altered the (western) world dramatically. The invention of printing with movable letters by Johannes Gutenberg (1400–1468) made knowledge in times thereafter slowly more accessible, while also offering the possibility of publishing one's own knowledge. The fundamental reforms in education beginning in the 16th century went hand in hand with the new technology. Medicine also profited from this development. In addition to the books that were used at the universities and in the medical faculties, publishers also produced numerous volumes about healing plants. These books, based in part on the works of ancient authors, gave a botanical description of numerous healing plants and explained how they worked. Moreover, the representations of the plants became ever more realistic.

The 16th century herbal book (*Kräuterbuch*) of Hieronymus Bock (1498–1554) was of great importance [42]. Bock tried to identify precisely the plants growing in Germany and to summarize their healing properties. Unlike most of his predecessors, he wrote in German.

For example, among healing plants for the cold, one finds helleborus. It works when it "is received in the nose with marjoram. It cleans the brain and makes you sneeze." The brain was still understood as the seat of mucus according to an understanding of the body based on humoral pathology. In analogy to Hildegard von Bingen, the expulsion of the bad parts of this humor is always the goal, in order to free the body from illnesses associated with mucus. Radish is also mentioned by Bock. Through its properties – hot and dry in the third degree – it was a good healing means for a 'moist-cold cold'.

The printed herbal books were at first only available to an educated public. With time they were expanded to include contemporary concepts alongside pharmacological knowledge from antiquity. Plants were added that were found in the New World discovered by Christopher Columbus (1451–1506) and later brought to Europe. Toward the beginning of the 16th/17th century, as shipping and other transportation improved, the exchange of goods including healing plants, minerals and medications from other cultures intensified and increased.

With tobacco and emetics: The 18th century

The 18th century is considered the era of the Enlightenment. It was characteristic of thought at the time to encourage people to use reason to free themselves from their "self-incurred immaturity" [43]. To achieve this end, the use of critical faculties is necessary. Criticism should be based on the natural sciences and aimed at authoritarian, irrational ideas, such as certain forms of Christian faith and superstition. This approach was picked up in the course of the century and echoed in the great European encyclopedias: The *Encyclopédie* (1751–80) or the *Encyclopaedia Britannica* (1768–71) represents the knowledge of their time in France and Great Britain. In Germany, enlightened contemporaries reached for Johann Heinrich Zedler's *Großes vollständiges Universal-Lexikon* (Great and complete universal lexicon) [44]. The most comprehensive encyclopedic work of the 18th century, it promised to illuminate all "sciences and arts which have hitherto been invented and improved by human reason and wit." The common cold also receives a place with extensive articles on "catarrh" and "gravedo" (cold in the head) [45]. Showing the critical spirit of the times, the articles distance themselves from the humoral pathological ideas of the 'ancients', who had localized the source of the illness in the head alone and had undertaken to differentiate according to qualities and elements. Modern medicine favored looking at only one 'humor': Diseases began in the blood, the cold as well. They then manifest themselves either in a location (runny nose, cough, hoarseness) or in the entire body (Catarrhus universalis), appear either sporadically or as an epidemic and influence the quality of the blood (fluid and hot, thick and slow). The traditional concept of a sluggish or corrupted humor, of too little or too much blood, remained valid: "The direct cause of a catarrh is of course without doubt the impeded movement of the seri [of the blood], which, if it begins to slow, causes growths and pain to ensue, such as to be seen with a growth in the salivary gland" [46]. Consequently, therapy must be aimed at getting the fluids to move again, to remove them or to add them. If the blood is too thick then it is advisable to drink a lot of tea or milk. Conversely, a reliable measure for 'evacuating' would involve administering a mild laxative. According to the encyclopedia, aches due to a cold can be treated by rubbing the limbs externally with frankincense and mastic gum, camphor or menthol [47].

Very traditional views, some from the Middle Ages, can also be found in Zedler's universal lexicon. The idea that sluggish blood can be stirred up artificially with mixtures such as snuff and castoreum appears to come in a direct line from Hildegard von Bingen – but without her cosmological framework! The advice to use surgical measures in the case of chronic colds that do not respond to any dietetic and pharmaceutical measures seems to be taken directly from medieval manuals on wound healing. Creating a fontanelle, i.e., an artificial wound in the skin that is then prevented from healing by applying a foreign substance, is supposed to allow corrupt fluids a channel by which to leave the body. An alternative was to set a setaceum, a string that was pulled through a fold of skin, and allowed to remain there until the pus that accumulated led to a discharge [48].

This reference work also reported about what makes colds contagious. The cause is sometimes "poisonous impurities in the air", so-called Miasma malignum, that are breathed in through the lungs. The illness can thus be avoided if one constantly spits. Otherwise, the damaging substances are mixed in the mouth with saliva after breathing and then swallowed and from there pass through the stomach and intestines into the "milk vessels" (lymph vessels) and from there into the blood. Salivants, such as myrrh, mastic gum, burnet or also tobacco smoke in the mouth should aid in spitting. If the miasmas have already reached the stomach, a light emetic should be administered [49].

Advisory literature developed in the 18th century parallel to the encyclopedias. Eventually, there were instructions and tips for all areas of life, including illnesses. When should one consult a doctor? What is the proper diet? What measures should one take and when?

> "Various preconceptions prevail in regard to the cold, all of which could have terrible effects. The first is that a cold can never be dangerous. This error has cost many people their lives every year.... In fact, you do not die of a cold, so long as it is a cold, but if you miss it, then it turns into a chest illness that can be deadly.... A further error is that people not only do not think a cold is dangerous, but also actually think it is healing. Of

> course it is better to have a cold than some worse disease; but it would be better, not to have any...." [50].

Thus wrote Samuel August Tissot (1728–1797), Swiss physician and scholar, in his work, *Gesundheitliche Ratschläge für das Volk oder Abhandlung der häufigsten Krankheiten* (Health Advice for the People or Treatise on the Most Common Illnesses), published in 1761. In this book he explains about illnesses and their symptoms, gives therapeutic advice and recommends when it would be necessary to visit a doctor. In the chapters, "Inflammation of the Chest", "About Sore Throats" and "About Colds", he expounds on the symptoms of the common cold. For Tissot, all of the symptoms in the nose, throat and chest have the same origin: the reason for the illness is an inflammation of the blood or an exhalation or perspiration that has been held back. As in 'Zedler', blood seems to be the central bodily fluid that causes illness.

The idea that a cold has something healing about it appears to have been widely believed and goes back to the concept that mucus is a waste product of the body. Tissot neither believed the cold to be dangerous in and of itself, nor did he understand it as a cleansing and healthy process of the body. Tissot saw how the entire breathing apparatus was interconnected and the signs of inflammation common to various illnesses. A light cold, together with a light cough and fever, lasting about 5 days, could therefore not be disregarded. With a severe cold, he recommended blood-letting. An evening footbath should help fight a cough, fever and headache. In addition to avoiding meat and an increased consumption of fruit and vegetables, he advised drinking an elderberry infusion with milk or barley soup. An enema should free the body of substances that were caught or stuck.

Cold and electricity, infections and microbes: The 19th century

In the first half of the 19th century, the general concepts of humoral pathology still dominated views of the common cold and the mechanism that caused it. However, the main point of attack for the illness changed to the skin. If the skin is exposed for shorter or longer periods of time to low temperatures or a draft, then the person will become chilled and get (a) cold. According to beliefs at the time, the function of the skin was to "evaporate moisture continuously and unnoticeably; if the necessary skin warmth is replaced too quickly by cold, then the pores of the skin close and perspiration is interrupted. Consequences: inflammations, rheumatism, catarrh." Quite obviously, wearing appropriate clothing protected from the illness. However, "the best means of keeping this great enemy of health at bay is hardening, since hardened skin is not kept from functioning when a little air blows in its direction". The "hardening" could be attained primarily by going outdoors in any weather, moderate heating in winter as well as washing in cold water in all seasons [51].

In the 19th century, if one still got a cold, advice for household use could be found in numerous medical guidebooks similar to Samuel Auguste Tissot's work. In the *Hauslexikon der Gesundheitslehre für Leib und Seele* (Household lexicon for a healthy body and soul) from 1873, individual illnesses are ordered alphabetically. The common cold can be found under the term 'catarrh'. Like the Ladies Lexicon, it gives the reason for the common cold as poor functioning of the skin through too much cold or great changes in temperature. The function of the skin is interrupted and the electricity in the skin is disturbed. The body reacts to this problem with an inflammation. If this reaction affects the mucus membranes of the air passages, then a cold is the result, a so-called 'good catarrh'. The following symptoms appear: "The feeling of a blocked nose is followed by a dry heat in the nose, sneezing and reddening of the eyes, frequently with feverish disquiet and headache, the senses of smell and taste are diminished, a prickly, watery discharge that irritates flows from the nasal openings, until finally, when the irritation lessens, mucus that is at first clear and then thicker is discharged and within 6 to 8 days normality has returned" [52]. The goal of therapy must be to restore the functioning of the skin. This can be brought about by the warmth of the bed, taking a tartar emetic mixture or Danish elixir (a mixture of licorice juice, fennel water, liquid ammonia and anise oil). Taking a walk in the fresh air is as important for regaining health as visiting a doctor if the symptoms continue.

In the guide book, influenza is clearly distinguished from the common cold. Influenza is an illness with fever that comes 'from the air', attacks primarily older and weak people and can even lead to death.

The physician Carl Hueter (1838–1882) already held the opinion in the early 1860s that colds were caused by a kind of infection, resulting from the intake of tiny organisms Hueter called "monads". Based on the prevailing humoral pathology, he believed the pressure of drafts squeezed the monads into the skin pores that, once opened by a strong secretion of sweat, offered an entry port for the harmful organisms. This theory led to treating colds prophylactically by dousing the skin with denatured salicylic acid [53].

As scientific methods in medicine became more accepted, researchers used physiological experiments in an effort to understand what local and systemic consequences attended large changes in body temperature. The resulting knowledge that cold stimuli could provoke temporary anemia, cramps in the vessels and inflammatory processes in the affected tissue, did not, however, help physicians further. The advice of the pastor Sebastian Kneipp (1821–1897), on the other hand, proved to be very successful. In the 1880s and early 1890s, his traditional humoral pathological ideas from folk medicine enjoyed exceeding popularity. The prescribed applications of cold and cold water procedures against a "Verwärmung" – as Kneipp called a cold – however, only followed the traditional opposition of a softened and a hardened human physique.

Although physiological experiments were known at this time that refuted a connection between a temporary cooling and a catarrh, there were physicians around 1900 who still "emphasized the possibility for the generation of a nose and throat cold, perhaps also tracheitis or bronchitis, completely as the result of a reflex." These authors believed they had frequently observed that a cold comes so hard on the heels of a cold stimulus, that it "would be difficult to imagine the whole path of a bacterial development and establishment of an inflammation in such a short time" [54]. Slowly it was recognized that colds could not merely be attributed to meteorological conditions, but rather to an acute infection. Proponents of the infection theory first associated the pathological microbes that caused illness with bacteria or simply called them "cold pathogens" [55]. From time to time, known pathogens were made responsible for the common cold: streptococcus and pneumococcus, which were frequently found in the air passages of patients with colds. The view that one could ward off a cold by taking measures to harden the body slowly but surely became untenable in medical circles (yet is still believed in wide parts of the population).

The basis for knowledge about the cold came from the new medical field of microbiology, where many new insights were being gained. Above all, the research of Robert Koch (1843–1910) led medical science to perceptions that allowed a closer understanding of the origin of infectious disease. Koch was able to prove the existence of tiny organisms in tissue samples of sick patients, to isolate them, to grow them in their pure form and then to prove that they caused infectious diseases. In this way he discovered the bacterial pathogen for anthrax (1876), tuberculosis (1882) and cholera (1883).

Despite all progress in making bacteria visible, there was increasing evidence for the existence of pathogens that were too small to see with an optical microscope. For the first time, in 1892, Dimitri Iwanowski (1864–1920) used the mosaic disease on the tobacco plant to confirm that a disease could be caused by a substance that could not be removed through filtration and whose particles must therefore be significantly smaller than bacteria [56]. The first proof of an animal virus succeeded in 1898 when Koch's former assistants, Friedrich Loeffler (1852–1915) and Paul Frosch (1860–1928), discovered the foot-and-mouth-disease virus [57].

The discovery of the rhinovirus that causes the common cold, however, was not to happen for several decades.

The rhinovirus: The 20th century

The search for the cause of the cold was difficult on two accounts. First, the cold could not command the attention of researchers because much more serious infectious diseases such as typhus or the frequently fatal influenza demanded research to find a cure for, as well as a way to eliminate or at least restrict, these diseases.

Second, the question about the pathogen responsible for coughs, colds and hoarseness turned out to be problematic. Up to the 1930s there was no consensus in medical research about which group of pathogens caused the cold. The idea that it could be a virus continued to circulate along with the assumption that aerobic or anaerobic bacteria were the cause, even though the first evidence for a viral infection had been found in 1914 [58].

The hygienist Walter Kruse (1864–1943) and his staff carried out experiments at his Leipzig University institute after one of his colleagues came to work with a cold. The secretion of the nose, generally free of the classic bacteria in the air passages, was prepared and given to other staff members to inhale into their noses. Many of them developed typical symptoms of a cold, so that it became clear to Kruse that only a virus could be the trigger since the bacterial components had been removed. Yet he could not prove his theory. Thus, his work remained unnoticed in research for some time. In addition, the outbreak of World War I diverted the attention of scientists to infections caused by wounds and the great epidemics. In the 1920s and 1930s in America and England, efforts were again made to find the cause of the common cold. Under the direction of Alphonse Dochez (1882–1964) in New York, the idea of a viral infection according to Kruse was reexamined. Experiments with chimpanzees and later with humans took place. The English virologist Christopher Andrewes (1906–1998) met Alphonse Dochez coincidentally in America and became very enthusiastic about his work. Back in England, he began his first experiments, but had to interrupt them because the money for his research was slashed due to the world economic crisis. Andrewes turned again to studying influenza. In the years 1918/19 it had claimed more fatalities in England than World War I and was, therefore, a more urgent matter [59].

The Common Cold Research Unit [60]

After World War II, new efforts, primarily in England, were again undertaken to research the cold. The focal point was the former Harvard Hospital in Salisbury/Wiltshire in the south of England. The institution had been established in 1939/40 by Harvard University in Boston and the American Red Cross to support Great Britain against the German Empire in World War II. It served to study infectious disease and as a hospital. Interest in research on the cold had not lapsed completely during wartime; as an economic factor it remained present consistently for a broad public. At peak times the illness incurred a high number of sick-days in the workplace that amounted to economic losses of many millions of pounds or dollars. During the war, the British government therefore started a campaign to alert people of the necessity for physical hygiene, the use of handkerchiefs and the danger of spreading infection.

After the end of the war, the American government gave the British government the building and its inventory. In 1946 the Common Cold Unit (CCU) was established.

The CCU thus served as the cornerstone for systematic research on the common cold. The researchers worked with volunteers who were willing to spend 10 days in isolation and be infected with the pathogen. Their lodging was paid and many were prepared to endure a simple cold in exchange for good, if temporary accommodations. Until the CCU was closed in 1989, more than 20000 volunteers took part in the experiments to identify and treat the cold.

The first years were plagued with many uncertainties, but in 1956 there was a decisive breakthrough. For a long time the existence of the pathogen had been known and had thus provided the conditions for specific experimentation. For the first time, it was possible to make a fragment of the so-called B 814 virus visible in tissue. The rhinovirus had been found. [61]

Over the years it became clear that there are many forms of the virus responsible for the common cold. Numerous subgroups of the so-called picornaviruses are the main cause of a cold.

Medical research today is still concerned primarily with the question of treatment and prevention of colds. In cooperation with the WHO, worldwide research and prevention programs are carried out with the aim of restricting the radius of action of cold viruses and preventing serious complications and secondary infections. The changeability of the rhinovirus makes it impossible to eradicate the common cold. But knowledge about the virus offers possibilities for new, innovative therapies.

Acknowledgements

We thank Dr. Mason Barnett, Berlin, for the translation of the German script and Bayer Health Care, especially Dr. Uwe Gessner, Leverkusen, for sponsoring the translation. We also thank Prof. Dr. Thomas Schnalke, Berlin, for the inspiring discussions on the topic.

References

1 Piek J, Terberger T (eds) (2006) *Frühe Spuren der Gewalt.* Landesamt für Kultur- und Denkmalpflege, Schwerin

2 Sjovold T (1994) Pathological conditions and medical treatment of the Tyrolean Late Neolithic Ice-man. *HOMO* 45: 119; Mariani-Constantini R, Capasso L, Capelli A, Frati L (1994) Paleopathology of the Copper Age Mummy from the Val Senales Glacier. *Medicina nei Secoli* 6 (1): 53–70

3 Dorfer L, Moser M, Bahr F (1999) A medical report from the stone age? *The Lancet* 354: 1023–1025

4 Unschuld PU (1980) *Medizin in China. Eine Ideengeschichte.* Beck, München; Porkert M (1982) *Die chinesische Medizin.* ECON, Düsseldorf/Wien; Kapchuk TJ (2003) *Das große Buch der chinesischen Medizin.* Barth, Wien
5 Unschuld PU (ed) (2003) *Huang Di nei jing su wen: nature, knowledge, imagery in an ancient Chinese medical text.* University of California Press, Berkeley
6 Mitchell C, Yè F, Wiseman N (eds) (1999) *Shang hán lùn* (*On cold damage*). Paradigm Publ., Brookline.
7 Herodotus *Historiai*, 2, 84
8 Porter R (2000) *Die Kunst des Heilens.* Spektrum, Heidelberg/Berlin, 47–51
9 Ebers Papyri, 763
10 Krug A (1993) *Heilkunst und Heilkult. Medizin in der Antike.* Beck, München; Kollesch J (2007) *Antike Heilkunst.* Reclam, Stuttgart; Steger F (2004) *Asklepiosmedizin. Medizinischer Alltag in der römischen Kaiserzeit.* Steiner, Stuttgart
11 Hippocrates *De natura hominis*, 7
12 Claudius Galenus *De facultatibus naturalibus*, II 9
13 Hippcrates *De natura hominis*, 7
14 Claudius Galenus *De facultatibus naturalibus*, II 9
15 Hippocrates *Aphorismi*, III, 19, 23
16 Dioscorides *Materia Medica*, II, 183
17 Dioscorides *Materia Medica*, III, 83
18 Edelstein L (1998) *Asclepius. A collection and interpretation of the testemonnies* I/II. John Hopkins University Press, Baltimore; Krug A (1993) *Heilkunst und Heilkult. Medizin in der Antike.* Beck, München: 120–187; Steger F (2004) *Asklepiosmedizin. Medizinischer Alltag in der römischen Kaiserzeit.* Steiner, Stuttgart
19 Quṣtā Ibn-Lūqā (1987) *Abhandlung über die Ansteckung.* Steiner, Wiesbaden/ Stuttgart, 13
20 Maimonides M et al. (1966) *Regimen sanitatis oder Diätetik für die Seele und den Körper.* Karger, Basel, 108
21 *Ibid.* 109–110
22 Dietrich A (ed) (1993) *Die Ergänzung Ibn Gulgul's zur Materia medica des Dioskurides.* Vandenhoek & Rupprecht, Göttingen, 51, 56–57
23 Spies O, Müller-Bütow H (1971) *Anatomie und Chirurgie des Schädels, insbesondere der Hals-, Nasen- und Ohrenkrankheiten nach Ibn al-Quff.* de Gruyter, Berlin/New York, 124
24 Jankrift KP (2003) *Krankheit und Heilkunde im Mittelalter.* Wiss. Buchgesellschaft, Darmstadt; Riha O (ed) (2005) *Heilkunde im Mittelalter.* Akademie-Verlag, Berlin
25 Stoll U (ed) (1992), *Das 'Lorscher Arzneibuch'. Ein medizinisches Kompendium des 8. Jahrhunderts* (*Codex Bambergensis medicinalis 1*). Steiner, Stuttgart
26 Hecht K (2005) *Der St. Galler Klosterplan.* VMA, Wiesbaden
27 Strabo W (2007) *De cultura hortorum* (*Hortulus*). Mattes, Heidelberg
28 Hildegard von Bingen (1997) *Heilkraft der Natur – Physica.* Pattloch, Augsburg, 128–129, 157–158
29 Hildegard von Bingen (1990) *Heilwissen – Causae et Curae.* Pattloch, Augsburg, 167

30 *Ibid.* 168
31 *Ibid.* 232, 292
32 Baader G (1978) Die Schule von Salerno. *Medizinhistorisches Journal* 13: 124–145; Jankrift KP (2003) Die Schule von Salerno. In: KP Jankrift: *Krankheit und Heilkunde im Mittelalter*. Wiss. Buchgesellschaft, Darmstadt, 41–45
33 Jacquart D (1996) Die scholastische Medizin. In: M Grmek (ed): *Die Geschichte des medizinischen Denkens: Antike und Mittelalter.* Beck, München, 216–259
34 Claudius Galenus *De simplicium medicamentorum temperamentis ac facultatibus*, II, 18
35 Plinius *Naturalis historia*, XXVIII, 31 & 53
36 Sextus Placitus *De medicamentis ex animalibus*, XXVII
37 Paullini CF (1696) *Heilsame Dreck-Apotheke, wie nemlich mit Koth und Urin fast alle … Kranckheiten … curirt worden*. Knoch, Frankfurt a. M.
38 Paullini CF (1700) Dass Dreck das allererste, älteste, edelste, vornehmste, nützlichste und nothwendigste unter allem in der gantzen Welt sey und ohne solchen nichts werden, leben, wachsen, noch bestehen könne. In: CF Paullini: *Philosophischer Feyerabend*. Knoch, Frankfurt a. M., 462–473
39 Bourke JG (1913) *Der Unrat in Sitte, Brauch, Glauben und Gewohnheitsrecht der Völker.* Ethnologischer Verlag, Leipzig, 479; Bächtold-Stäubli H (ed) (2000) *Handwörterbuch des deutschen Aberglaubens*. de Gruyter, Berlin/New York, V, 330–350
40 Glorez A (1700) *Des Mährischen Albertus Magnus … Eröffnetes Wunderbuch von Waffensalben*. Regensburg, Stadtamhof, 57
41 Thomas C (1993) *Ein ganz besonderer Saft – Urin*. vgs, Köln
42 Hoppe B (1969) *Das Kräuterbuch des Hieronymus Bock*. Hiersemann, Stuttgart
43 Kant I (1983) Beantwortung der Frage: Was ist Aufklärung? In: I Kant: *Werke in sechs Bänden*. Wiss. Buchgesellschaft, Darmstadt, VI, 53
44 Zedler JH (ed) (1732–1754) *Grosses vollständiges Universal-Lexicon aller Wissenschafften und Künste: welche bißhero durch menschlichen Verstand und Witz erfunden und verbessert worden*. Zedler, Leipzig/Halle
45 *Ibid.* V, 1440–1454; XI, 637–643
46 *Ibid.* V, 1442
47 *Ibid.* V, 1451
48 *Ibid.* V, 1451–1452
49 *Ibid.* XXXV, 610–611
50 Tissot SA (1789) *Gesundheitliche Ratschläge für das Volk oder Abhandlung der häufigsten Krankheiten*. Augsburg
51 Herloßsohn C (ed) (1834–1838) *Damen Conversations Lexikon*. Verlags-Bureau, Adorf, III, 480
52 Klencke H (1873) *Hauslexicon der Gesundheitslehre für Leib und Seele*. Kummer, Leipzig
53 Eschle (1902) *Die Erkältung. Eine historisch-kritische Studie*. Gmelin, München, 5
54 Strasser A (1903) Erkältung und Abhärtung. *Deutsche Klinik* 1: 629; cf. Chodounsky K (1911) *Erkältung als Krankheitsursache*. J. Šafář, Wien/Leipzig

55 Ruhemann J (1904) Über das Wesen der Erkältung. *Zeitschrift für diätetische und physikalische Therapie* 7: 334

56 Iwanowski D (1892) O dvuch boleznjach tabaka. Tabacnaja pepliza. Mozatcnaja bolezn´ tabaka. *Sel`skoje chozaistvo i lesovodstvo St. Petersburg* 169: 104–121

57 Loeffler F, Frosch P (1897) Berichte der Kommission zur Erforschung der Maul- und Klauenseuche bei dem Institut für Infektionskrankheiten in Berlin. *Zentralblatt für Bakteriologie, Parasitenkunde und Infektionskrankheiten (Abt. I, Originale)* 22: 257–259; (1898) 23: 371–391

58 Kruse W (1914) Der Erreger von Husten und Schnupfen. *Münchener medizinische Wochenschrift* 61: 1547; Tyrell D, Fielder M (2002) *Cold Wars. The fight against the common cold.* Oxford University Press, New York, 16–22

59 Tyrell D, Fielder M (2002) *Cold Wars. The fight against the common cold.* Oxford University Press, New York

60 Tyrell D, Fielder M (2002) *Cold Wars. The fight against the common cold.* Oxford University Press, New York, 159–201

61 For the initial isolations see for example Price WH (1956) The isolation of a new virus associated with respiratory clinical disease in humans. *Proc Natl Acad Sci USA* 42: 892–896

Common Cold
ed. by R. Eccles and O. Weber

Mechanisms of symptoms of common cold and flu

Ronald Eccles

Common Cold Centre, Cardiff School of Biosciences, Cardiff University, Museum Avenue, Cardiff CF10 3AX, UK

Abstract

It is the familiar symptoms of sore throat, runny nose, sneezing, and nasal congestion, muscle aches, chilliness and fever, etc., that define the common cold and flu syndromes as self-diagnosed illnesses. Although there is much information about the molecular biology of the viruses that cause the common cold and flu syndromes, there is relatively little research on the immunological, physiological and pathophysiological mechanisms involved in generating the symptoms. This chapter studies the mechanisms that cause local symptoms associated with local inflammation of the airway (sore throat, sneezing, rhinorrhoea and purulent nasal discharge, nasal congestion, sinus pain, watery eyes and cough), and the mechanisms that cause systemic symptoms associated with release of cytokines from leukocytes (headache, chilliness and fever, psychological effects, malaise and mood changes, loss of appetite, and muscle aches and pains).

Introduction

Common cold and flu are common syndromes of illness that are self-diagnosed on the basis of a grouping of familiar symptoms such as sore throat, runny nose, sneezing, nasal congestion, fever and muscle aches [1]. In terms of common knowledge, the common cold is associated with a mild illness with symptoms usually restricted to the nose and throat (a head cold), whereas flu is perceived as a more severe systemic illness with fever and muscle aches. People often go to work with a cold but phone in sick with flu. This chapter focuses on the physiological mechanisms that generate the symptoms of common cold and flu, rather than the viruses involved in the syndromes, as these are discussed elsewhere in the book. The common cold and flu syndromes are related to viral infection of the upper respiratory tract (URTI) and, although they are commonly self-diagnosed, they are difficult to define exactly because of the great variation in the severity, duration and types of symptoms. Although common cold viruses are responsible for a lot of morbidity and mortality, especially in developing countries where malnutrition may weaken the host response to infection, the common cold syndrome is usually understood as a self-limiting mild illness, and complications of common cold infections are usually described by other terms such as sinusitis, otitis media, laryngitis, tonsillitis, pharyngitis, etc. The common cold syndrome has been defined in terms of experimental colds, as a short mild illness with early symptoms of headache, sneezing, chilliness and sore throat and later symptoms of nasal discharge, nasal obstruction, cough and malaise [2].

In a study on common cold symptoms induced by challenge with infected nasal secretions, the symptoms of URTI were classified as either 'early' or 'later' symptoms [2]. The early symptoms consisted of headache, sneezing, chilliness and malaise and they developed quickly and also declined rapidly after 1 or 2 days of duration, whereas the later symptoms consisted of malaise, nasal discharge, nasal obstruction and cough, and these symptoms developed slowly over several days and they were still present 1 week after challenge. The time course of an early symptom (sneezing) is compared with that of a later symptom (cough) in Figure 1. The early development of sneezing compared to cough in cases of common cold may be explained on the basis that URTI develops in the upper airways first and subsequently

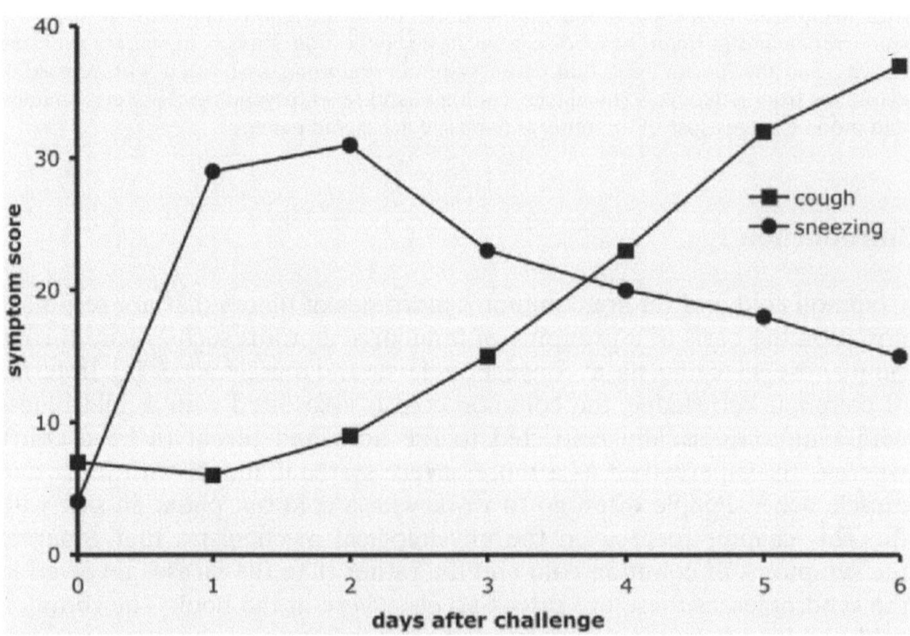

Figure 1. Time course of symptoms of sneezing and cough using challenge with infected nasal secretions to infect human volunteers. Results redrawn from the study by Jackson et al. [2].

spreads to the lower airways. The upper airways are innervated by the trigeminal nerves that mediate sneezing, whereas the airways below the larynx are innervated by the vagus nerves that mediate cough.

Generally, the severity of symptoms increases rapidly, peaks within 2–3 days after infection, with a mean duration of symptoms of 7–10 days but with some symptoms persisting for more than 3 weeks [3]. Experimental colds in adults are rarely associated with fever, and some subjects have a transient depression of the oral temperature during the early phases of a cold [2]. Studies on the symptoms generated by different common cold viruses indicate that it is not possible to identify the virus on the basis of the symptoms, as similar symptoms are caused by different viruses [4].

The flu syndrome is typically of sudden onset and is characterised by fever, headache, cough, sore throat, myalgia (muscle aches), nasal congestion, weakness and loss of appetite [5]. The clinical expression of symptoms is variable and is partly influenced by the nature of the infecting virus, and is modulated to a great extent by the immunological experience of the host and other factors such as age, and nutritional status. The syndromes of common cold and flu may be discussed as separate syndromes but the term acute upper respiratory tract infection (URTI) is used here to include both these syndromes.

Symptoms, pathogenesis, transmission

The symptoms of common cold and flu syndromes in normal healthy subjects are, by definition, conditions that are more of a nuisance rather than life-threatening illnesses. Pathogenesis is based on physiological, biochemical or molecular mechanisms that lead to harmful effects for the host, for example depletion of its resources, tissue destruction and detrimental changes in behaviour [6]. Common cold can be considered a mildly pathogenic illness as there is little evidence of any tissue destruction in the airways associated with colds [7], but there can be effects on behaviour and mood [8] that reduce performance and may cause loss of work days or school days. The presence of systemic symptoms such as fever, muscle aches and pains, tiredness and anorexia is associated with the flu syndrome, and this may be caused by both common cold viruses and influenza viruses as there is much overlap in the clinical presentation of these infections. The best predictors for influenza are cough and fever, as this combination of symptoms has been shown to have a positive predictive value of around 80% in differentiating influenza from a population suffering from flu-like symptoms [5].

Common cold is a mild illness and the idea that well-adapted parasites are relatively harmless to their hosts [9] may mean that humans have been interacting with these viruses for a long period. However, it seems unlikely that the parasite-host interaction will finally evolve to a completely harmless infection without any symptoms, as the symptoms may be important in aiding transmission of common cold and influenza viruses. A common cold or flu virus that causes a sub-clinical infection is unlikely to succeed in transmission to other hosts, as viruses spread in airway mucus, and in order for the chain of transmission to be complete, virus-laden mucus must pass from one airway to another [10]. The most successful common cold viruses are likely to be those that cause the most nasal mucus secretions, and coughs and sneezes may also aid in transmission of this mucus, although hand to hand contact is also an important mechanism of infection [11]. Symptomatic medicines that reduce mucus secretions and coughs and sneezing in colds and flu such as antihistamines, anticholinergics, and antitussives, may have a role in reducing transmission of colds but at present there are no studies to test this idea.

Common cold and flu symptoms are caused by the immune response to the infection rather than by tissue damage [12, 13]. Histological surveys of the nasal epithelium during experimental rhinovirus infections have not been able to find any morphological changes in the nasal epithelium of infected volunteers apart from a significant increase in polymorphonuclear leukocytes early in the course of the infection [7]. The major cell monitoring the host for viral infection is the macrophage and this cell has the ability to trigger an acute-phase response when stimulated with components of viruses such as viral RNA. The surface of the macrophage exhibits Toll-like receptors that combine with the components of viral and bacterial pathogens and trigger the production of cytokines [14]. The cytokines act to recruit other immune cells, trigger inflammation, and generate systemic symptoms such as fever [15]. A complex mix of pro-inflammatory cytokines and mediators generates the symptoms of URTI [16]. The inflammatory mediator bradykinin is believed to play a major role in generating the local symptoms of URTI, such as sore throat and nasal congestion [17, 18], and cytokines are believed to be responsible for the systemic symptoms such as fever [19]. The mechanisms generating symptoms of URTI are illustrated in Figure 2. They can be divided into two pathways: one for systemic symptoms generated by cytokines and the other for local symptoms generated by a local inflammatory response in the infected airway. A discussion of the mechanisms that generate the symptoms of common cold and flu is the topic of this chapter and each symptom is discussed in turn.

Sensory perception of symptoms

A symptom by definition is a condition that the patient feels or senses, and in order for the patient to feel the symptom it must in some way stimulate sensory nerves to be perceived by the patient. The cranial nerves that supply sensory nerves to the nose and throat such as the maxillary and ophthalmic divisions of the trigeminal nerves are important pathways for generating the symptoms of URTI [16]. The modalities of sensation detected by the

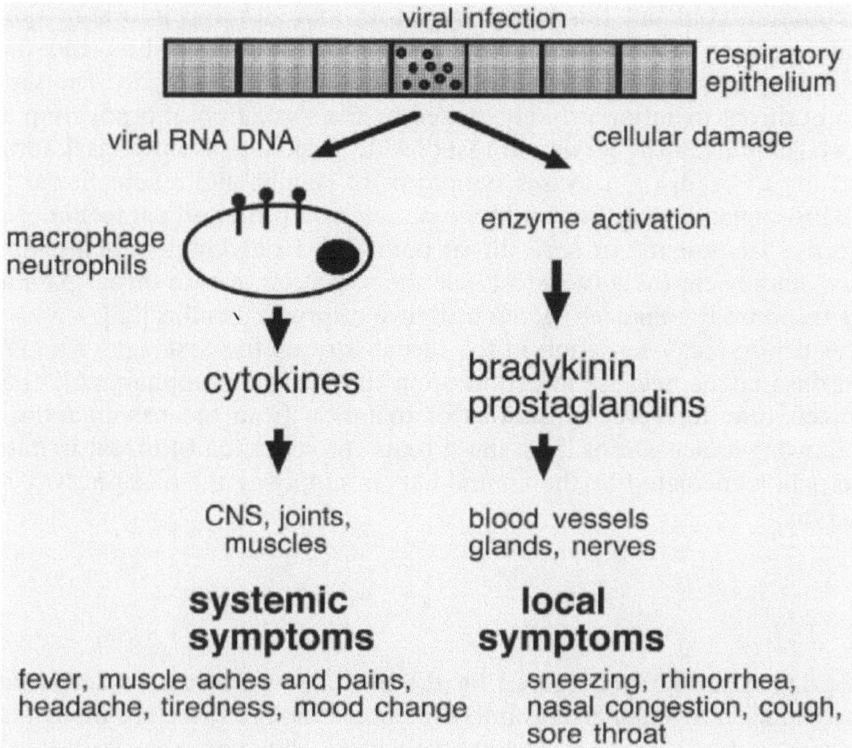

Figure 2. Mechanisms of symptoms. Viral infection triggers symptoms by two pathways. Local symptoms are caused by the generation of bradykinin and prostaglandins in the nasal epithelium. Systemic symptoms are caused by the release of cytokines from macrophages, neutrophil and dendritic cells upon stimulation of Toll-like receptors.

cranial nerves include pain in conditions such as sore throat and sinus pain, pressure in the case of nasal congestion, and irritation in the case of sneezing. However, some of the sensations associated with URTI symptoms are poorly understood, such as the sensation of irritation associated with cough, and the urge to cough, and the sensation of chilliness that is commonly felt with URTI. Tiredness and malaise are also poorly understood as regards the central mechanisms that generate these sensations.

Local symptoms

Sore throat

Sore throat is caused by inflammation of the upper airway triggered by the viral infection. The sensation of throat irritation is an early symptom of common cold but this minor symptom may develop into sore throat pain associated with nasopharyngitis, pharyngitis or tonsillitis, and these conditions may also be associated with bacterial infection [20]. The sensation of throat irritation is likely caused by the formation of bradykinin and prostaglandins in the airway in response to infection, as intranasal administration of bradykinin causes symptoms of rhinitis and a sore throat [17, 21]. Prostaglandin synthesis inhibitors such as aspirin and paracetamol are effective treatments for sore throat pain [22]. Bradykinin stimulates pain nerve endings in the airway to cause the sensation of sore throat pain and this response is enhanced by the presence of prostaglandins [23].

A dry scratchy sensation in the throat is often the first sign of a URTI and this may be because infection often starts in the nasopharynx [24] and subjects may interpret sensations of irritation from the nasopharynx on swallowing as sensations from the throat. The sensation of throat irritation and pain is mediated by the cranial nerves supplying the nasopharynx and pharynx.

Sneezing

Sneezing is normally triggered by the presence of dust or other inhaled material such as small insects into the nose, although there are many other triggers such as exposure to light, urination, shivering, gastric distension and sexual excitement [25]. Sneezing is a reflex that, unlike cough, cannot be initiated voluntarily and it consists of nasal congestion accompanied by a watery secretion and a violent expiration through the mouth and nose. Sneezing is related to inflammatory responses in the nose and nasopharynx that stimulate the trigeminal nerves. The sneeze response may be mediated *via* histamine receptors on the trigeminal nerves as intranasal administration of histamine causes sneezing [26]. A sneeze is an all-or-nothing patterned response generated from the sneeze centre in the brainstem. The trigeminal nerves relay information to the sneeze centre and cause reflex activation of motor and parasympathetic branches of the facial nerve, and activate respiratory muscles. A model of the sneeze reflex is illustrated in Figure 3. The sneeze centre coordinates the patterned inspiratory and expiratory actions of sneezing *via* respiratory muscles, and lacrimation, nasal secretion *via* parasympathetic branches of the facial nerve. The eyes are always closed during sneezing by the activation of facial muscles, and this indicates a close relationship between the protective reflexes of the nose and eyes. A common phenomenon is the 'photic sneeze' caused by a sudden increase in light intensity that again highlights the overlap of protective nasal and eye reflexes [27, 28]. Sneezing activates parasympathetic pathways to nasal glands to cause a watery nasal secretion that may help to cleanse the nose of irritants, and there appears to be some cholinergic central control of

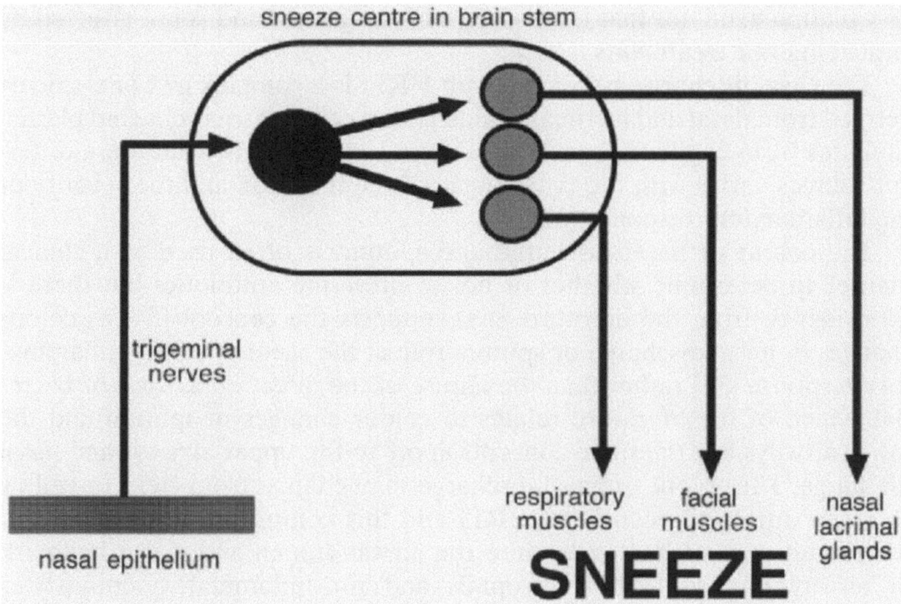

Figure 3. Sneeze reflex. Irritation of sensory nerves in the nose is relayed to the sneeze centre by branches of the trigeminal nerves. The sneeze centre can be thought of as a pattern generator that initiates a patterned sneeze once the sensory stimulation exceeds a threshold point. The sneeze involves inspiratory and expiratory respiratory muscles, facial muscles and nasal and lacrimal glands.

sneezing, as anticholinergics such as ipratropium [29] and first generation antihistamines [30] have been shown to inhibit sneezing.

Sneezing is a more common symptom in allergic rhinitis than URTI, and this may be because histamine, which triggers sneezing, is a major mediator of allergy but not so important in the inflammatory response associated with URTI [31].

Rhinorrhoea and purulent nasal discharge

Rhinorrhoea or 'runny nose' refers to the watery nasal secretions that are associated with common cold. These watery nasal secretions are secreted from nasal glands, and much of the secretion is produced from nasal ducts that enter the anterior part of the nose [32]. Rhinorrhoea is an early symptom of common cold and is associated with sneezing and reflex activation of parasympathetic nerves that stimulate nasal secretions from nasal glands as described above. The early symptom of rhinorrhoea can be controlled by anticholinergic treatments such as intranasal ipratropium [29, 33] but these medicines are only effective in first 4 days of common cold symptoms as the later nasal fluid issuing from the nose becomes dominated by an inflammatory plasma exudates that is not derived from glands and is not affected by anticholinergic treatments.

The nasal discharge associated with URTI is a complex mix of elements derived from nasal and lacrimal glands, goblet cells, plasma cells, and plasma exudates from capillaries, and the relative contributions from these different sources varies with the time course of the infection and the severity of the inflammatory response [32].

The colour of nasal discharge and sputum is often used as a clinical marker to determine whether or not to prescribe antibiotics but there is no evidence from the literature that supports the concept [34] as colour changes in nasal discharge or sputum reflect the severity of the inflammatory response [35] rather than the nature of the infection as viral or bacterial. Much of the literature relates to colour changes in sputum and the lower airways but the same concepts apply to the upper airways and nasal discharge. The colour of nasal discharge may change from clear to yellow to green during the course of URTI and this colour change is related to the recruitment of leukocytes into the airway lumen and it is a hallmark of airway disease [35]. Neutrophils and pro-inflammatory monocytes have azurophil granules that owe their green colour to the green protein myeloperoxidase. Nasal discharge with few leukocytes is white or clear, with increasing numbers of leukocytes the nasal discharge appears yellow (pale green) and with large numbers of leukocytes the colour becomes green [35].

Evidence-based research indicates that antibiotics have no benefit in the treatment of URTI and that they should not routinely be prescribed to those presenting with purulent rhinitis [36].

Nasal congestion

A blocked nose due to congestion of nasal blood vessels is a later symptom of common cold that increases in severity during the first week of symptoms [2]. Nasal congestion is caused by dilation of large capacitance veins that are sometimes referred to as 'erectile tissue' because of they can swell and block the nose [37]. The venous erectile tissue is particularly well developed at the anterior end of the inferior turbinate and nasal septum. Swelling in this narrow 'nasal valve' region acts to regulate nasal airway resistance to airflow. The ostia of the paranasal sinuses are also surrounded by a lip of venous erectile tissue, and swelling of these blood vessels in association with a generalised nasal congestion may cause obstruction of the paranasal sinuses and lead to sinusitis as discussed below.

The nasal venous erectile tissue exhibits phases of congestion and decongestion under the influence of the sympathetic vasoconstrictor nerves that supply the nose, and this causes reciprocal changes in nasal airflow (often termed the 'nasal cycle') [38]. The asymmetry of nasal airflow associated

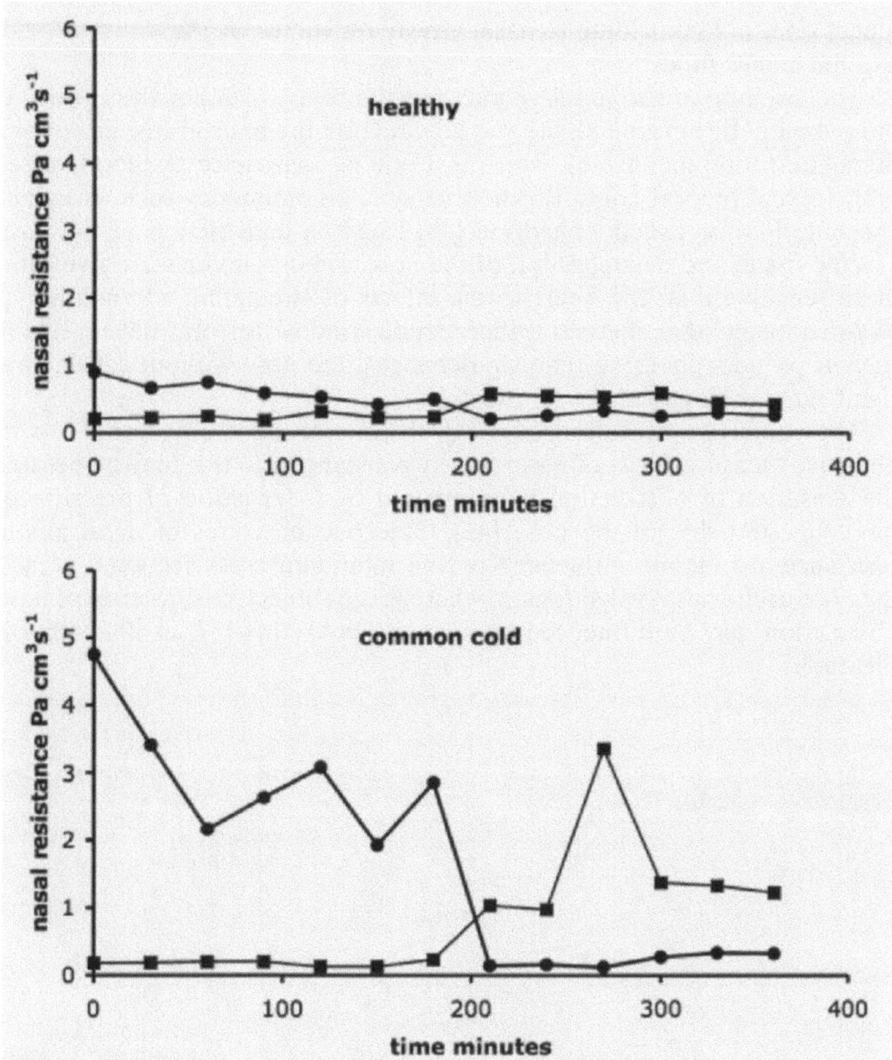

Figure 4. Spontaneous changes in unilateral nasal airway resistance recorded in one subject with symptoms of common cold (below), and 6–8 weeks later when healthy (above). Round symbols are left nasal airway resistance and square symbols right nasal airway resistance. Redrawn from Eccles et al. [39].

with the nasal cycle is increased with URTI and this may result in one nasal passage being open while the other is completely obstructed [39]. Figure 4 illustrates the changes in nasal airflow associated with the nasal cycle in health and with URTI [37, 38].

Nasal mucus may contribute to nasal blockage when there is nasal congestion, as the viscous mucus blocks the narrowed airway and this may lead to total nasal obstruction. However, under normal conditions the nasal mucus does not contribute to nasal airway resistance, as the airway is wide and the mucus fluid.

The swelling of the nasal venous erectile tissue is under the control of the sympathetic nerves [40, 41] and they release the neurotransmitter noradrenaline (norepinephrine), which is a potent constrictor of blood vessels [42]. Topical or oral administration of sympathomimetics such as xylometazaline [43] or pseudoephedrine [44] causes a constriction of the nasal erectile tissue and decongestion of the nose. The nasal veins are five times more sensitive than the heart to the effects of circulating adrenaline [40] and this means that there is a therapeutic window for oral decongestants such as pseudoephedrine that can decongest the nose without causing any significant cardiovascular side effects.

The subjective sensation of nasal obstruction does not correlate with objective measurements of nasal airway resistance and this may be because the sensation of obstruction is dominated by a sensation of pressure on the congested side of the nose [45]. Objective measures of nasal airway resistance are mainly influenced by the minimum cross sectional area of the nose at the nasal valve region, whereas the subjective sensation of nasal obstruction may be influenced by many other factors [37] as illustrated in Figure 5.

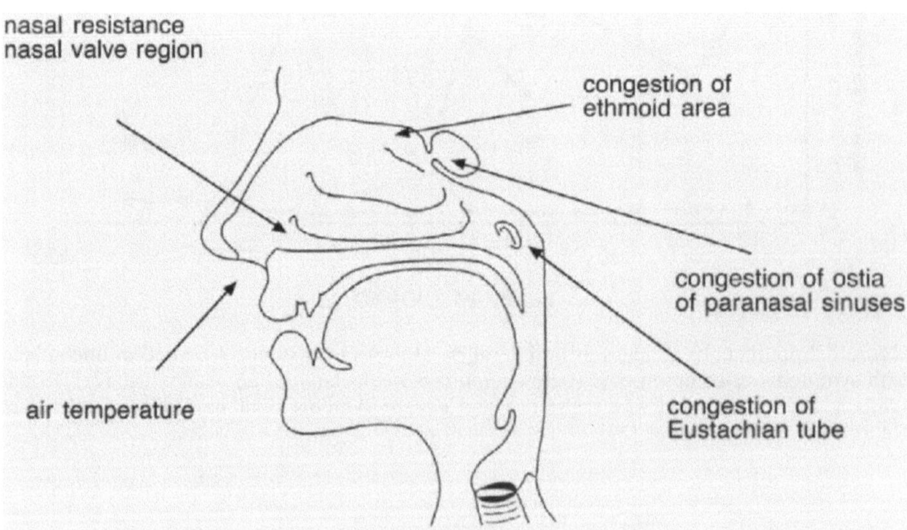

Figure 5. Factors that influence the patient's perception of nasal congestion. Nasal resistance to airflow is mainly determined by the cross-sectional area of the nasal valve region at the tip of the inferior turbinate. The patient's perception of nasal congestion may be influenced by air temperature and stimulation of cold receptors in the airway. Congestion in the ethmoid area, ostia of paranasal sinuses and Eustachian tube causes a perception of congestion and obstruction that is unrelated to any change in nasal airway resistance as these areas are distant from the nasal valve.

Sinus pain

The paranasal sinuses surround the nasal airway, and any URTI will always involve the sinuses, causing inflammation and a fluid level in the sinuses, especially the maxillary sinuses [46], as illustrated in Figure 6. Figure 6 also illustrates the asymmetry of congestion of the nasal turbinates associated with the nasal cycle and the asymmetrical nasal obstruction associated with URTI. The origin of sinus pain may be related to several factors such as pressure changes in the sinus air space, and pressure changes in the blood vessels draining the sinus [47]. The ostia of the paranasal sinuses are often occluded as the nasal epithelium becomes inflamed and congested with URTI, and this may result in gas absorption from the sinus and 'vacuum maxillary sinusitis' [37, 48]. Sinus pain may also be caused by the presence of inflammatory mediators such as bradykinin that stimulate pain nerve endings in the lining of the sinus or cause distension of blood vessels in the wall of the sinus [49].

Sinus pain can be treated with analgesics and sometimes these are combined with an oral decongestant such as pseudoephedrine, which is believed to decongest the nasal venous sinuses and open up the ostia of the sinuses to aid drainage and ventilation of the sinuses.

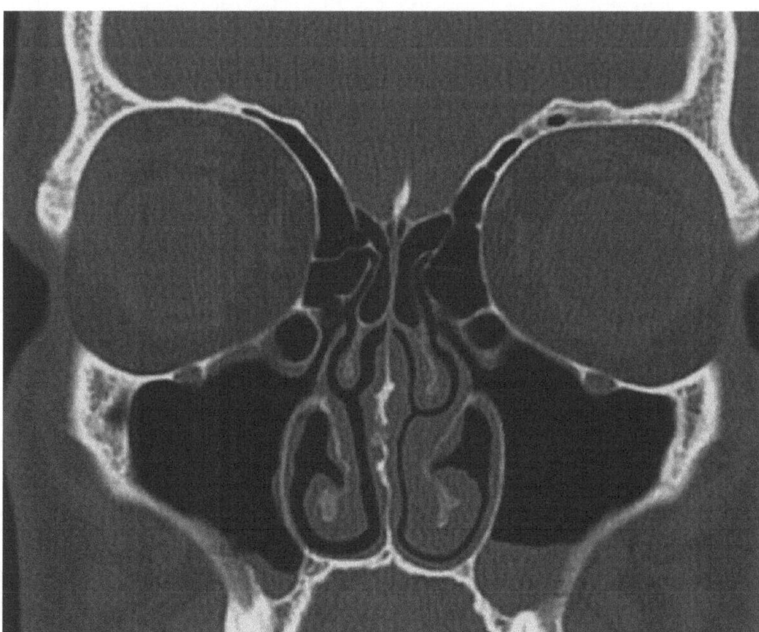

Figure 6. A 2-mm thick coronal CT scan of nose with patient prone and neck extended, simulating erect posture. Fluid levels are apparent in the maxillary sinuses, probably due to a common cold. Note the asymmetry in the size and degree of congestion of the nasal turbinates due to the nasal cycle.

Watery eyes

Watery eyes (epiphora) is due to accumulation of tear fluid in the eye and it may be caused by a combination of increased tear secretion and decreased drainage of tears *via* the nasolacrimal duct. Nasal irritation and sneezing leads to increased tearing as the protective reflexes of the nose and eye are closely linked. Any irritant that enters the nose is likely to enter the eyes, hence the closure of the eyes and increased tearing associated with sneezing. The nasolacrimal duct may be obstructed at its opening into the nose by inflammation and congestion of blood vessels in the nasal epithelium around the opening of the duct, and this will cause an accumulation of tears and the symptom of watery eyes. The nasolacrimal duct has been shown to have a vascular plexus of veins (cavernous tissue) similar to the venous sinuses of the nasal epithelium, and congestion of this plexus causes obstruction of the duct [50]. The nasolacrimal duct cavernous tissue is supplied by autonomic nerves that may control the patency of the duct [51], so that during sneezing and tearing the parasympathetic nerves lead to duct congestion that restricts the drainage of tears and causes watery eyes.

Cough

Cough is a vital protective reflex that prevents aspiration of food and fluid, and any inhibition of this reflex such as may occur in motor neurone disease may lead to aspiration of food and fluid and serious lower respiratory tract infections [52]. URTI may be associated with a dry unproductive cough that serves no useful function and may cause loss of sleep and exhaustion. The unproductive cough may be caused by the inflammatory response in the nose and throat spreading to the larynx and trachea. Cough associated with URTI is believed to be caused by a hyperreactivity of the cough reflex, and this may be due to the effects of inflammatory mediators such as bradykinin and prostaglandins on airway sensory nerve endings [53, 54].

In health, cough is readily induced by mechanical stimulation of the larynx, and when the larynx is inflamed and hyperreactive cough may occur spontaneously or in response to stimuli that would not normally cause cough, such as the mildly irritating effects of cold air or airway vibration [53]. Cough occurs spontaneously with URTI, and some cough may be voluntary rather than reflex, and this voluntary cough may be related to a sensation of airway irritation [55] and an urge to cough [56]. Productive cough usually occurs later in the course of URTI and may be related to the inflammation and infection spreading to the lower airways and triggering mucus production and expectoration. Common cold viruses usually do not cause any significant damage to the airway epithelium, whereas influenza

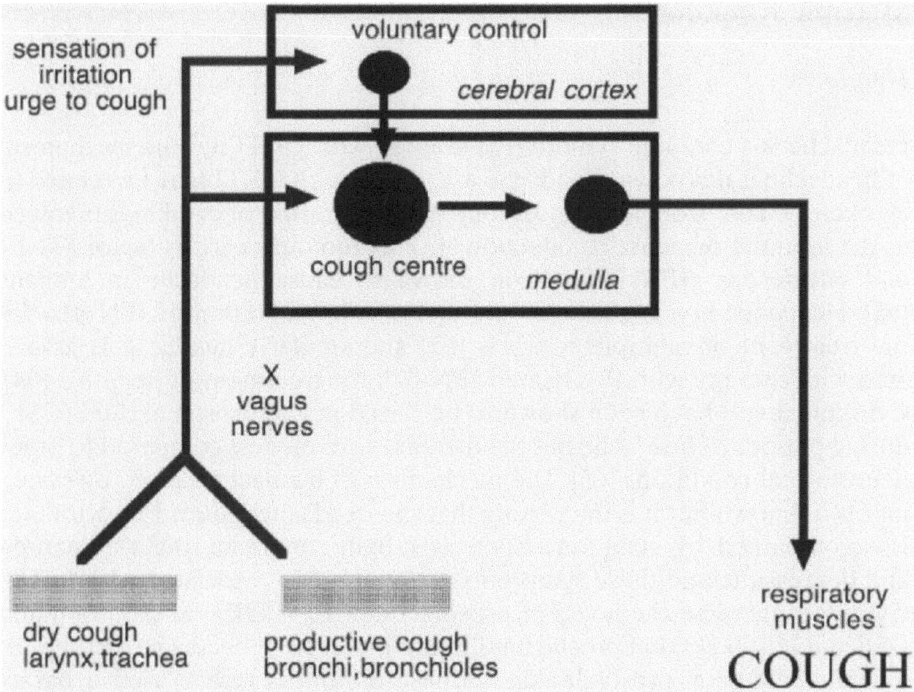

Figure 7. Cough associated with URTI is usually a dry cough associated with inflammation of the larynx and trachea. Inflammation of the lower airway may result in a productive cough with expectoration. Both types of cough are mediated by sensory branches of the vagus nerve that supply the respiratory epithelium. Cough is controlled from the brainstem region but it is not just a simple reflex as a sense of irritation may cause an urge to cough and voluntary cough *via* the cerebral cortex.

may cause substantial cellular damage to the respiratory epithelium, and this may be why influenza infection is usually associated with cough [5], whereas common cold often occurs as a 'head cold' with little if any symptom of cough.

The control of cough is illustrated in Figure 7, which shows that cough can be initiated by stimuli from both the upper (larynx and trachea) and lower airways (bronchi and bronchioles). Cough is controlled from the medulla region of the brainstem but can also be initiated voluntarily from areas of the cerebral cortex [55, 57, 58]. Cough can be voluntarily suppressed, and studies have demonstrated that cough due to URTI [59] or inhalation of irritants such as capsaicin [60] can be almost abolished by voluntary control. The voluntary initiation of cough and voluntary suppression, together with the sensitivity of cough to a placebo effect [61], makes it very difficult to conduct clinical trials on cough medicines.

Systemic symptoms

Headache

Headache is a common symptom associated with URTI but the mechanism of headache is unknown. Headache associated with URTI may be related to cytokine release from leukocytes [62]. Administration of cytokines involved in the immune response to infection such as tumour necrosis factor (TNF) and interferons (IFNs) has been shown to cause headache in humans [62]. Headache is a common side effect of administration of IFN-α1a for the treatment of multiple sclerosis [63] and similarly headache is associated with therapy with PEGylated IFN-β2b for treatment of hepatitis [64]. Cytokine levels have been shown to be raised in cerebrospinal fluid (CSF) during periods of headache but the increases are modest compared to other neurological conditions [65]. The mechanism of headache caused by cytokines is unknown but it is interesting that the headache induced by cytokines is accompanied by symptoms such as fatigue, anorexia, malaise, nausea and depression, and these symptoms are commonly associated with URTI. Cytokines increase the levels of prostaglandin E_2 (PGE_2) in the brain and CSF and it is likely that prostaglandins are involved in headache, perhaps as a final mediator, as prostaglandin synthesis inhibitors such as aspirin, paracetamol and ibuprofen are the standard treatments for headache.

Chilliness and fever

The common cold may have been so named because of the sensation of chilliness that accompanies URTI. In most folklore, the common cold is associated with chilliness and the standard antidote is some warm therapy such as a hot drink [66, 67]. A sensation of chilliness may be the first stage in the development of fever associated with skin vasoconstriction and shivering that tend to raise body temperature. Common cold in an adult is rarely accompanied by fever and some subjects have a transient fall in oral temperature during the early stages of common cold. In a study on 272 patients with sore throat associated with URTI, the mean aural temperature was 36.8°C and around 35% of these patients said they were suffering from ‘chills’ and ‘feverish discomfort’ [22]. Although it is generally accepted that skin cold-receptors signal the sensation of cold, the sensation of chilliness associated with URTI may be due to a central effect of cytokines and be unrelated to skin temperature. In a study on human volunteers, a sensation of chill still developed on administration of exogenous pyrogen even though the volunteers were immersed in a water bath that maintained a neutral skin temperature (34.5°C) [68]. The sensation of chilliness occurred after visible signs of shivering in the volunteers. Chilliness and shivering occurred even though there was no change in skin temperature and body temperature was actually rising in response to skin vasoconstriction. This finding indicates that the sensation of chilliness may be a central sensation closely linked to control of shivering. Chilliness and shivering are most likely induced by the effects of cytokines on the temperature regulating centres of the hypothalamus, and perceived at the level of the cerebral cortex.

Fever in response to infection is found in a wide range of animals and is believed to be beneficial as regards the host response to infection [69]. Fever is usually associated with novel or severe viral infections, especially emerging viral infections where the virus is novel to the host, as in influenza epidemics and SARS [5, 70]. Fever is uncommon in adult cases of common cold, but is common in infants, presumably because the adult has been exposed to numerous common cold viruses and subsequent infections do not trigger a strong immune response, whereas the viruses are novel to the infant and cause a greater release of fever-inducing cytokines than in the adult.

Cytokines have been implicated as endogenous pyrogens that are released from macrophages and other leukocytes in response to infection, and there is considerable evidence for pyretic and antipyretic effects of cytokines [19]. The pro-inflammatory cytokines interleukin 1 (IL-1), interleukin 6 (IL-6) and TNF-α as well as the anti-inflammatory cytokines interleukin 1 receptor antagonist (IL-1ra) and IL-10, have been mostly investigated for their pyrogenic or antipyretic action [19]. IL-1 and IL-6 are believed to be the most important cytokines for inducing fever [71]. Cytokines are believed to cross the blood-brain barrier or interact with the vagus nerve endings to signal the temperature control centre in the ventromedial preoptic area (VPMO) of the hypothalamus to increase the thermal set point [71, 72]. The cytokines induce cyclooxygenase (COX)-2-dependent prostaglandin synthesis in the VPMO. The hypothalamus then initiates shivering, constriction of skin blood vessels, and a sensation of chilliness as illustrated in Figure 8. Peripheral stimulation of intraperitoneal vagal nerve endings by inflammatory mediators such as prostaglandins may also initiate fever *via* pathways in the nucleus tractus solitarius that link directly with the VPMO without the need for cytokines to penetrate the CNS [73].

Psychological effects, malaise, and mood changes

Common cold and flu are associated with tiredness and lack of 'energy' and these infections have been shown to lead to a reduction in subjective alertness and impaired psychomotor functioning [8].

Cytokines released from leukocytes are believed to be responsible for the behavioural and mood changes associated with infection but the relative contribution of different cytokines to these changes is poorly understood. Cytokine-induced 'sickness behaviour' associated with infection has been proposed as an adaptive behaviour response to reduce energy consumption

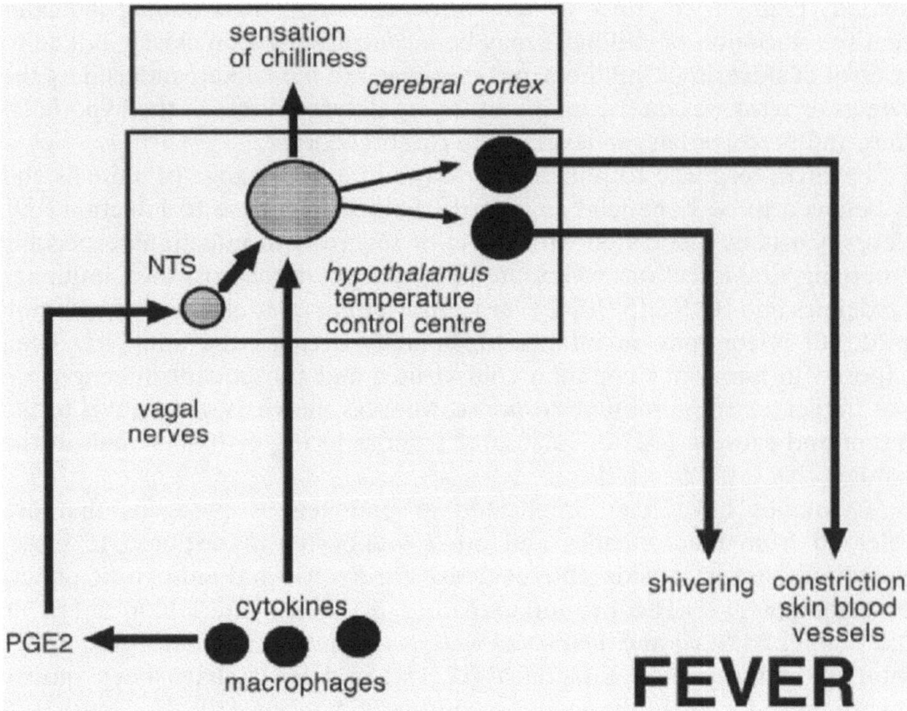

Figure 8. Fever associated with URTI is caused by cytokines released from macrophages and other immune cells. The cytokines enter the brain to cause a resetting of the temperature control centre in the hypothalamus. The hypothalamus causes shivering and constriction of skin blood vessels and also initiates a sensation of chilliness that is perceived at the level of the cerebral cortex. Direct stimulation of intraperitoneal vagal nerve endings by PGE_2 in bacterial infections may also initiate fever via the nucleus tractus solitarius (NTS).

at a time of high-energy demand, that is necessary to maintain fever and to fight infection, and that sickness behaviour is a motivational state that has important implications in terms of homeostasis [74]. The behavioural and mood changes associated with infection are just as normal and beneficial to the organism as the state of arousal that occurs in response to perceived harm [74]. IL-1β and IL-6 have been shown to be implicated in the development of sickness behaviour associated with viral infections [75] but at present it is difficult to determine the relative importance of any particular cytokine in inducing sickness behaviour.

IFNs are a group of cytokines that are involved in the immune response to viral infection and intranasal IFNs have been tested in clinical trials as a treatment for common cold [76, 77]. Exogenous administration of cytokine IFN-α is used as a therapy for chronic viral diseases such as hepatitis B and C, and therapy is associated with flu-like side effects similar to those observed with URTI, such as fatigue, fever, chills, myalgia, nausea and mood changes [78, 79], and these observations support the idea that cytokines such as IFNs are responsible for the mood changes and tiredness associated with URTI. Psychiatric side effects such as depression, irritability, lack of motivation, impaired concentration, psychoses and confusional states have been reported to occur in some patients after therapy with IFN-α [79, 80]. The present state of knowledge indicates that cytokine-induced alterations in serotonin metabolism and dopamine in the basal ganglia play an important role in the development of depression and fatigue [79] and this may be the mechanism responsible for mood changes and tiredness in URTI.

Loss of appetite

Loss of appetite and decreased intake of food and fluid is often associated with URTI, especially with flu and fever, and this symptom has entered the folklore [66] as advice to "feed a cold and starve a fever", although the word "starve" may have been substituted for "stave" which means to prevent. Indicating that a good diet during a cold could help to prevent a more serious infection with fever.

While some of the symptoms associated with URTI, such as fever, have been shown to be of adaptive value in host resistance to infection, the suppression of food intake during infection seems to be a paradoxical response, especially at a time when the metabolic rate may be increased due to elevation of body temperature, and protein intake is needed to sustain the increase in leukocytes and immunoglobulins that help to fight infection. Metabolic rate, oxygen consumption and protein catabolism are all raised during infection and nursing interventions to increase the intake of high calorie or high protein foods would seem to be indicated [81].

Anorexia associated with infection can be studied in healthy animals by injecting components of the cell wall of bacteria such as lipopolysaccharide (LPS). The LPS model of anorexia has demonstrated that the loss of appetite associated with infection is due to the release of cytokines from leukocytes and, as in fever, these cytokines can influence appetite by entering the brain or influencing the activity of vagal nerve endings [81] as illustrated in Figure 7. The literature indicates that a range of cytokines, such as TNF, IL-6 IL-1, IL-1α and IL-1β, may be involved in the anorexia associated with infection, and as with most cytokine responses there is much overlap of cytokine activity, and interference with any single cytokine only has a limited effect on the control of appetite [81].

As mentioned above, the loss of appetite associated with common cold is not usually as great as in flu where fever may also occur. One idea that has been put forward to explain the loss of appetite associated with infection is that the rise in temperature suppresses appetite in the same way that a postprandial rise in total body heat content contributes to a sensation of satiety [82].

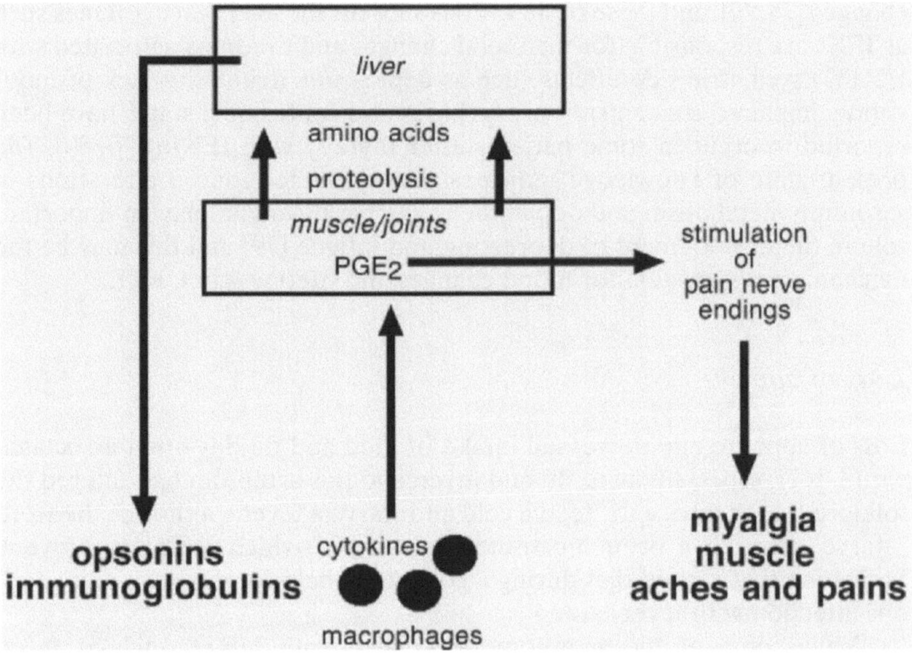

Figure 9. Myalgia. Muscle aches and pains are caused by the breakdown of muscle and joint proteins caused by PGE_2, which also stimulates pain nerve endings. PGE_2 production in muscles and joints is stimulated by cytokines released from macrophages and neutrophils in the airway epithelium.

Anorexia may aid in eliminating infection in several ways; by saving energy that would be otherwise used in finding food, by reducing heat loss from the body that would be lost by convection, by reducing the availability of micronutrients such as iron and zinc that are essential for the growth of pathogens, and by enhancing monocyte and macrophage activity [14, 83].

At present our understanding of changes in appetite and food intake associated with URTI is very limited, but there may well be insights into controlling food intake that can be obtained from research on the mechanisms of anorexia and URTI.

Muscle aches and pains

Around 50% of subjects with common cold symptoms may experience some muscle aches and pains [22]. Myalgia is a symptom of the acute-phase response to infection and there is evidence that this symptom is caused by the effects of cytokines on skeletal muscle [84]. Pro-inflammatory cytokines have been implicated as inducing the breakdown of muscle proteins, and TNF was initially referred to as 'cachetin' because of its role in causing muscle wasting or 'cachexia' [85]. The breakdown of muscle protein in response to URTI can be viewed as beneficial as it mobilises proteins and amino acids that can be converted in the liver to opsonins and other components of the immune response [85] as illustrated in Figure 9. There is some evidence to indicate that myalgia associated with infection is related to the formation of PGE_2 in muscles and joints in response to circulating cytokines [84]. The cytokine-induced generation of PGE_2 and the breakdown of skeletal muscle *in vitro* is inhibited by indomethacin [84] and similarly myalgia associated with URTI is relieved with acetylsalicylic acid [22].

References

1 Eccles R (2005) Understanding the symptoms of the common cold and influenza. *Lancet Infect Dis* 5: 718–725
2 Jackson G, Dowling H, Spiesman I, Boand A (1958) Transmission of the common cold to volunteers under controlled conditions. 1. The common cold as a clinical entity. *Arch Intern Med* 101: 267–278
3 Heikkinen T, Jarvinen A (2003) The common cold. *Lancet* 361: 51–59
4 Tyrrell DA, Cohen S, Schlarb JE (1993) Signs and symptoms in common colds. *Epidemiol Infect* 111: 143–156
5 Monto AS, Gravenstein S, Elliott M, Colopy M, Schweinle J (2000) Clinical signs and symptoms predicting influenza infection. *Arch Intern Med* 160: 3243–3247
6 Schmid-Hempel P (2009) Immune defence, parasite evasion strategies and their relevance for 'macroscopic phenomena' such as virulence. *Philos Trans R Soc Lond* 364: 85–98
7 Winther B, Farr B, Turner RB, Hendley JO, Gwaltney JM Jr, Mygind N (1984) Histopathologic examination and enumeration of polymorphonuclear leukocytes in the nasal mucosa during experimental rhinovirus colds. *Acta Otolaryngol* Suppl 413: 19–24
8 Smith A, Thomas M, Kent J, Nicholson K (1998) Effects of the common cold on mood and performance. *Psychoneuroendocrinology* 23: 733–739
9 Weiss RA (2002) Virulence and pathogenesis. *Trends Microbiol* 10: 314–317
10 Eccles R (2005) Asymptomatic spread of flu is not proved. *BMJ* 331: 1145
11 Turner RB, Hendley JO (2005) Virucidal hand treatments for prevention of rhinovirus infection. *J Antimicrob Chemother* 56: 805–807
12 Turner RB (1997) Epidemiology, pathogenesis, and treatment of the common cold. *Ann Allergy Asthma Immunol* 78: 531–539
13 Hendley JO (1998) The host response, not the virus, causes the symptoms of the common cold. *Clin Infect Dis* 26: 847–848
14 Beutler B (2003) Science review: Key inflammatory and stress pathways in critical illness – The central role of the Toll-like receptors. *Crit Care* 7: 39–46
15 Exton MS (1997) Infection-induced anorexia: active host defence strategy. *Appetite* 29: 369–383
16 Eccles R (2000) Pathophysiology of nasal symptoms. *Am J Rhinol* 14: 335–338
17 Proud D, Reynolds CJ, Lacapra S, Kagey-Sobotka A, Lichenstein LM, Naclerio

RM (1988) Nasal provocation with bradykinin induces symptoms of rhinitis and a sore throat. *Am Rev Respir Dis* 173: 613–616
18 Shibayama Y, Skoner D, Suehiro S, Konishi JE, Fireman P, Kaplan AP (1996) Bradykinin levels during experimental nasal infection with rhinovirus and attenuated influenza virus. *Immunopharmacology* 33: 311–313
19 Conti B, Tabarean I, Andrei C, Bartfai T (2004) Cytokines and fever. *Front Biosci* 9: 1433–1449
20 Georgitis JW (1993) Nasopharyngitis, pharyngitis, and tonsillitis. *Immunol Allergy Clin North Am* 13: 109–118
21 Rees GL, Eccles R (1994) Sore throat following nasal and oropharyngeal bradykinin challenge. *Acta Otolaryngol* 114: 311–314
22 Eccles R, Loose I, Jawad M, Nyman L (2003) Effects of acetylsalicylic acid on sore throat pain and other pain symptoms associated with acute upper respiratory tract infection. *Pain Med* 4: 118–124
23 Eccles R (2006) Efficacy and safety of over-the-counter analgesics in the treatment of common cold and flu. *J Clin Pharm Ther* 31: 309–319
24 Winther B, Gwaltney JM, Mygind N, Turner RB, Hendley O (1986) Sites of rhinovirus recovery after point inoculation of the upper airway. *J Am Med Assoc* 256: 1763–1767
25 Leung AKC, Robson WLM (1994) Sneezing. *J Otolaryngol* 23: 125–129
26 Mygind N, Secher C, Kirkegaard J (1983) Role of histamine and antihistamines in the nose. *Eur J Respir Dis* Suppl 128: 16–20
27 Askenasy JJM (1990) The photic sneeze. *Postgrad Med J* 66: 892–893
28 Whitman BW, Packer RJ (1993) The photic sneeze: Literature review and discussion. *Neurology* 43: 868–871
29 Hayden FG, Diamond L, Wood PB, Korts DC, Wecker MT (1996) Effectiveness and safety of intranasal ipratropium bromide in common colds. A randomized, double-blind, placebo-controlled trial. *Ann Intern Med* 125: 89–97
30 Eccles R, Vancauwenberge P, Tetzloff W, Borum P (1995) A clinical study to evaluate the efficacy of the antihistamine doxylamine succinate in the relief of runny nose and sneezing associated with upper respiratory-tract infection. *J Pharm Pharmacol* 47: 990–993
31 Gwaltney JM, Winther B (1984) Symposium on rhinovirus pathogenesis. *Acta Otolaryngol (Stockholm)* Suppl 413: 45p
32 Eccles R (1983) Physiology of nasal secretion. *Eur J Respir Dis* 62: 115–119
33 Eccles R, Pedersen A, Regberg D, Tulento H, Borum P, Stjarne P (2007) Efficacy and safety of topical combinations of ipratropium and xylometazoline for the treatment of symptoms of runny nose and nasal congestion associated with acute upper respiratory tract infection. *Am J Rhinol* 21: 40–45
34 Murray S, Del Mar C, O'Rourke P (2000) Predictors of an antibiotic prescription by GPs for respiratory tract infections: A pilot. *Fam Pract* 17: 386–388
35 Stockley RA, Bayley D, Hill SL, Hill AT, Crooks S, Campbell EJ (2001) Assessment of airway neutrophils by sputum colour: Correlation with airways inflammation. *Thorax* 56: 366–372
36 Arroll B, Kenealy T (2005) Antibiotics for the common cold and acute purulent rhinitis. *Cochrane Database of Systematic Reviews* (Online): CD000247

37 Davis SS, Eccles R (2004) Nasal congestion: Mechanisms, measurement and medications. Core information for the clinician. *Clin Otolaryngol* 29: 659–666
38 Eccles R (2000) Nasal airflow in health and disease. *Acta Otolaryngol (Stockholm)* 120: 580–595
39 Eccles R, Reilly M, Eccles KSJ (1996) Changes in the amplitude of the nasal cycle associated with symptoms of acute upper respiratory tract infection. *Acta Otolaryngol* 116: 77–81
40 Malcolmson KG (1959) The vasomotor activities of the nasal mucous membrane. *J Laryngol Otol* 37: 73–98
41 Eccles R (1983) Sympathetic control of nasal erectile tissue. *Eur J Respir Dis* 64: 150–154
42 Lacroix JS, Stjarne P, Anggard A, Lundberg JM (1989) Sympathetic vascular control of the pig nasal mucosa (III): Co-release of noradrenaline and neuropeptide Y. *Acta Physiol Scand* 135: 17–28
43 Eccles R, Eriksson M, Garreffa S, Chen SC (2008) The nasal decongestant effect of xylometazoline in the common cold. *Am J Rhinol* 22: 491–496
44 Eccles R, Jawad MS, Jawad SS, Angello JT, Druce HM (2005) Efficacy and safety of single and multiple doses of pseudoephedrine in the treatment of nasal congestion associated with common cold. *Am J Rhinol* 19: 25–31
45 Clarke JD, Eccles R (2005) Paradoxical sensation of nasal airflow in patients with common cold. Are we measuring the correct modality? *Acta Otolaryngol* 125: 1307–1311
46 Gwaltney JM, Phillips CD, Miller RD, Riker DK (1994) Computed tomographic study of the common cold. *N Engl J Med* 330: 25–30
47 Falck B, Svanholm H, Aust R, Backlund L (1989) The relationship between body posture and pressure in occluded maxillary sinus of man. *Rhinology* 27: 161–167
48 Whittet HB (1992) Infraorbital nerve dehiscence: The anatomic cause of maxillary sinus "vacuum headache"? *Otolaryngol Head Neck Surg* 107: 21–28
49 Falck B, Svanholm H, Aust R, Backlund L (1990) Blood flow and pulse amplitude in the mucosa of the human maxillary sinus in relation to body posture. *Rhinology* 28: 169–176
50 Ayub M, Thale AB, Hedderich J, Tillmann BN, Paulsen FP (2003) The cavernous body of the human efferent tear ducts contributes to regulation of tear outflow. *Invest Ophthalmol Vis Sci* 44: 4900–4907
51 Paulsen F, Hallmann U, Paulsen J, Thale A (2000) Innervation of the cavernous body of the human efferent tear ducts and function in tear outflow mechanism. *J Anat* 197: 177–187
52 Hadjikoutis S, Eccles R, Wiles CM (2000) Coughing and choking in motor neuron disease. *J Neurol Neurosurg Psychiatry* 68: 601–604
53 Eccles R, Lee PC (2004) Cough induced by airway vibration as a model of airway hyperreactivity in patients with acute upper respiratory tract infection. *Pulm Pharmacol Ther* 17: 337–342
54 Jacoby DB (2004) Pathophysiology of airway viral infections. *Pulm Pharmacol Ther* 17: 333–336
55 Lee P, Cotterill-Jones C, Eccles R (2002) Voluntary control of cough. *Pulm Pharmacol Ther* 15: 317–320

56 Davenport PW (2008) Urge-to-cough: What can it teach us about cough? *Lung* 186 (Suppl 1): S107–111
57 Widdicombe J, Eccles R, Fontana G (2006) Supramedullary influences on cough. *Respir Physiol Neurobiol* 152: 320–328
58 Simonyan K, Saad ZS, Loucks TM, Poletto CJ, Ludlow CL (2007) Functional neuroanatomy of human voluntary cough and sniff production. *NeuroImage* 37: 401–409
59 Hutchings HA, Eccles R, Smith AP, Jawad M (1993) Voluntary cough suppression as an indication of symptom severity in upper respiratory tract infections. *Eur Respir J* 6: 1449–1454
60 Hutchings HA, Morris S, Eccles R, Jawad M (1993) Voluntary suppression of cough induced by inhalation of capsaicin in healthy volunteers. *Respir Med* 87: 379–382
61 Eccles R (2006) Mechanisms of the placebo effect of sweet cough syrups. *Respir Physiol Neurobiol* 152: 340–348
62 Smith RS (1992) The cytokine theory of headache. *Med Hypotheses* 39: 168–174
63 Gold R, Rieckmann P, Chang P, Abdalla J (2005) The long-term safety and tolerability of high-dose interferon beta-1a in relapsing-remitting multiple sclerosis: 4-year data from the PRISMS study. *Eur J Neurol* 12: 649–656
64 van Zonneveld M, Flink HJ, Verhey E, Senturk H, Zeuzem S, Akarca US, Cakaloglu Y, Simon C, So TM, Gerken G et al. (2005) The safety of pegylated interferon alpha-2b in the treatment of chronic hepatitis B: Predictive factors for dose reduction and treatment discontinuation. *Aliment Pharmacol Ther* 21: 1163–1171
65 Bo SH, Davidsen EM, Gulbrandsen P, Dietrichs E, Bovim G, Stovner LJ, White LR (2009) Cerebrospinal fluid cytokine levels in migraine, tension-type headache and cervicogenic headache. *Cephalalgia* 29: 365–372
66 Helman CG (1978) "Feed a cold, starve a fever". Folk models of infection in an English suburban community, and their relation to medical treatment. *Cult Med Psychiatry* 2: 107–137
67 Sanu A, Eccles R (2008) The effects of a hot drink on nasal airflow and symptoms of common cold and flu. *Rhinology* 46: 271–275
68 Guieu JD, Hellon RF (1980) The chill sensation in fever. *Pflugers Arch* 384: 103–104
69 Cabanac M (1990) Phylogeny of fever. In: J Bligh, K Voigt (eds): *Thermoreception and temperature regulation*. Springer, Berlin, 284–296
70 Booth CM, Matukas LM, Tomlinson GA, Rachlis AR, Rose DB, Dwosh HA, Walmsley SL, Mazzulli T, Avendano M, Derkach P et al. (2003) Clinical features and short-term outcomes of 144 patients with SARS in the greater Toronto area. *JAMA* 289: 2801–2809
71 Leon LR (2002) Invited review: Cytokine regulation of fever: Studies using gene knockout mice. *J Appl Physiol* 92: 2648–2655
72 Netea MG, Kullberg BJ, Van der Meer JW (2000) Circulating cytokines as mediators of fever. *Clin Infect Dis* 31 (Suppl 5): S178–184
73 Blatteis CM (2007) The onset of fever: New insights into its mechanism. *Prog Brain Res* 162: 3–14

74 Dantzer R, Kelley KW (2007) Twenty years of research on cytokine-induced sickness behavior. *Brain Behav Immun* 21: 153–160
75 Vollmer-Conna U, Fazou C, Cameron B, Li H, Brennan C, Luck L, Davenport T, Wakefield D, Hickie I, Lloyd A (2004) Production of pro-inflammatory cytokines correlates with the symptoms of acute sickness behaviour in humans. *Psychological Medicine* 34: 1289–1297
76 Herzog C, Berger R, Fernex M, Friesecke K, Havas L, Just M, Dubach UC (1986) What dose of intranasal interferon for the common cold? *Lancet* 1: 1089–1090
77 Gwaltney JM Jr, Winther B, Patrie JT, Hendley JO (2002) Combined antiviral-antimediator treatment for the common cold. *J Infect Dis* 186: 147–154
78 Schaefer M, Schmidt F, Neumer R, Scholler G, Schwarz M (2002) Interferon-alpha, cytokines and possible implications for mood disorders. *Bipolar Disord* 4 (Suppl 1): 111–113
79 Miller AH (2009) Norman Cousins Lecture. Mechanisms of cytokine-induced behavioral changes: psychoneuroimmunology at the translational interface. *Brain Behav Immun* 23: 149–158
80 Raison CL, Borisov AS, Majer M, Drake DF, Pagnoni G, Woolwine BJ, Vogt GJ, Massung B, Miller AH (2009) Activation of central nervous system inflammatory pathways by interferon-alpha: relationship to monoamines and depression. *Biol Psychiatry* 65: 296–303
81 McCarthy DO (2000) Cytokines and the anorexia of infection: Potential mechanisms and treatments. *Biol Res Nurs* 1: 287–298
82 Brobeck JR (1948) Food intake as a mechanism of temperature regulation. *Yale J Biol Med* 20: 545–552
83 Mahoney T, Ball P (2002) Common respiratory tract infections as psychological entities: A review of the mood and performance effects of being ill. *Aust Psychol* 37: 86–94
84 Baracos V, Rodemann HP, Dinarello CA, Goldberg AL (1983) Stimulation of muscle protein degradation and prostaglandin E2 release by leukocytic pyrogen (interleukin-1). A mechanism for the increased degradation of muscle proteins during fever. *N Engl J Med* 308: 553–558
85 Kotler DP (2000) Cachexia. *Ann Intern Med* 133: 622–634

Common Cold
ed. by R. Eccles and O. Weber

Common respiratory infections diagnosed in general practice

Alex J. Elliot[1,2] and Douglas M. Fleming[1]

[1] *Royal College of General Practitioners Research and Surveillance Centre, Lordswood House, 54 Lordswood Road, Harborne, Birmingham B17 9DB, UK*
[2] *Real-Time Syndromic Surveillance Team, Health Protection Agency, 6th Floor, 5 St Philip's Place, Birmingham B3 2PW, UK*

Abstract

Acute respiratory infections are one of the most common causes for presentation to a general practitioner. The range of symptoms associated with each infection can be wide ranging in both presentation and severity, depending on age of the patient, underlying co-morbidities and other confounding factors. In this chapter we describe the most common respiratory infections ranging from relatively mild infections such as the common cold, through to more serious presentations including pneumonia. Data are presented from a general practitioner morbidity surveillance system based in England and Wales. Each acute respiratory syndrome is described in respect of seasonality, secular trends and microbiological aetiology providing an insight into the complex nature of these acute respiratory episodes. The more serious endpoints of acute respiratory infections are hospitalisation and death. Many acute respiratory infections are mild in nature and generally self-limiting and therefore do not commonly require further medical interventions. However, despite major advances in the prevention and treatment of acute respiratory infections in recent years, hospitalisation and deaths continue to exert pressures on national health resources and provide an economic burden in countries across the world on an annual basis.

Introduction

Acute respiratory infections present one of the most common reasons for consulting a general practitioner (GP) in England and Wales [1]. Approximately 30% of the general population consulted at least once because of a respiratory illness during the 1991/92 GP-based National Morbidity Survey: by 2001, the proportion had fallen to 25% and by 2007 to 21% [2]. Eighty five per cent of all episodes of illness classified to the International Classification of Diseases (ICD) chapter on respiratory disorders are due to acute respiratory infections. The Royal College of General Practitioners (RCGP) Weekly Returns Service (WRS), a sentinel

GP surveillance network located across England and Wales has monitored the incidence of acute respiratory infections since 1966 [3]. In 1991 approximately 18% of all consultations were attributable to the respiratory chapter of the ICD9; the vast majority of these were acute respiratory infections [4]. In recent years this proportion has decreased due to reducing numbers of respiratory infections diagnosed, and increasing numbers of total consultations [5, 6]. There are large age-related differences in the illness episode and consultation rates with children reporting much higher rates of upper respiratory tract infection (URTI) and older persons higher rates of lower respiratory tract infection (LRTI). In pre-school children (aged less than 5 years), the incidence of respiratory infections is higher in males than females; in school children and the elderly there is no gender difference; in most adult years reported incidence is higher in females, partly because of gender bias in consultation but also partly because of a greater potential of spread from children.

In this chapter, we address the most commonly diagnosed URTI and LRTI, starting with the organisms that are responsible for the presenting symptoms. We then address the presenting clinical syndromes and diagnoses; these are ordered in degree of severity, starting with mild episodes encountered in general practice, finishing with severe episodes that result in hospital admission and/or death. We relate these to long-term and secular trends, the microbiological aetiology of the diagnoses, and possible prevention strategies in the primary care setting.

The viruses

In this chapter, the majority of the clinical syndromes described are primarily of a viral cause. In this section, a short introduction to the viruses responsible is provided with an emphasis on the clinical aspects of infection. A more detailed summary including the taxonomy, structure, replication, transmission and immunology of each virus is provided in the chapter by Olaf Weber.

Influenza virus

The influenza viruses are grouped into three distinctive classes: A, B and C. Influenza B and C are found almost exclusively in humans with sporadic isolations in seals and pigs [7, 8] and cause relatively mild seasonal outbreaks of disease [9]. The natural reservoir of influenza A is in aquatic birds [10]. There are further subgroups of influenza A [10, 11]. The ability of influenza A viruses to undergo major genetic reassortments (antigenic shift) makes them ideal candidates for causing major outbreaks of disease on a global scale. Over the last century, three influenza pandemics have led to the introduction of novel variants into the human population: H1N1 (1918/19); H2N2 (1957/58); and H3N2 (1968/69) [12]. Currently, two influenza A subtypes H3N2 and H1N1 (reintroduced in 1977/78) circulate in the human population. Despite recent scares involving highly pathogenic avian influenza viruses, e.g. H5N1, H7N7 causing severe disease and high mortality rates in humans, efficient human-to-human transmission has yet to be confirmed and therefore these isolated incidents have not developed into potential pandemic strains.

In the Northern Hemisphere, during each winter, influenza A and B strains cause annual outbreaks of respiratory illness in the community. Continual evolution of these viruses allows them to evade of the immune response, thus enabling new epidemics of disease to occur from year to year.

Respiratory syncytial virus

There is an increasing awareness that human respiratory syncytial virus (RSV) is a major cause of serious lower respiratory illness. It has been shown that RSV can cause significant respiratory disease across all age groups [13]; however, the effect of RSV has been most frequently recorded in young children [14–16]. Despite the association with severe disease in the elderly, the exact role that RSV plays is not clearly understood partly due to the difficulty in recognising the clinical symptoms presented by RSV and influenza A infections in the elderly [17].

Similar to the influenza viruses, RSV is classified into subgroups (RSV A and B) and is also subject to annual evolution [18]. Despite the serious burden of RSV in respect of morbidity and mortality, there are currently no licensed vaccines, although there are candidate vaccines that are undergoing early safety and immunogenicity studies [19]. There were major setbacks during early RSV vaccine trials in the late 1960s: children administered formalin-inactivated RSV vaccines suffered severe LRTI following subsequent exposure to wild-type RSV leading to hospitalisation rates of up to 80% and the deaths of two patients [20].

Human parainfluenza virus

There are four distinct human parainfluenza virus (HPIV) serotypes that have been identified (types 1–4) and are important causes of URTI and LRTI, especially in children [21, 22]. Circulation in summer is unusual for a respiratory virus: HPIV type 3 activity typically peaks during May–June. HPIV type 1 has circulation from September to December (i.e. earlier than common winter respiratory viruses) and HPIV 2 has typical winter circulation peaking December/January [23].

Human coronavirus

Human coronaviruses (HCoV) can be divided into two distinct groups, those that cause respiratory infections and those causing gastrointestinal disease. Respiratory HCoV were originally isolated from the respiratory tract of an adult with a common cold. Until recently, respiratory HCoV were thought to cause relatively minor upper respiratory tract illnesses. However, the emergence of Severe Acute Respiratory Syndrome (SARS) in 2002, which was subsequently shown to be caused by a new variant of a HCoV, changed opinion on the relative importance of these viruses on public health [24–26].

Rhinovirus

Rhinovirus (RV) is known to cause common cold symptoms and due to the large number of serotypes can cause repeated infections throughout an individual's life. In children, RV infections are commonly associated with recurrent wheeze, or exacerbations of asthma [27, 28]. The role of RV in the development of more severe disease in adults is not clear, but there is growing evidence of a link between RV infections and lower respiratory tract disease, especially in the elderly [29–31].

Human metapneumovirus

Human metapneumovirus (HMPV) is a relatively newly detected respiratory pathogen discovered in a group of young children in the Netherlands presenting with respiratory tract infections [32]. The virus is classified in the same *Pneumovirus* subfamily as human RSV. Hospital-based studies have demonstrated that HMPV is a common respiratory pathogen often implicated in respiratory admissions of young children [15, 33]. Community-based studies have shown that HMPV is the cause of acute respiratory tract infections across many age groups [34]. Although infection in adults is common and often asymptomatic, infections can cause serious illness and lead to hospitalisation [35, 36].

Human bocavirus

Human bocavirus (HBoV) is a parvovirus recently identified in Sweden, and now independently identified in children presenting with acute LRTI in several other countries [37]. The prevalence of viral detection in LRTI ranges from 3.1% to 10.3% with a relatively high rate of co-infection with other viruses [37–40].

Microbiological aetiology

The underlying microbiological aetiology of URTI and LRTI is complex due to the potential number of pathogens involved. The majority of acute uncomplicated respiratory infections are caused by viral pathogens, with further secondary complications induced by bacterial colonisation of damaged cells lining the respiratory tract. Each viral pathogen has a distinct seasonality, although some are more predictable in their nature (Fig. 1). Influenza viruses are not consistent in their circulation; however, one can generalise their circulation as peaking during winter months, mainly between November and February. It has been noted that the more severe epidemics (for example in 1989/90) have started earlier in the winter, and peaked well before the Christmas/New Year period. Influenza B virus circulation is distinct from influenza A as these viruses commonly circulate later in the winter. Typically, influenza B circulation follows that of influenza A, and viruses can be isolated from cases during February and into March.

RSV is much more predictable in its circulation. Laboratory reports peak during weeks 50–52 (mid to late December) [41]. One of the most useful clinical markers of RSV activity is acute bronchitis in young children aged 0–4 years [42]. Over 90% of all RSV laboratory reports are from children aged less than 5 years. A comparison of RSV reports and acute bronchitis in young children demonstrates a remarkable association (Fig. 2).

During periods of concurrent circulation of influenza and RSV, it can be difficult to disentangle the effects of each virus. We have defined virus active periods of influenza and RSV and introduced a combined period, where we have tried to apportion the effects of each virus. From the studies, it is clear

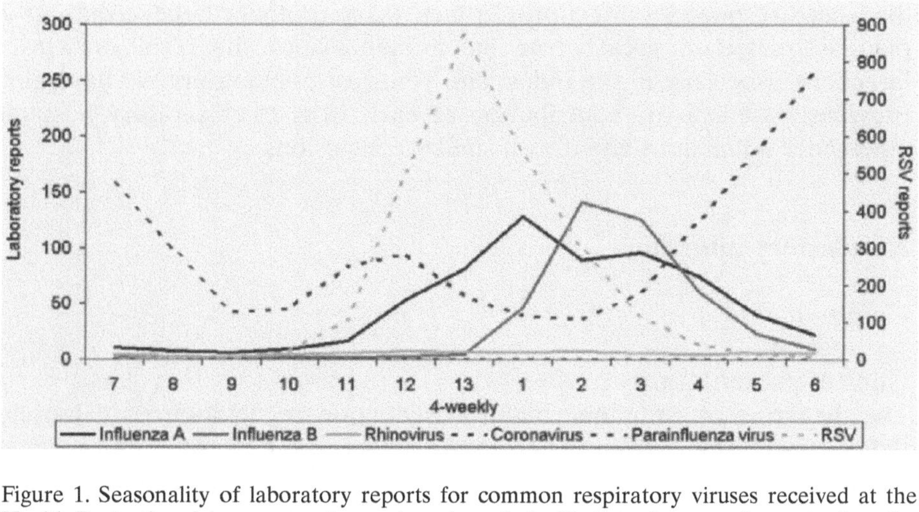

Figure 1. Seasonality of laboratory reports for common respiratory viruses received at the Health Protection Agency; reports per 4-week period with the winter weeks centred on the horizontal axis on mid winter (data averaged over years 1993–2001) [42].

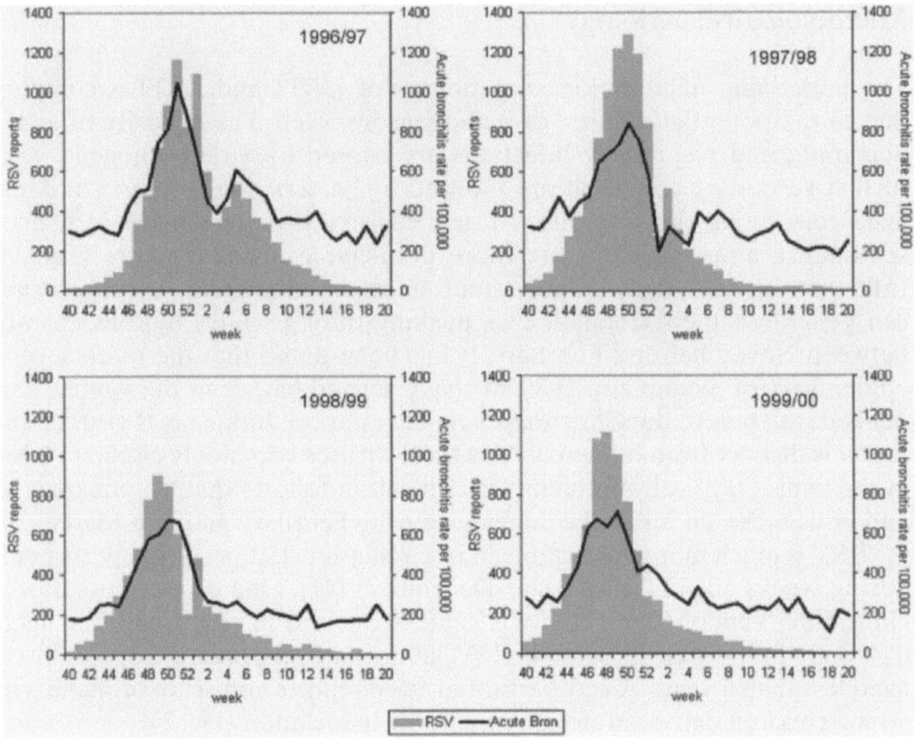

Figure 2. Incidence rate per 100 000 population of acute bronchitis in young children aged 0–4 years compared with laboratory reports for respiratory syncytial virus (RSV) over selected winters [42].

that RSV plays an important role in the burden of a number of commonly diagnosed respiratory infections. In fact, we, and others, believe that RSV plays as great, if not greater role than influenza in causing respiratory tract infections, especially in the oldest and youngest populations. We have also previously studied the contribution of each virus to respiratory hospital emergency admissions and drawn similar conclusions.

Respiratory infections

Common cold

Clinical presentation

The diagnosis of common cold is based upon recognition of a loosely defined syndrome rather than specific symptoms. Generally, the term is taken to mean an acute URTI with rhinitis and variable degrees of pharyngitis. Other presenting symptoms may include sneezing, runny nose, sore throat, chills; the presence of a mild fever is common but, except in young

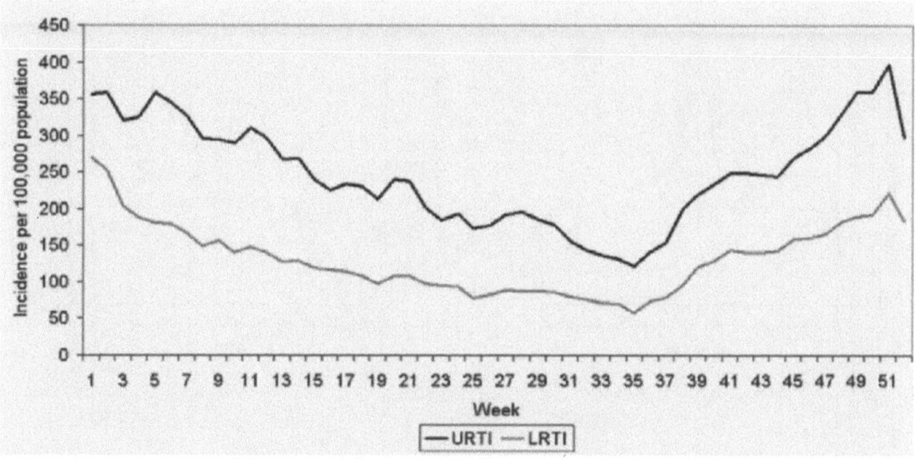

Figure 3. Mean weekly incidence rate per 100000 population over the period 2002–2007 of upper and lower respiratory tract infections (URTI and LRTI).

children, the fever tends to be less than that associated with influenza. Colds are caused by a range of viruses such as RV, adenovirus and HCoV. Viruses such as influenza and RSV may also cause symptoms that are commonly described as a cold, although we tend to associate these viruses with more severe respiratory symptoms. A plot of the weekly incidence of URTI and LRTI averaged over a 6-year period (2002–2007) shows how the two types of illness show the same trend, suggesting a common aetiology (Fig. 3). The incidence of acute otitis media (AOM) and the common cold in children aged 0–4 years is plotted over 4 selected winters in Figure 4, again suggesting a common aetiology [43]. The common cold is usually a mild self-limiting acute respiratory illness; however, symptoms may be more severe in younger children. The duration of illness is mostly about 7 days but the acute phase lasts 3–4 days. In addition to AOM, the common cold may trigger exacerbations of asthma and cause sinusitis [27]. The mild self-limiting nature of URTI prompts only limited collection of clinical specimens for virological investigation from routine disease management and thus it is difficult to be specific about aetiology in the majority of cases of common cold and URTI.

Secular trends

Similar to other acute respiratory infections, the incidence of diagnosed common cold infections has gradually fallen over previous years. The reduction in young children is particularly significant and has been accompanied by a similar reduction in AOM. Whereas in older age groups these reductions may be attributable in part to changes in consulting behaviour, the decrease in young children with acute ear problems suggests a real decrease

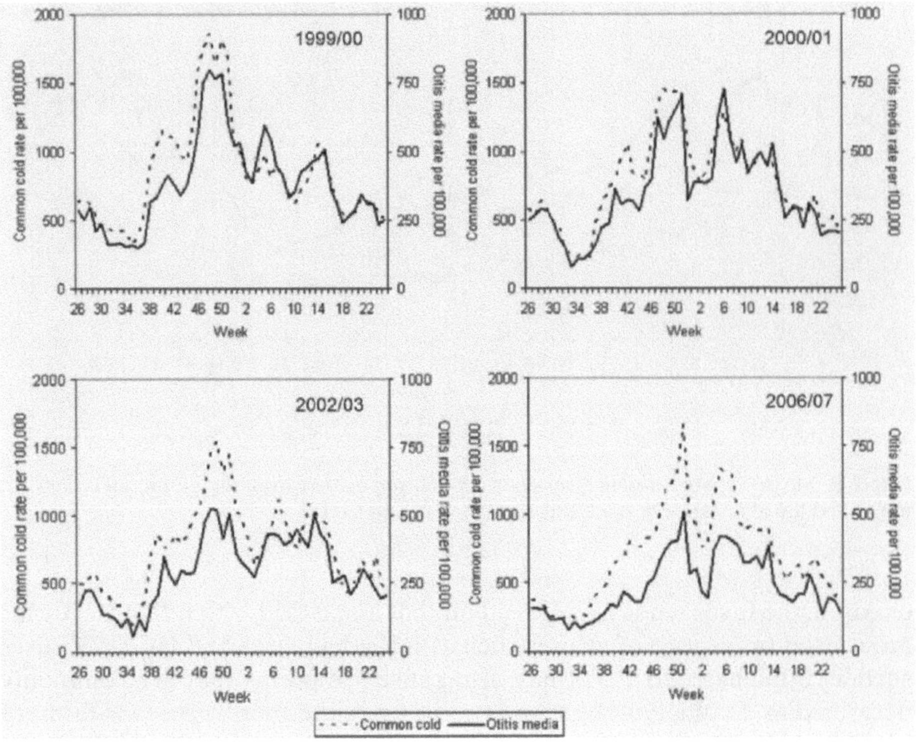

Figure 4. Weekly incidence rate per 100000 of common cold and acute otitis media in young children aged 0–4 years over selected years (horizontal axes centred on turn of year: note differing scales on vertical axes) [87].

since patient health care expectations on behalf of children are more likely to be higher than lower.

Seasonality

As with most acute respiratory infections, the common cold is more frequent in winter. Peak incidence rates occur between weeks 48 and 02. Incidence is much higher in young children with the highest incidence recorded in children aged 0–4 years (Fig. 5).

Herpes simplex and cold sores

Cold sores are commonly associated with the common cold but these are due to specific herpes viruses. The constitutional symptoms experienced by persons with cold sores are similar to the common cold and often confused with it. It is possible that a common cold infection increases the likelihood

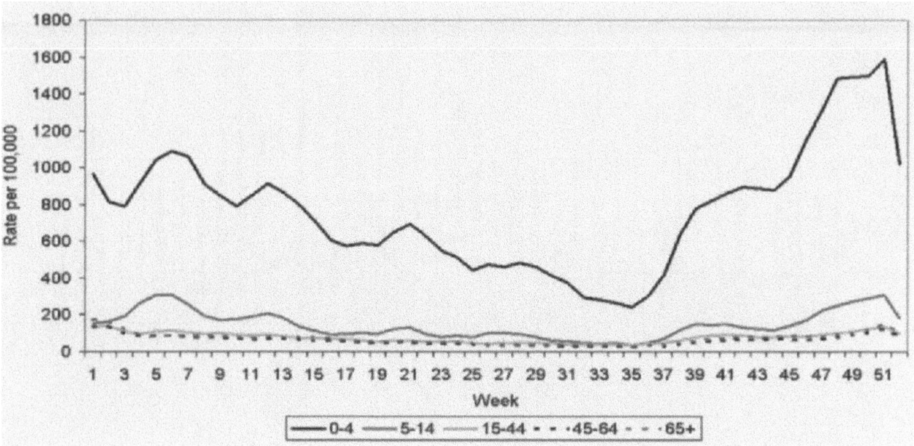

Figure 5. Weekly incidence rate of common cold over the period 1999–2008 by age group.

of a herpes simplex infection and the development of the typical cold sores, particularly on the lips and around the mouth.

There are two types of herpes simplex virus: type 1, which is implicated in the commonly encountered facial cold sore, but less frequently in genital herpes [44]; and type 2, which is more commonly a cause of genital herpes [45]. Both conditions are more common in females than males [46]. There are specific antiviral treatments for herpes simplex infections and they include acyclovir, either given orally or topically applied [47]. The topical application is commonly prescribed for persons with cold sores, but to be effective it must be given immediately the first symptoms appear [48].

Acute otitis media

Clinical presentation

AOM is the inflammation of the middle ear involving the Eustachian tube and is a common reason for presentation of young children with earache. AOM may be suppurative or non-suppurative. It is often thought of as a secondary complication of acute respiratory infections: however, data from the RCGP WRS for common cold and AOM demonstrate a close association, suggesting that AOM is as likely a direct result of the respiratory infection rather than an associated complication (Fig. 4).

Secular trends

Contrary to the trends of influenza-like illness (ILI), the incidence of AOM increased steadily from 1967 to a peak during the late 1990s, since when rates have steadily declined (Fig. 6).

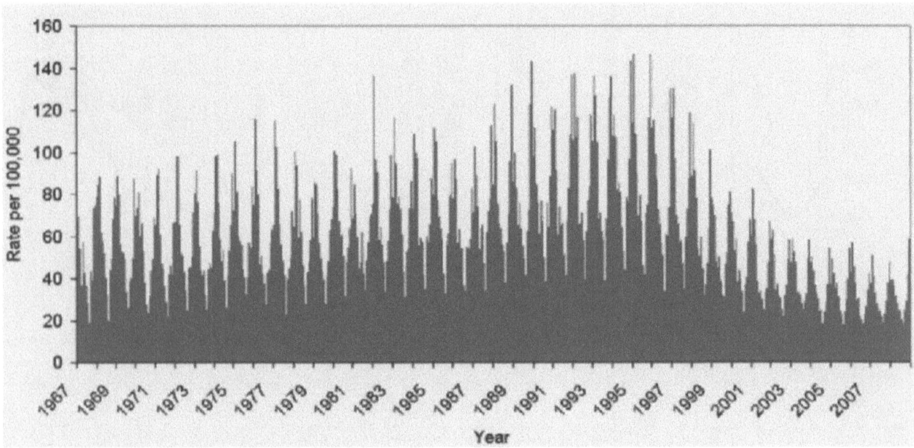

Figure 6. Mean weekly incidence rate in 4-week periods per 100000 population of acute otitis media over the period 1967–2008 [53].

We have recorded data separately for suppurative otitis media since 1994; incidence of suppurative otitis media is generally lower with rates among all age groups about half those of total non-suppurative otitis media. These data show a similar trend to AOM with incidence falling from 1995 and then stabilising from 2003/2004 onwards. This trend is also seen in data for pneumonia (Fig. 12). The peak of AOM during the 1990s has been recorded for a number of other respiratory infections, including acute bronchitis and asthma.

Although uncommon now, mastoiditis as a complication of AOM was a serious problem fifty and more years ago [49]. The lingering fear of a recurrence of mastoiditis is a major reason for the continued excessive use of antibiotics for the treatment of AOM. Mastoiditis is not always a complication of a viral URTI: it is sometimes a complication of streptococcal infections [49]. Intensive (probably intravenous) treatment with antibiotics and appropriate surgical intervention remains necessary for the treatment of this condition [50]. Clinically, it presents with acute pain and tenderness over the mastoid process usually accompanied by aural discharge.

Seasonality

The seasonality of AOM demonstrates a close association with the diagnosis of common cold (Fig. 4). In children aged 0–4 years, both clinical diagnoses peak during winter weeks 50–52; the diagnosis of common cold is more frequent than AOM, at a ratio of ~2:1 [43]. It is also interesting that there are six main peaks of AOM during the year, and the troughs between these peaks coincide with school holidays, providing evidence again that infections are concurrent with the increase in acute respiratory infections associated with the return of children to school after holiday periods.

Acute sinusitis

Clinical presentation

Acute sinusitis usually presents with a background of recent URTI [51]. The mucosal lining of the paranasal sinuses is continuous with the upper respiratory tract and is subject to the catarrhal oedema and mucosal congestion affecting the entire upper respiratory tract when subject to infection or to pollen sensitisation. The label acute sinusitis describes infection in any of the paranasal sinuses (frontal, ethmoidal, maxillary) but is usually reserved to describe secondary bacterial infection [52]. This arises because sinus drainage becomes blocked and the relevant sinus fills up with pus that does not drain properly. The increased pressure created causes local pain and tenderness, which is usually readily apparent on percussion of the area. It is commonly accompanied by a sensation of blockage and by pus in the nose. The sense of smell is impaired or lost. The diagnosis is prompted by the history and local tenderness but can be confirmed by X-ray. Treatment includes nasal decongestants and antibiotics with surgical drainage in non-responding cases. Some people get particularly frequent episodes and develop nasal polyps. Nasal polypectomy and surgical measures to improve drainage are sometimes needed for these patients.

Seasonality

The incidence of acute sinusitis roughly follows that of URTI generally. Experience in the WRS has shown that this condition is reported more frequently in females than males (by a factor of 2 to 1) [2]. At one time we thought this may be part of a well-recognized gender-based consultation bias. However, the magnitude of the difference and the fact that it is not seen in most other respiratory infections suggest that this is not a sufficient explanation for the difference. We speculate that the anatomical architecture in females is more prone to blockage than that in males. It could also be partly explained by the difficulty of distinguishing the head pain from a migraine attack, which is well recognized as commoner in females. Incidence of acute sinusitis is maximal in the 25–64-year age group [53].

Croup

Clinical presentation

Croup is an infection associated with inflammation and swelling of the larynx and trachea; it is a clinically distinct illness and is more prevalent in children under 3 years of age [54]. Clinical presentation is commonly characterised by the sudden onset of the distinctive harsh "barking" cough and sore throat [55]. Symptom onset most usually happens at night and is accompanied by stridor, hoarse voice and respiratory distress [55]. Upon examination of the patient, inspiratory stridor may be present, with prolonged inspiration and chest wall retraction. When considering the diagnosis of croup, it is important to exclude other causes of shortness of breath or stridor such as foreign bodies and epiglottitis.

Epiglottitis is a frightening condition especially in young children where the lumen of the upper airways is small. It can be rapidly progressive leading to virtual asphyxiation from a very swollen epiglottis, obstructing the laryngeal opening [56]. Clinical features are classically those of an acute tonsillitis plus signs of progressive airway obstruction. The condition needs to be recognised as a serious emergency and dealt with promptly. Tracheostomy may well be necessary. *Haemophilus influenzae* type B (HIB) is one of the most common pathogens implicated with this condition and incidence has decreased since the introduction of the HIB vaccine [56, 57].

Pertussis infection or whooping cough can be confused with croup, but, whereas in croup the respiratory obstruction appears almost at the beginning of the illness, it takes some time to build up in whooping cough. In pre-vaccination days whooping cough was described as a condition which was 3 weeks coming, 3 weeks of significant symptoms and 3 months in which symptoms recurred with every respiratory virus infection. Although this was useful advice and a suitable warning for an anxious parent, it is a limited view of this illness in young children (less than 12 months of age), where the illness is particularly serious because of the small airways. The disease in this age group commonly progresses more rapidly than in older children and adults. Clinically, it is diagnosed on hearing the classical paroxysmal cough which leaves the sufferer gasping for breath and often quite cyanosed. The coughing paroxysms and terminal stridor are caused by laryngeal oedema. Retching or sometimes vomiting commonly follows the paroxysm.

Whooping cough is a bacterial infection mainly caused by *Bordetella pertussis*. The organism can be isolated from posterior nasal specimens (per nasal swab) obtained in the early stages of the illness. Management of whooping cough is essentially preventive by immunization [58]. However, the immunisation schedule only starts at 3 months of age and the protective response is variable and wanes with advancing age. Management of the acute condition involves the use of cough and spasm suppressants, plus a course of erythromycin, provided it can be started early in the course of the illness (it is of less use if administered later than 2 weeks after onset). Erythromycin should also be considered in infant contacts who have not yet received primary immunisation. Any decrease in the uptake of pertussis vaccination is likely to lead to an increased possibility of transmission from an older sibling to vulnerable young babies sometimes before there has been an opportunity to offer them immunisation. In older children and adults, whooping cough may present as an acute spasmodic cough with increasing intensity over 3 weeks, but these symptoms can be very protracted.

Secular trends

Historically, whooping cough used to occur with a secular trend about every 3 or 4 years [53]. That pattern no longer exists: 1997 was the most recent year in which there were a substantial number of cases reported to the WRS [59].

The long-term complications of *B. pertussis* infection include bronchiectasis, and here it is relevant specifically to mention measles [60]. Most doctors primarily associate measles with its classical morbilliform rash, which incidentally is often preceded by Koplik's spots on the buccal mucosa [61]. However, in terms of the clinical impact of measles the respiratory component is more significant. Indeed, if a suspicious rash is not accompanied by a cough it is very unlikely to be measles. Pre-immunisation, measles was often complicated by pneumonia and to a lesser extent by measles encephalitis. The long-term damage caused by pneumonia as a complication of measles was sometimes further complicated by the development of bronchiectasis [60].

Sore throat and tonsillitis

Clinical presentation

The presenting symptom of sore throat is often one of a constellation of symptoms associated with almost any viral URTI or LRTI. It is aggravated by any obstruction of the nasal passages. For some patients, however, a sore throat is a very specific symptom. It may be accompanied by substantial fever and difficulty in swallowing. In most viral respiratory infections the patient also complains of cough but the absence of cough and other respiratory symptoms makes bacterial tonsillitis more likely. On examination there is commonly a purulent exudate over the tonsils or pharynx but tender enlarged tonsillar lymph nodes are a clue to bacterial cause (commonly haemolytic streptococcus) [62]. In cases with enlarged or tender tonsillar nodes it is worth trying to confirm the diagnosis by throat swab culture or using one of the streptococcal rapid tests.

In former years streptococcal throat infections were often complicated by a skin rash (scarlet fever or in its mild form scarlatina), arthropathy and cardiac manifestations (rheumatic fever) or by renal problems (acute nephritis) [63]. Although these manifestations are now rare, it does not follow that they will not return and we need to be alert to noticing critical symptoms such as joint pain and swelling or blood in the urine. Occasionally, tonsillitis may progress to cause a peritonsillar abscess which may even require surgical drainage. Although it is no longer fashionable to give penicillin to everyone with a sore or even streptococcal sore throat, patients with any of these complications should be treated with a 10-day course of Penicillin V administered intramuscularly if there is any difficulty with oral administration [64].

Glandular fever is often confused with acute tonsillitis. It occurs less frequently and is concentrated in the age group 15–24 years. It is caused by the Epstein-Barr virus. Clinically, the throat often has much more extensive exudates but is not always as painful as in streptococcal tonsillitis. It differs from tonsillitis with the extensive distribution of lymphadenopathy and the presence of an enlarged or tender spleen. However, in mild cases it is not always easy to distinguish the two conditions. The diagnosis should be established by the Paul-Bunnell blood test or by culture of the Epstein-Barr virus from a throat swab specimen. Antibiotics do not help in the management of this condition and in particular, the use of amoxicillin or ampicillin can prompt an unpleasant rash.

Secular trends

Examined over 40 years there has been a decline in the incidence of acute tonsillitis. An all age incidence rate of 100–150 per 100000 population per week was usual in the 1970s but now this rate is more commonly around 60–80 per 100000. These trends have been observed separately in all age groups, although rates in childrenof 0–4 and 5–14 are approximately twice those found in adults 15–44 years and five times those seen in older adults. The incidence of glandular fever has also declined [65].

Influenza-like illness

Clinical presentation

Traditionally, the diagnostic label "influenza-like illness" (ILI) has always been associated with an infection with one of the many influenza viruses circulating in the community. The name 'influenza' originates in Italy and was used to describe epidemics of cough and fever, which were thought to be influenced by the disposition of the planets and heavenly bodies in the winter sky [66]. In the late nineteenth century it was thought to be caused by *Haemophilus influenzae* but in 1933 it was clearly attributed to the influenza virus [67]. ILI as a diagnostic label covers a wide range of symptoms and it is now apparent that these symptoms can be caused by numerous other respiratory pathogens that circulate at the same time as the influenza viruses.

The clinical term ILI is classically defined as a collection of presenting symptoms including myalgia, fever, chills, sore throat and cough, which typically appear with sudden onset [9]. A non-productive cough is more common at a later stage in the illness, and is often the main reason for subsequent consultation with a GP. Other symptoms may be present during the acute phase of the illness including rhinitis, pharyngitis, conjunctivitis and AOM (especially in children). The acute febrile phase of illness tends to resolve within 3–5 days; however, malaise and general fatigue may persist for several days and sometimes weeks post infection.

The data collected in the WRS for surveillance purposes are not based on a precise case definition of ILI, although GPs are given guidance on the appropriate use of respiratory diagnostic terminology based on their judgement at the time of consultation. The symptomatology differs according to age; the elderly often present without fever; young children may present with AOM; patients immunised with seasonal influenza vaccine may present with less severe symptoms.

Secular trends

The RCGP WRS has provided continuous monitoring of ILI in the community since 1966 [68]. Figure 7 displays the weekly incidence per 100000 population of new cases of ILI diagnosed by GPs in the WRS. The clinical impact of the 1968/69 pandemic was felt in the winter of 1969/70 in the United Kingdom (UK), demonstrating the spread of global pandemics and the delay of subsequent waves [69]. During the 1969/70 winter all age rates of ILI reached 1252 per 100000 in week 1 of 1970. In the following decade, rates of ILI remained relatively high. During subsequent decades the clinical incidence of ILI has gradually fallen, a trend seen with other common respiratory infections [6]. The last major epidemic occurred in 1989/90, when the prevailing influenza A H3 virus infected persons of all ages but particularly children aged 0–4 years in whom the recorded incidence exceeded that seen in the pandemic which hit the UK in the winter of 1969/70 (Fig. 8). During

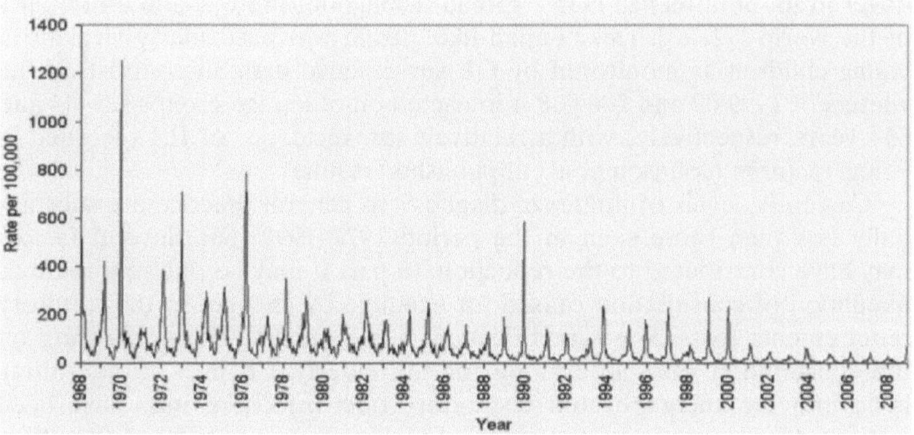

Figure 7. Weekly incidence rate per 100000 population of influenza-like illness (ILI) over the period 1968–2008 [68].

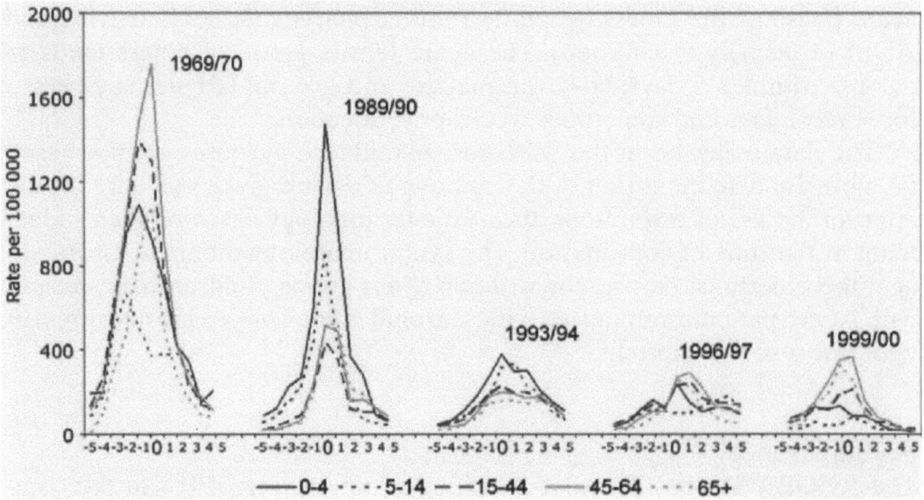

Figure 8. Age-specific incidence rate per 100 000 of influenza-like illness (ILI) over selected winters. Incidence rates are centred around the peak week (week 0) ±5 weeks.

the Millennium winter (1999/00) the National Health Service in England was severely stretched due to an influenza epidemic and there were dramatic news stories of persons spending several hours on trolleys in corridors while a hospital bed could be found [70]. Although the ILI activity was not particularly great in magnitude, it impacted on the 45–64 and 65+ years age groups (Fig. 8): respiratory infections in these age groups are more likely to result in hospital admission, and longer stays in hospital [71]. The hospital admission pressures in the Millennium winter came partly also from persons requiring admission for acute bronchitis, which was likely due to viruses other than influenza, in particular to RSV [70]. During the winter 2003/04 a novel strain of influenza H3N2 spread throughout the UK and other parts of the world [72, 73]. This "Fujian-like" strain was particularly virulent in young children as monitored by GP surveillance data; in contrast, in the winters of 1999/00 and 2007/08 it impacted on older age groups (25–44 and 65+ years, respectively) with a relatively low incidence of ILI recorded in young children (Johnson et al., unpublished results).

Currently, levels of influenza diagnosis in general practice are substantially less than those seen in the period 1970–1999 [68]. Several factors may have contributed to the reduction. In part it may be due to a reduced likelihood of consultation caused for example by changes in the statutory requirements for sickness certification; however, that has no bearing on the consultation rates in children or the elderly. Changes in consulting behaviour for uncomplicated respiratory tract infections may have been instigated by promotional campaigns discouraging patients from consulting doctors for "colds and the 'flu". The introduction of the tele-health service NHS Direct may also have had an effect by, in effect, providing a triage service, advising uncomplicated and low risk respiratory cases to self-treat at home [74]. Other potential factors reducing the incidence of ILI include: the overall health of the general population has improved in recent decades due to reductions in pollution/smoking, and smaller family sizes, providing less opportunity for virus spread. Viewed over a 40-year period, however, changes in the incidence of respiratory infections are not the same for all conditions, suggesting that the changes are more complex, probably relating to changes in the circulating viruses and in their transmission characteristics [75]. For influenza in particular, the more severe epidemics over the last years have been caused by influenza A H3N2 viruses and have involved numerous mutations [76]: perhaps we are reaching an evolutionary end point.

Seasonality

In the Northern Hemisphere influenza circulates during the winter months. A feature of influenza epidemics is the unpredictability of its appearance in winter [70]. WRS data demonstrate that annual influenza epidemic periods can range from early November (e.g. 1993) through to late March/April (e.g. 1988), although the most common period of circulation is around December/January. Influenza B tends to appear later in the winter than influenza A. Accordingly, national surveillance systems designed to monitor the burden of ILI in the community have a wide window of enhanced surveillance activities in order to capture any unusually early or late activity. Public health surveillance systems such as the WRS, NHS Direct and QSurveillance® specifically monitor ILI activity from October to May [77].

Acute bronchitis

Clinical presentation

Acute bronchitis is one of the most common infections reported in general practice, especially in the youngest and oldest age groups. Using routine incidence data collected from the RCGP WRS, we have estimated that 6.2% of children (aged 0–14 years) presented to their GP with one or more episodes of acute bronchitis during 2001. The presentation and diagnosis of acute bronchitis is usually associated with cough as the chief symptom sometimes accompanied by wheeze and pain on coughing and by fever. The diagnosis is usually made when the cough is productive and rales are heard on auscultation of the chest. The diagnosis of acute bronchitis is often problematic due to the difficulty in differentiating from asthma. This differentiation presents the GP with problems, especially in young children, where there is no satisfactory distinction between asthma and acute bronchitis when it first appears. Mostly, the diagnosis of asthma follows a series of ill-

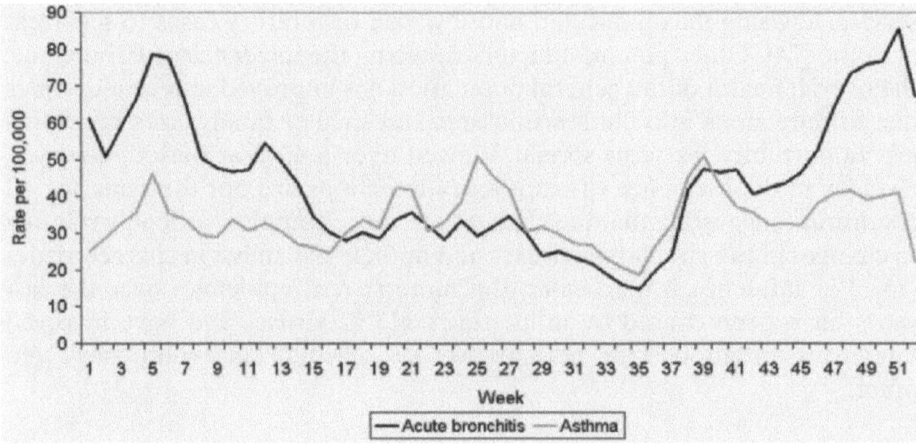

Figure 9. Mean weekly incidence rate per 100000 of asthma and acute bronchitis over the period 1999–2008 in children aged 5–14 years.

nesses described variously as wheezy or acute bronchitis. For some persons, there is a strong tendency of respiratory infections to prompt attacks of asthma. In Figure 9 a comparison is made between WRS weekly incidence data averaged over 10 years for asthma attacks and for acute bronchitis in children of 5–14 years. These conditions follow the same seasonal pattern. The duration of illness varies considerably and is not clearly related to the causative pathogen.

Acute bronchiolitis is a particular problem in young children where the pathological damage is concentrated at the smaller bronchiole and alveolar level. It cannot be clinically differentiated from broncho-pneumonia. Cough may be less prominent than shortness of breath and respiratory distress may occur. It is commonly caused by RSV and is highly consistent in its seasonal appearance in December in almost all winters. It is very common in children under 5 years; it has been estimated that there are on average 25 respiratory deaths and 79 deaths from all causes attributed to RSV in this age group, estimates similar to those attributed to influenza [78].

The conditions described as trachea-bronchitis and laryngitis imply an emphasis of symptoms based on epithelial damage in the major tracheal and laryngeal airways. Coughing is usually more intense when these parts of the airways are affected and in some cases quite prolonged. Whooping cough and croup are particular examples of such infections.

Secular trends

The RCGP WRS has collected clinical incidence data on acute bronchitis since 1967. In comparison to ILI, the long-term secular trend of acute bronchitis is remarkably different (Fig. 10). During the 1990s the incidence of

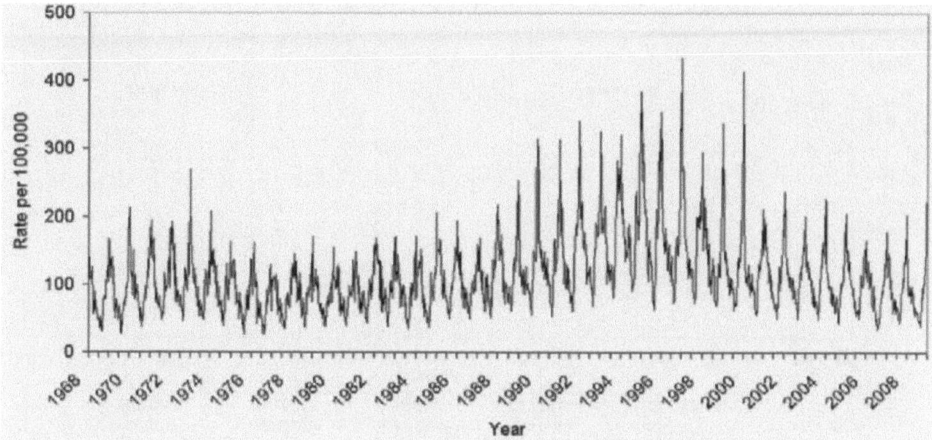

Figure 10. Weekly incidence rate of acute bronchitis per 100000 population over the period 1968–2008.

acute bronchitis increased, peaking during 1994 and then gradually decreasing to present day. The differences between the two respiratory conditions are indicative of differing aetiologies. Interestingly, the trend of acute bronchitis is mirrored by that of asthma with the peak occurring during the mid-1990s demonstrating the close relationship between the two conditions.

Seasonality

Acute bronchitis demonstrates a clear seasonal peak during the last weeks of the year. Interestingly, there are differences in the peak between age groups as previously reported. The incidence of acute bronchitis in young children (0–4 years) peaks during week 48; the peak in the elderly (65+ years) is approximately 2–3 weeks later; this finding is consistent from season to season and probably represents the mode of spread from young children to the elderly during the holiday period at Christmas and New Year (Fig. 11). Interestingly, this is not replicated in ILI data; a similar analysis reveals no lag between these age groups suggesting that ILI infections start and spread through all age groups at an equal rate. These findings for ILI have been replicated in other sentinel networks across Europe [79].

Pneumonia

Clinical presentation

Pneumonia can be defined as an illness of the lung involving alveolar and parenchyma inflammation, which results in abnormalities of alveolar gas exchange. Although often a secondary complication of viral or bacte-

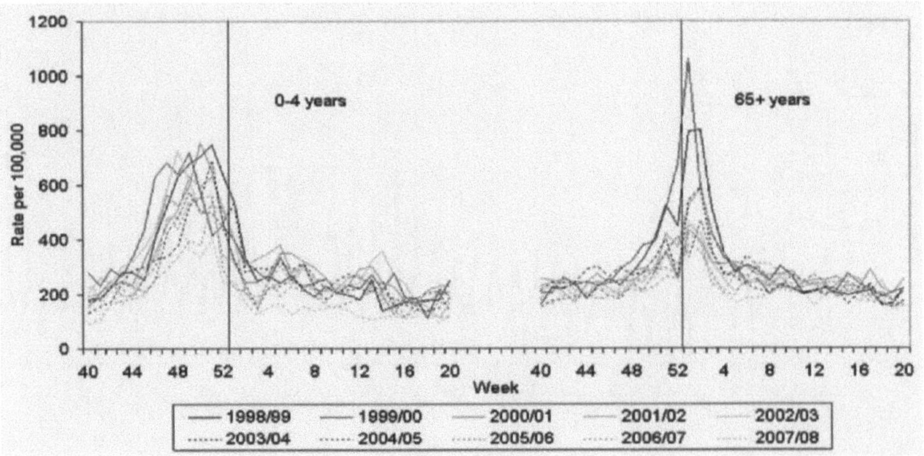

Figure 11. Weekly incidence rate per 100000 of acute bronchitis in young children aged 0–4 years and the elderly aged 65+ years over selected winter weeks 40–20. The vertical lines mark the year end.

rial infections, primary viral pneumonia is associated with clinical features including non-productive cough, and in more severely ill patients, cyanosis and hypoxemia. Viral causes of pneumonia are mainly associated with influenza and RSV infection, although more recent literature suggest that serious LRTI including pneumonia can be caused by a wide range of viral pathogens and the seasonality of pneumonia suggests that even though caused by a bacterial pathogen it is often consequent on a viral infection [30].

Secular trends

Incidence rates of pneumonia peaked at their highest rate during the winter of 1969/70; this was when the last influenza pandemic occurred and is most likely a reflection of complications of primary influenza infection. Rates steadily declined over the 1970s, but then stabilised during the 1980s and 1990s. Since the turn of the Millennium, the incidence of pneumonia again decreased, although data from the last couple of years suggest that this decrease has once again stabilised.

Seasonality

The seasonality of pneumonia as recorded by the RCGP WRS suggests a close association with acute respiratory infections. Comparing the incidence of pneumonia and that of ILI over the last 40 years shows that the highest incidence of pneumonia occurs at the same time as the highest incidence of ILI (Fig. 12). We performed a cross-correlation of the weekly data for pneu-

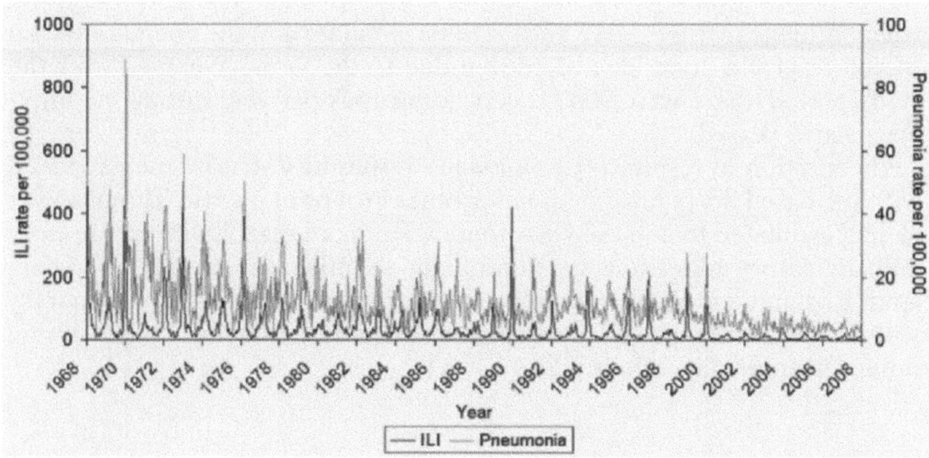

Figure 12. Weekly incidence rate per 100 000 of influenza-like illness (ILI) and pneumonia over the period 1968–2008 in elderly persons aged 65+ years (smoothed 3-week rolling average).

monia and ILI over this 40-year period, demonstrating that the incidence of ILI and pneumonia were maximally correlated in week 0, strongly supporting (although not proving) a casual relationship.

Hospital admissions

Acute respiratory infections place an annual burden on secondary health care facilities. Although these 'winter pressures' are not a new phenomenon, in the UK they received more prominence during the winter of 1999/2000 when the National Health Service was severely crippled, producing a national crisis during which many hospitals were unable to meet the demand.

Influenza and RSV are the two pathogens most notably associated with the pressures. Although there are numerous other pathogens potentially capable of causing disease severe enough to prompt admission (especially in elderly or other at-risk groups), these two pathogens have previously been associated with hospitalisations for respiratory and other causes [70, 80–82]. Using hospital admission data accessed from the Hospital Episode Statistics database, there were approximately 4.7 million emergency admissions for all causes and all ages to hospitals in England during 2006/07 (May–April), of which approximately 530 000 were labelled as a respiratory cause (J Chapter ICD10) [83].

Admissions due to respiratory causes were estimated over the winters 1989/90 to 1997/98 [84]. During winters where serious influenza epidemics occurred, e.g. 1997/98, there were an estimated 21 000 excess admissions. These estimates were made during influenza epidemic periods, i.e., periods when influenza viruses were known to be circulating in the community and therefore give a good idea of burden due to the virus. Averaged over the study period, there were 9000 excess admissions per year during the influenza active period.

In addition to respiratory admissions, respiratory viruses are associated with increased hospital admission for other groups of disease. Thompson et al. [82] estimated that in the USA there were more than 200000 respiratory and circulatory admissions per annum due to influenza. A study using data from England and Wales found increased circulatory deaths contemporary with new episodes of respiratory disease diagnosed by sentinel GPs during influenza epidemic periods [85].

Deaths

Despite the range of pathogens that circulate in the community causing respiratory tract infections each season, influenza and RSV remain the two main causes of respiratory mortality. Therefore, in respect of estimating numbers of deaths resulting from these infections, this work is predominantly concentrated on these two pathogens. It has been estimated that during the 1990s in England and Wales an average of 12000 deaths (all-cause mortality) were attributable to influenza each winter [84]. However, it is important to remember that these estimates were made using data collected at a time when there were much higher rates of community-based influenza activity than at present: therefore, current estimates would probably be lower. In the USA, Thompson et al. [76] studied age-specific pneumonia and influenza deaths and estimated those attributable to influenza and RSV. Over the winters 1990/91 to 1998/99 there were 8097 and 2707 underlying pneumonia and influenza deaths associated with influenza and RSV, respectively. In the age-specific analysis, 90% of influenza and 78% of RSV-related respiratory and circulatory deaths occurred in the 65+ years age group [76]: a similar study based on mortality data from England provided similar estimates of deaths [85]. These data highlight the severe impact of respiratory infections, in particular influenza and RSV, on the elderly population. We have recently undertaken an analysis of admissions due to ILI and acute bronchitis with respiratory emergency and all deaths against a background of influenza and RSV 'active periods' [80]. Clinical incidence rates of ILI and acute bronchitis both peak during virus active periods; however, it is clear that the greatest impact occurs during periods of RSV activity. In winters where both virus active periods coincide, e.g. 1999/00, this impact is greatest [70]. In the years where there is good separation between periods of virus activity, it is easier to disentangle the associated effects from each virus, and again it is clear that the clinical, admission and death statistics all increase more during periods of RSV activity (Fig. 13). The active period for RSV, as it affects persons over 65 years, is based on a 3-week lag behind RSV reports

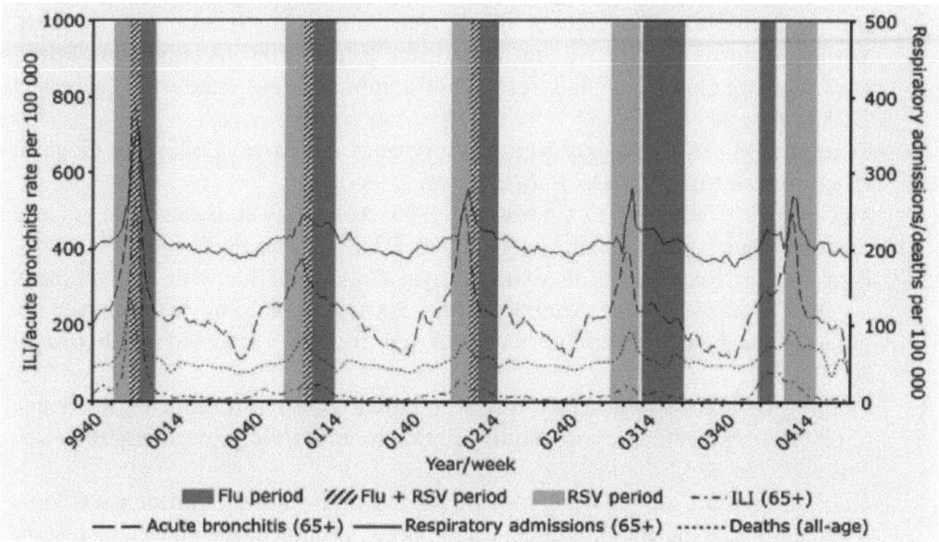

Figure 13. Weekly incidence rate of influenza-like illness (ILI) and acute bronchitis, emergency hospital admissions for respiratory causes and all-cause mortality against influenza and respiratory syncytial virus (RSV) active periods over the period 1999/00–2003/04.

in infants, which in turn is taken from the lag in clinical incidence between acute bronchitis as diagnosed in young children and in adults.

It is important to note that the elderly population is increasing. In England and Wales, the population aged over 65 years has increased from 5.5 million in 1961 to over 8.5 million in 2007, and is projected to increase to over 11 million by 2020 [86]. These population estimates imply that health care services that are particularly pressurised by respiratory infections in the elderly population will come under increasing pressure in the future as this burden increases.

Acknowledgement

We are grateful to the GPs involved in the Royal College of General Practitioners Weekly Returns Service for providing the morbidity data used in this chapter.

References

1 Fleming DM, Smith GE, Charlton JR, Charlton J, Nicoll A (2002) Impact of infections on primary care – Greater than expected. *Commun Dis Public Health* 5: 7–12

2 Birmingham Research Unit of the Royal College of General Practitioners. Weekly Returns Service Annual Prevalence Report 2007. Available at: http://www.rcgp.org.uk/clinical_and_research/bru/annual_prevalence.aspx (accessed 27 February 2009)

3 Fleming DM (1999) Weekly Returns Service of the Royal College of General Practitioners. *Commun Dis Public Health* 2: 96–100

4 McCormick A, Fleming D, Charlton J (1995) Morbidity statistics from general practice. Fourth national study 1991–1992. HMSO, London

5 Birmingham Research Unit of the Royal College of General Practitioners. Weekly Returns Service Annual Report 2006. Available at: http://www.rcgp.org.uk/clinical_and_research/bru/annual_reports.aspx (accessed 27 February 2009)

6 Fleming DM, Ross AM, Cross KW, Kendall H (2003) The reducing incidence of respiratory tract infection and its relation to antibiotic prescribing. *Br J Gen Pract* 53: 778–783

7 Guo YJ, Jin FG, Wang P, Wang M, Zhu JM (1983) Isolation of influenza C virus from pigs and experimental infection of pigs with influenza C virus. *J Gen Virol* 64: 177–182

8 Osterhaus AD, Rimmelzwaan GF, Martina BE, Bestebroer TM, Fouchier RA (2000) Influenza B virus in seals. *Science* 288: 1051–1053

9 Nicholson KG (1998) Human Influenza. In: KG Nicholson, RG Webster, AJ Hay (eds): *Textbook of Influenza*. Blackwell Sciences, Oxford, 219–264

10 Webster RG, Bean WJ, Gorman OT, Chambers TM, Kawaoka Y (1992) Evolution and ecology of influenza A viruses. *Microbiol Rev* 56: 152–179

11 Fouchier RA, Munster V, Wallensten A, Bestebroer TM, Herfst S, Smith D, Rimmelzwaan GF, Olsen B, Osterhaus AD (2005) Characterization of a novel influenza A virus hemagglutinin subtype (H16) obtained from black-headed gulls. *J Virol* 79: 2814–2822

12 Monto AS, Comanor L, Shay DK, Thompson WW (2006) Epidemiology of pandemic influenza: Use of surveillance and modeling for pandemic preparedness. *J Infect Dis* 194 (Suppl 2): S92-S97

13 Zambon MC, Stockton JD, Clewley JP, Fleming DM (2001) Contribution of influenza and respiratory syncytial virus to community cases of influenza-like illness: An observational study. *Lancet* 358: 1410–1416

14 Mufson MA, Levine HD, Wasil RE, Mocega-Gonzalez HE, Krause HE (1973) Epidemiology of respiratory syncytial virus infection among infants and children in Chicago. *Am J Epidemiol* 98: 88–95

15 Nicholson KG, McNally T, Silverman M, Simons P, Stockton JD, Zambon MC (2006) Rates of hospitalisation for influenza, respiratory syncytial virus and human metapneumovirus among infants and young children. *Vaccine* 24: 102–108

16 Parrott RH, Kim HW, Arrobio JO, Hodes DS, Murphy BR, Brandt CD, Camargo E, Chanock RM (1973) Epidemiology of respiratory syncytial virus infection in Washington, D.C. II. Infection and disease with respect to age, immunologic status, race and sex. *Am J Epidemiol* 98: 289–300

17 Walsh EE, Peterson DR, Falsey AR (2007) Is clinical recognition of respiratory

syncytial virus infection in hospitalized elderly and high-risk adults possible? *J Infect Dis* 195: 1046–1051
18 Cane PA (2001) Molecular epidemiology of respiratory syncytial virus. *Rev Med Virol* 11: 103–116
19 Falsey AR, Walsh EE, Capellan J, Gravenstein S, Zambon M, Yau E, Gorse GJ, Edelman R, Hayden FG, McElhaney JE et al. (2008) Comparison of the safety and immunogenicity of 2 respiratory syncytial virus (RSV) vaccines – nonadjuvanted vaccine or vaccine adjuvanted with alum – given concomitantly with influenza vaccine to high-risk elderly individuals. *J Infect Dis* 198: 1317–1326
20 Kim HW, Canchola JG, Brandt CD, Pyles G, Chanock RM, Jensen K, Parrott RH (1969) Respiratory syncytial virus disease in infants despite prior administration of antigenic inactivated vaccine. *Am J Epidemiol* 89: 422–434
21 Hall CB (2001) Respiratory syncytial virus and parainfluenza virus. *N Engl J Med* 344: 1917–1928
22 Jartti T, Lehtinen P, Vuorinen T, Osterback R, van den Hoogen B, Osterhaus AD, Ruuskanen O (2004) Respiratory picornaviruses and respiratory syncytial virus as causative agents of acute expiratory wheezing in children. *Emerg Infect Dis* 10: 1095–1101
23 Fry AM, Curns AT, Harbour K, Hutwagner L, Holman RC, Anderson LJ (2006) Seasonal trends of human parainfluenza viral infections: United States, 1990–2004. *Clin Infect Dis* 43: 1016–1022
24 (2003) Severe acute respiratory syndrome (SARS). *Wkly Epidemiol Rec* 78: 81–83
25 Drosten C, Gunther S, Preiser W, van der Werf S, Brodt HR, Becker S, Rabenau H, Panning M, Kolesnikova L, Fouchier RA et al. (2003) Identification of a novel coronavirus in patients with severe acute respiratory syndrome. *N Engl J Med* 348: 1967–1976
26 Ksiazek TG, Erdman D, Goldsmith CS, Zaki SR, Peret T, Emery S, Tong S, Urbani C, Comer JA, Lim W et al. (2003) A novel coronavirus associated with severe acute respiratory syndrome. *N Engl J Med* 348: 1953–1966
27 Message SD, Johnston SL (2002) Viruses in asthma. *Br Med Bull* 61: 29–43
28 Nicholson KG, Kent J, Ireland DC (1993) Respiratory viruses and exacerbations of asthma in adults. *BMJ* 307: 982–986
29 Hicks LA, Shepard CW, Britz PH, Erdman DD, Fischer M, Flannery BL, Peck AJ, Lu X, Thacker WL, Benson RF et al. (2006) Two outbreaks of severe respiratory disease in nursing homes associated with rhinovirus. *J Am Geriatr Soc* 54: 284–289
30 Jennings LC, Anderson TP, Beynon KA, Chua A, Laing RT, Werno AM, Young SA, Chambers ST, Murdoch DR (2008) Incidence and characteristics of viral community-acquired pneumonia in adults. *Thorax* 63: 42–48
31 Louie JK, Yagi S, Nelson FA, Kiang D, Glaser CA, Rosenberg J, Cahill CK, Schnurr DP (2005) Rhinovirus outbreak in a long term care facility for elderly persons associated with unusually high mortality. *Clin Infect Dis* 41: 262–265
32 van den Hoogen BG, de Jong JC, Groen J, Kuiken T, de Groot R, Fouchier RA, Osterhaus AD (2001) A newly discovered human pneumovirus isolated from young children with respiratory tract disease. *Nat Med* 7: 719–724

33 Camps M, Ricart S, Dimova V, Rovira N, Munoz-Almagro C, Garcia JJ, Pons-Odena M, Marcos MA, Pumarola T (2008) Prevalence of human metapneumovirus among hospitalized children younger than 1 year in Catalonia, Spain. *J Med Virol* 80: 1452–1460

34 Stockton J, Stephenson I, Fleming D, Zambon M (2002) Human metapneumovirus as a cause of community-acquired respiratory illness. *Emerg Infect Dis* 8: 897–901

35 Johnstone J, Majumdar SR, Fox JD, Marrie TJ (2008) Viral infection in adults hospitalized with community-acquired pneumonia: Prevalence, pathogens, and presentation. *Chest* 134: 1141–1148

36 Walsh EE, Peterson DR, Falsey AR (2008) Human metapneumovirus infections in adults: Another piece of the puzzle. *Arch Intern Med* 168: 2489–2496

37 Allander T, Tammi MT, Eriksson M, Bjerkner A, Tiveljung-Lindell A, Andersson B (2005) Cloning of a human parvovirus by molecular screening of respiratory tract samples. *Proc Natl Acad Sci USA* 102: 12891–12896

38 Ma X, Endo R, Ishiguro N, Ebihara T, Ishiko H, Ariga T, Kikuta H (2006) Detection of human bocavirus in Japanese children with lower respiratory tract infections. *J Clin Microbiol* 44: 1132–1134

39 Sloots TP, McErlean P, Speicher DJ, Arden KE, Nissen MD, Mackay IM (2006) Evidence of human coronavirus HKU1 and human bocavirus in Australian children. *J Clin Virol* 35: 99–102

40 Weissbrich B, Neske F, Schubert J, Tollmann F, Blath K, Blessing K, Kreth HW (2006) Frequent detection of bocavirus DNA in German children with respiratory tract infections. *BMC Infect Dis* 6: 109

41 Goddard NL, Cooke MC, Gupta RK, Nguyen-Van-Tam JS (2007) Timing of monoclonal antibody for seasonal RSV prophylaxis in the United Kingdom. *Epidemiol Infect* 135: 159–162

42 Fleming DM, Elliot AJ, Nguyen-van Tam JS, Watson JM, Wise R (2005) *A Winter's Tale: Coming to terms with winter respiratory illnesses*. Health Protection Agency, London

43 Elliot AJ, Fleming DM (2008) Viral infections and acute otitis media in young children. *Clin Infect Dis* 47: 146–147

44 Fatahzadeh M, Schwartz RA (2007) Human herpes simplex labialis. *Clin Exp Dermatol* 32: 625–630

45 Gupta R, Warren T, Wald A (2007) Genital herpes. *Lancet* 370: 2127–2137

46 Fleming DM, Cross KW, Cobb WA, Chapman RS (2004) Gender difference in the incidence of shingles. *Epidemiol Infect* 132: 1–5

47 Nasser M, Fedorowicz Z, Khoshnevisan MH, Shahiri Tabarestani M (2008) Acyclovir for treating primary herpetic gingivostomatitis. *Cochrane Database Syst Rev*: CD006700

48 Amir J, Harel L, Smetana Z, Varsano I (1997) Treatment of herpes simplex gingivostomatitis with aciclovir in children: a randomised double blind placebo controlled study. *BMJ* 314: 1800–1803

49 Spratley J, Silveira H, Alvarez I, Pais-Clemente M (2000) Acute mastoiditis in children: Review of the current status. *Int J Pediatr Otorhinolaryngol* 56: 33–40

50 Zanetti D, Nassif N (2006) Indications for surgery in acute mastoiditis and their complications in children. *Int J Pediatr Otorhinolaryngol* 70: 1175–1182

51 Gill JM, Fleischut P, Haas S, Pellini B, Crawford A, Nash DB (2006) Use of antibiotics for adult upper respiratory infections in outpatient settings: A national ambulatory network study. *Fam Med* 38: 349–354

52 Dykewicz MS (2003) 7. Rhinitis and sinusitis. *J Allergy Clin Immunol* 111: S520-S529

53 Birmingham Research Unit of the Royal College of General Practitioners. Weekly Returns Service Annual Report 2007. Available at: http://www.rcgp.org.uk/clinical_and_research/bru/annual_reports.aspx (accessed 27 February 2009)

54 Denny FW, Murphy TF, Clyde WA Jr, Collier AM, Henderson FW (1983) Croup: An 11-year study in a pediatric practice. *Pediatrics* 71: 871–876

55 Bjornson CL, Johnson DW (2008) Croup. *Lancet* 371: 329–339

56 Stroud RH, Friedman NR (2001) An update on inflammatory disorders of the pediatric airway: Epiglottitis, croup, and tracheitis. *Am J Otolaryngol* 22: 268–275

57 Guldfred LA, Lyhne D, Becker BC (2008) Acute epiglottitis: Epidemiology, clinical presentation, management and outcome. *J Laryngol Otol* 122: 818–823

58 McIntyre P (2004) Vaccines for other neonatal infections: vaccination strategies for the prevention of neonatal pertussis. *Expert Rev Vaccines* 3: 375–378

59 Miller E, Fleming DM, Ashworth LA, Mabbett DA, Vurdien JE, Elliott TS (2000) Serological evidence of pertussis in patients presenting with cough in general practice in Birmingham. *Commun Dis Public Health* 3: 132–134

60 Montella S, De Stefano S, Sperli F, Barbarano F, Santamaria F (2007) Increased risk of chronic suppurative lung disease after measles or pertussis in non-vaccinated children. *Vaccine* 25: 402–403

61 Gershon AA (2005) Measles virus (Rubeola). In: GL Mandell, JE Bennett, R Dolin (eds): *Principles and Practice of Infectious Diseases*. Elsevier, Philadelphia, 2031–2038

62 Fleming DM (1994) Facts for audit and facts from an audit of throat swabs. *Audit Trends* 2: 137–141

63 Martin JM, Green M (2006) Group A streptococcus. *Semin Pediatr Infect Dis* 17: 140–148

64 Dunn N, Lane D, Everitt H, Little P (2007) Use of antibiotics for sore throat and incidence of quinsy. *Br J Gen Pract* 57: 45–49

65 Morris MC, Edmunds WJ (2002) The changing epidemiology of infectious mononucleosis? *J Infect* 45: 107–109

66 di Camugliano GN (1933) *The chronicles of a Florentine family, 1200–1470*. J. Cape, London

67 Smith W, Andrewes CH, Laidlaw PP (1933) A virus obtained from influenza patients. *Lancet* ii: 66–68

68 Elliot AJ, Fleming DM (2006) Surveillance of influenza-like illness in England and Wales during 1966–2006. *Euro Surveill* 11: 249–250

69 Kilbourne ED (2006) Influenza pandemics of the 20th century. *Emerg Infect Dis* 12: 9–14

70 Elliot AJ, Cross KW, Fleming DM (2007) Acute respiratory infections and winter pressures on hospital admissions in England and Wales 1990–2005. *J Public Health (Oxf)* 30: 91–98
71 Fleming D, Harcourt S, Smith G (2003) Influenza and adult hospital admissions for respiratory conditions in England 1989–2001. *Commun Dis Public Health* 6: 231–237
72 Bhat N, Wright JG, Broder KR, Murray EL, Greenberg ME, Glover MJ, Likos AM, Posey DL, Klimov A, Lindstrom SE et al. (2005) Influenza-associated deaths among children in the United States, 2003–2004. *N Engl J Med* 353: 2559–2567
73 Health Protection Agency (2003) Influenza in the United Kingdom. CDR Weekly 13: 6
74 Chapman RS, Smith GE, Warburton F, Mayon-White RT, Fleming DM (2002) Impact of NHS Direct on general practice consultations during the winter of 1999–2000: Analysis of routinely collected data. *BMJ* 325: 1397–1398
75 Fleming DM, Elliot AJ (2006) Changing disease incidence: The consulting room perspective. *Br J Gen Pract* 56: 820–824
76 Thompson WW, Shay DK, Weintraub E, Brammer L, Cox N, Anderson LJ, Fukuda K (2003) Mortality associated with influenza and respiratory syncytial virus in the United States. *JAMA* 289: 179–186
77 Health Protection Agency. Seasonal Influenza. Available at: http://www.hpa.org.uk/web/HPAweb&Page&HPAwebAutoListName/Page/1191942171468 (accessed 27 February 2009)
78 Fleming DM, Pannell RS, Cross KW (2005) Mortality in children from influenza and respiratory syncytial virus. *J Epidemiol Community Health* 59: 586–590
79 Elliot AJ, Paget WJ, Donker G, Falcao JM, Falcao I, Fleming DM (2008) Are children the main transmitters of influenza-like illness in the community; an analysis of data from European sentinel networks: *The Third European Influenza Conference*. European Scientific Working Group on Influenza, Vilamoura, Portugal
80 Fleming DM, Elliot AJ, Cross KW (2007) Morbidity profiles of patients consulting during influenza and respiratory syncytial virus active periods. *Epidemiol Infect* 135: 1099–1108
81 Mangtani P, Hajat S, Kovats S, Wilkinson P, Armstrong B (2006) The association of respiratory syncytial virus infection and influenza with emergency admissions for respiratory disease in London: an analysis of routine surveillance data. *Clin Infect Dis* 42: 640–646
82 Thompson WW, Shay DK, Weintraub E, Brammer L, Bridges CB, Cox NJ, Fukuda K (2004) Influenza-associated hospitalizations in the United States. *JAMA* 292: 1333–1340
83 Hospital Episode Statistics Online. Hospital Episode Statistics: Primary diagnosis 3 character – 2006/07. Available at: http://www.hesonline.org.uk/ (accessed 27 February 2009)
84 Fleming DM (2000) The contribution of influenza to combined acute respiratory infections, hospital admissions, and deaths in winter. *Commun Dis Public Health* 3: 32–38

85 Fleming DM, Cross KW, Pannell RS (2005) Influenza and its relationship to circulatory disorders. *Epidemiol Infect* 133: 255–262
86 National Statisitcs Online. Population estimates for UK, England and Wales, Scotland and Northern Ireland. Available at: http://www.statistics.gov.uk/StatBase/Product.asp?vlnk=601 (accessed 27 February 2009)
87 Elliot AJ, Cross KW, Smith GE, Fleming DM (2007) Do children drive the spread of influenza-like illness in the community? Presented at: *Options for the Control of Influenza VI.* MediTech Media Conferencing, Inc., Toronto, Canada, Abstract P1311

Common Cold
ed. by R. Eccles and O. Weber

Epidemiology

Ian M. Mackay[1,2], Katherine E. Arden[1,2] and Stephen B. Lambert[1,2]

[1]*Queensland Paediatric Infectious Diseases Laboratory, Sir Albert Sakzewski Virus Research Centre, Queensland Children's Medical Research Institute, Royal Children's Hospital, Brisbane, Australia*
[2]*Clinical Medical Virology Centre, University of Queensland, Brisbane, Australia*

Abstract

The common cold is the result of an upper respiratory tract infection causing an acute syndrome characterised by a combination of non-specific symptoms, including sore throat, cough, fever, rhinorrhoea, malaise, headache, and myalgia. Respiratory viruses, alone or in combination, are the most common cause. The course of illness can be complicated by bacterial agents, causing pharyngitis or sinusitis, but they are a rare cause of cold and flu-like illnesses (CFLIs). Our understanding of CFLI epidemiology has been enhanced by molecular detection methods, particularly polymerase chain reaction (PCR) testing. PCR has not only improved detection of previously known viruses, but within the last decade has resulted in the detection of many divergent novel respiratory virus species. Human rhinovirus (HRV) infections cause nearly all CFLIs and they can be responsible for asthma and chronic obstructive pulmonary disease exacerbations. HRVs are co-detected with other respiratory viruses in statistically significant patterns, with HRVs occurring in the lowest proportion of co-detections, compared to most other respiratory viruses. Some recently identified rhinoviruses may populate an entirely new putative HRV species; HRV C. Further work is required to confirm a causal role for these newly identified viruses in CFLIs. The burden of illness associated with CFLIs is poorly documented, but where data are available, the impact of CFLIs is considerable. Individual infections, although they do not commonly result in more severe respiratory tract illness, are associated with substantial direct and indirect resource use. The product of frequency and burden for CFLIs is likely to be greater in magnitude than for any other respiratory syndrome, but further work is required to document this. Our understanding of the viral causes of CLFIs, although incomplete, has improved in recent years. Documenting burden is also an important step in progress towards improved control and management of these illnesses.

Introduction

The common cold is the result of an upper respiratory tract infection (URTI) resulting in an acute syndrome best described as cold and flu-like illness (CFLI). It is characterised by a combination of non-specific symptoms, including sore throat, cough, fever, rhinorrhoea, malaise, headache and myalgia. It is usually due to infection by one or more of many viruses detected in the respiratory tract [1]. Bacterial commensals or those causing pharyngitis or sinusitis may complicate clinical CFLI diagnoses due to an overlap in detection or symptoms but overall, bacteria are rare causes of CFLI [2, 3] and are not reviewed here.

In 2001, the first of many divergent novel respiratory virus species were described for the first time with the aid of polymerase chain reaction (PCR)-based molecular techniques. Discovery of human metapneumovirus (HMPV) [4] was followed by other newly identified viruses (NIVs) including the human coronaviruses (HCoVs) NL63 [5] and HKU1 [6], human bocavirus (HBoV) [7] and many new human rhinovirus (HRV) strains [8, 9] populating an entirely new putative HRV species; HRV C [10, 11]. Some NIVs are yet to be clearly associated with specific clinical syndromes, but all have been detected in patients with CFLIs [12]. Because there have been no case-controlled studies of the common cold for some time, it is unclear what the combined impact of molecular diagnostic testing for respiratory viruses and the increasing number of NIVs will be for our understanding of the syndrome, but it is likely to be significant.

In this chapter we review the epidemiology of the common cold. This includes several aspects of the incidence and disease distribution of the common cold by discussing which, when and how the viral causative agents are detected, focussing on the HRVs. We briefly examine causal association of some complications following CFLIs which include asthma [13] and chronic obstructive pulmonary disease (COPD) [14] and describe the impact and cost of CFLIs.

Epidemiology of viral causes of CFLIs

The viruses consistently causing most CFLIs are HRVs [15] comprising 50–80% [3, 16] of relevant symptomatic respiratory illnesses. However, the human influenza viruses (IFVs; IFAV, IFBV and IFCV), the human parainfluenza viruses (HPIVs, 1–4), the HCoVs, 229E and OC43, human respiratory syncytial virus (HRSV), human adenoviruses (HAdV) and human enteroviruses (HEV) [17] have also been associated with 8–15% of CFLIs [18–20], despite some being traditionally considered more 'serious' causes of respiratory syndromes, including acute lower respiratory tract illnesses (LRTIs).

Factors affecting the circulation patterns and clinical impact of respiratory viruses

The reported peak activity and rate of different viral infections associated with CFLIs varies with the manner in which illnesses are defined, recorded, documented aetiologically, and tracked longitudinally [21]. However, historical detection rate data do not comprehensively represent HRV circulation patterns because sequential infections by different strains occur and may appear as unbroken symptomatic episodes during a single observation period [22, 23]; an occurrence which is rarely examined. In other instances, multiple HRV strains can be isolated [24, 25] or detected [26–28] from a single specimen, indicating a capacity for HRV co-infection which is similarly overlooked.

Studies seeking to explain epidemics of the colloquially termed 'respiratory viruses' often attribute them to the season [29]. Commonly, the circulation pattern for each virus that can recur annually is dominated by a different strain or species, which changes each year depending on the nature of pre-existing immunity within that location's population. When we documented the seasonal characteristics of HMPV detections over 4 years, we found that among over 700 HMPV-positive specimens, the four genetically defined HMPV subtypes exchanged dominance each year and detection frequencies cycled up to, or down from, their peak at other times [30, 31]. Herd immunity contributes to controlling epidemics of viruses, especially those which elicit strong and long-lasting immune responses in their hosts. The age of a population is therefore a significant factor in the epidemiology of respiratory viruses. In general terms, adults suffer fewest severe outcomes from respiratory virus infection and children most. In the very young a portion of the pathology of severe illness can be attributed to the small and developing airways. Individual immunity is accrued over time for the adults but is relatively weak among neonates and young children since it is during the early years of life that this response is developed by repeated exposure to infection. A relative increase in the prevalence of symptomatic illnesses is also seen among the elderly, often attributed to the waning of immunity with age.

For some respiratory viruses, including IFV and HRSV, a strict pattern of peak activity occurring with colder or wetter weather is common [33–35]. Exceptions can occur during which higher temperatures and greater daily temperature fluctuations parallel the respiratory virus epidemic period [34]. Some of these epidemic peaks can be seen in Figure 1 exemplified by HRSV, HMPV and IFAV detected in a paediatric hospital-based population during 2003. The defined peaks usually recur at a similar time each year, whereas HEVs and HAdVs are more consistently present and the HRVs, apart from dominating the overall number of detections in this population, often peak in spring and autumn. HRSV activity also correlates with complex interactions of latitude, temperature, humidity and UVB radiance [29]. Apart from weather conditions, cohorting of populations can also occur during return from long school or university holidays, which is a particularly common trigger for HRV epidemics in the young [36–39]. The accompanying increased risk of transmission due to aerosols in close quarters and shared contact with contaminated surfaces are implicated as the cause of

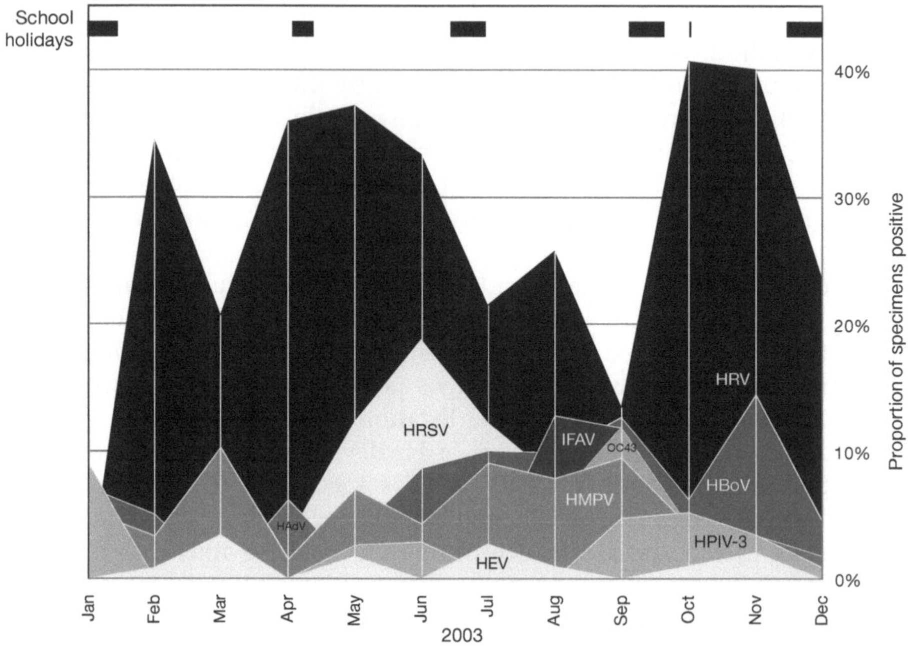

Figure 1. Virus detections plotted by month for 2003. The virus detected is indicated, as are school holidays in Queensland, Australia, during the year of the study at this location. Data were derived from a paediatric hospital-based, in- and outpatient population [8, 32].

rapid increases in the numbers of symptomatic illnesses. Susceptibility to CFLIs may also be directly influenced by weather conditions affecting the respiratory epithelium [40].

HRV detections occur throughout the year but are usually seen to peak in spring and autumn [41–48] depending on the method of detection, the length of the study period and the type of population investigated [22, 49]. One study indicated that HRVs of any given strain might be sporadically detected ahead of an epidemic, providing warning of the impending widespread activity by that strain [50]. Few studies examine whether every strain recurs each year at a single location or whether herd immunity protects against reinfection by a previous epidemic strain, and if so, how long such an effect might last. In Brisbane (Queensland, Australia) during 2003, HRV B strains circulated during winter and HRV C strains predominantly circulated during spring [8]. In contrast, the HRV As occurred in all seasons.

The role of common cold viruses in potentiating bacterial infections

It has long been known that bacterial adherence is enhanced by preceding infection of a respiratory virus [51], particularly HRSV and IFAV [51]. Such studies began after the influenza pandemic of 1918 [52] during which death due to secondary bacterial infection was a significant contributor to total morbidity. Since then, prior infection by IFAV and HRV has been shown to increase the number of staphylococci, streptococci and pneumococci adhering to a pharyngeal cell line, while measles virus decreased adherence and HAdV had no effect [53]. Possible mechanisms, identified using animal studies, include IFV neuraminidase-mediated removal of sialic acid moieties permitting bacteria access to otherwise hidden receptor molecules [52, 54] on the cell surface, and expression of haemagglutinin which enhances group A streptococcal binding [55]. HRV-14 infection can also increase subsequent bacterial adherence by up-regulating streptococcal receptor expression on human tracheal cells, partly mediated by transcription factor activation after HRV infection [56]. Both infectious HRV-16 and HRV-2 reduced the capacity of human alveolar macrophages to respond to lipopolysaccharide and lipoteichoic acids *in vitro* [57], which may, *in vivo*, permit worsening of an HRV infection *via* concomitant bacterial superinfection. In children, but not adults, peak HRSV activity was significantly and positively correlated with peak *Streptococcus pneumoniae*-mediated pneumococcal disease activity in Australia and New Zealand [58, 59]. In the Netherlands, both children and adults were found to have higher rates of pneumococcal and meningococcal disease during peak IFV and HRSV seasons [35]. Vaccination to prevent pneumococcal disease successfully prevented nearly one third of cases of pneumonia associated with the major respiratory viruses [60], presumably by preventing bacterial super infections.

Methods of detecting viruses in CFLIs

Robust detection methods that are kept up-to-date have been of paramount importance to our evolving understanding of the epidemiology of the CFLIs. Co-culture of patient secretions with “permissive” cells lines has been the longest serving method of detection but it is now well known for being insensitive [48, 61, 62]. Examples of previously unknown respiratory viruses believed to be endemic rather than recently emerged are being reported with increasing frequency. For the HRVs this was exemplified by the molecular identification of a large number of highly divergent, and at writing, unculturable HRV C strains [8, 10, 11, 32]. Insensitive and inefficient testing of the HRV super-group is to be blamed for delaying characterisation of the rhinoviruses, thus leading to a significant underestimation of the total number and nature of strains, which has been undeniably detrimental for all previous epidemiology studies of CFLI. With the introduction of nucleic acid testing and improvements to PCR product detection methods, a quantum leap in respiratory virus detection frequencies has been achieved. Even so, no single assay has been shown to robustly detect all HRVs and no panel of assays has achieved 100% laboratory diagnoses. Time to specimen delivery was once thought to be a cause for reduced aetiologies but even the use of PCR, not requiring infectious pathogens, still misses a large proportion of suspected infections [63].

Cell culture methods

Cell culture techniques are limited by poor sensitivity due to slow growth or poorly cytopathic viruses, reduced viability due to poor specimen handling, narrow detection windows, complex result interpretation requiring high levels of operator expertise, host immunosuppression, antimicrobial therapies, high levels of background signal and non-specific cross-reactions [64, 65]. Nonetheless, both microbial culture and rapid immunofluorescence assays can be used to produce valuable epidemiological data, reveal new, uncharacterised or atypical microbes and yield intact or infectious organisms for further study [66].

Viruses have been isolated in cell cultures since the 1950s but diagnostic services were limited for a further two decades [67]. Microscopic examination of degenerative changes brought about by virus replication (cytopathic effects), a sometimes slow and always technically demanding skill, was later augmented by haemadsorption tests to identify the extent of haemagglutinating protein expression, which indicates the replication of certain respiratory viruses. Subsequently, shell vial methods were employed, which, when used with specific antibodies, identified viral antigens in 1–2 days compared to 2–10 days for haemagglutination methods [68]. In 1953 Andrewes and colleagues at the Common Cold Unit (Salisbury, UK) described the first isolation of an HRV strain [69, 70]. Later, improved culture systems permitted viral replication to be more easily identified and maintained [71, 72]. Nonetheless, even using cell-culture conditions normally favouring the appearance of cytopathicity, instances of non-cytopathic HRV strains have been found by other methods [73], which may have included HRV C-like viruses.

Because the respiratory tract is a cellularly diverse environment and because a wide variety of viruses with diverse tropism cause CFLIs, cell culture methods require the use of a broad range of cell types. For methods to be useful, they must encompass virus concentrations ranging from 10^1 to 10^5 $TCID_{50}$/ml [74–77]. Additionally, successful isolation and higher viral yields require monitoring of cell age after plating (< 72 h), inoculum volume, culture medium pH (6.8–7.3) and cell density [78–81]. Therefore, culture can be expensive, not just for the labour required to inoculate, maintain under sometimes fastidious conditions [70, 80, 82–84] and monitor the cultures, but also to ensure that the diverse range of cell stocks and culture media are available and fresh. Even with these criteria met, HRVs and most of the respiratory NIVs have proven to be very poor targets for isolation methods based on cell culture [67]. Despite the challenges [85], virus isolation is reportedly a more sensitive indicator of infection than an antibody rise in paired sera [86].

Antibody-based methods

To date, antibody-based methods have proven the most diversely commercialised and robust diagnostic format either for the indirect detection of a host response to a respiratory virus, or the direct detection of viral antigen in culture or from infected cells present in specimens, such as nasopharyngeal aspirates or bronchoalveolar lavage. Antibody-based results augment both general diagnostic molecular data and those data provided by research studies aiming at better characterising respiratory viruses. Apart from speed, cost-benefit and familiarity, an obvious advantage derived from use of a protein-based system is the existence of conserved antigenic regions among related viruses; regions that do not vary significantly among strains of the same species or other relevant taxonomic grouping. Such conservation is infrequently reflected at the nucleotide level making these regions troublesome targets for nucleic acid-based systems but ideal for antibodies. Unfortunately, antigenic conservation can also be manifested as cross-reaction; difficulty discriminating between infections caused by closely related viruses. Such discrimination is important when searching for the role of each individual respiratory virus in illness [87].

Antigen detection methods may be performed with or without a biological amplification step such as *in vitro* cell culture. If culture is not being employed, then it is necessary to collect cellular specimens since the cells confine virions to a small, easily identified space that aids/allows immunofluorescent detection; but such cellular specimens are not always available. Rapid respiratory virus antigen detection is relatively insensitive and, depending on the clinical priorities for the particular virus, negative results may need to be confirmed using another assay, which largely abrogates the benefits of speed [88, 89]. Furthermore, antibody-based methods have not kept up with the recent flurry of NIVs and so reliable diagnostic reagents are not available for the latest viral discoveries [67].

Seroclassification or 'serotyping' of an HRV infection was once the gold standard for strain identification of the 'common cold viruses' but serotyping became impractical as the number of distinct strains grew beyond convenience [79, 90]. Antibodies are essential for strain-specific neutralisation of infection [91], techniques around which the HRV nomenclature system evolved in 1967 [92]. These determine whether co-incubation of a characterised antibody with a preparation of an unknown virus can preclude its cellular entry and replication. If successful, the antibody chosen confers some degree of identification upon the unknown virus. Such techniques have found that a large number of distinct strains circulate each year and that a selection of them predominate in a given season, replaced by others in subsequent years [70, 93]. Today, PCR-based sequencing methods can do the same job at the genetic level with increased objectivity and speed compared to the complex and lengthy neutralisation methods [94, 95].

Polymerase chain reaction

The improved sensitivity of PCR-based assays dramatically increased the frequency of viral detection compared to cultivation methods [96], which has meant that many previous studies are incomparable to today's findings. This improvement is especially noticeable for the HRVs [3, 26, 42, 97–99] but also for other viruses that are fastidious or, to date, impossible, to culture. Because of PCR it is becoming commonplace to find reports of HRVs predominating in CFLIs [100–102], despite the incomplete validation of published assays against all picornavirus (HRV and HEV) strains using clinical material. Nonetheless, many assays successfully detect the currently circulating HRV strains at levels as low as 10^2 $TCID_{50}$/sample. This amount is commonly shed during experimental infections [103, 104]. Because HRV strains are now being detected beyond their traditionally understood symptomatic context of the CFLI syndrome [16, 105], it is becoming more important to define a qualitative and quantitative correlation between HRV nucleic acid detection and the presence of infectious virus at the sampling site. Unfortunately, the latter is problematic when using PCR to study respiratory viruses because of the inability to normalise the amount of starting RNA template [106].

Improved detection by PCR compared with traditional methods means that less invasive specimen types can be used for research, and in most circumstances, diagnostic testing. For example, prior to PCR, there were problems with the sensitivity of RSV detection using less-invasive specimen types. Using antigen detection, a reduction in positives by approximately one-third was seen when nasal swabs were used, compared with nasopharyngeal aspirates [107, 108]. Use of PCR has largely overcome this issue [109], to the point where less-invasive specimen types can be easily collected by lay people in community settings for research purposes [47, 110], or used instead of invasive techniques in clinic or outpatient settings [109].

When they are included in the PCR testing menu, HRVs raise the frequency of pathogen detection above one per sample [111]. Studies find that HRV strains are very frequent contributors to co-infections [112] and co-detections [113], sometimes presenting this in terms of their minor contributing role in serious respiratory disease [112, 113]. More likely this reflects the insensitivity of old cell culture-based methods that simply failed to propagate many HRV strains and in the process created paradigms for the HRVs that reduced their profile for further study. In one study, half of all HRV detections were found concurrently with another virus, on the surface, a significant fraction, and yet 80% or more of HRSV, HMPV, HEV and IFV detections and 71% of HCoV-NL63 detections were found in the company of another virus [114].

The use of a multiplex real-time PCR (m-rtPCR) or a suite of individual rtPCR assays [113] that encompass the majority of regularly detected viral targets is being steadily embraced by diagnostic laboratories that receive respiratory secretions and a number of these panels include a capacity to detect HRVs [115]. Multiplexing PCRs increases result throughput and reduces costs associated with labour and time but also requires significant research and developmental time and may still perform at a reduced clinical sensitivity compared to individual assays.

Innovative, but less well evaluated, multitarget molecular laboratory tools now exist including the MultiCode-PLx system, which employs a synthetic nucleobase pair, multiplex PCR and microsphere flow cytometry [116]. It permits the discrete detection of 17 respiratory viral targets and two assay controls, although it returns an unusually low HRV detection rate. Similar technology also provides a sensitive, 20-target, 2-step RT-PCR-based assay [117]. The Seeplex® respiratory virus detection kit targets 12 respiratory viruses [118] using dual priming oligonucleotides [119] and detecting the amplicon by capillary electrophoresis (Seegene Inc.). It has compared favourably to culture-based testing [120]. The ResPlex II assay (Qiagen) employs a proprietary multiplex RT-nPCR [121] approach followed by amplicon detection using a Luminex suspension array to identify 12 targets [122, 123]. The xTAG™ respiratory viral panel combines PCR and the Luminex array system and detects more than 20 different targets including controls (Luminex Corporation). PCR amplicon detection by MassTag technology can discriminate 20–30 viral and bacterial agents of illness [124] using oligonucleotides tagged with a unique compound that is released *via* a photolabile link (Qiagen). The MassTag approach has been able to detect HRV C strains [9, 26, 125]. Microarrays can detect thousands of viral targets (US$ 30–300 per sample) but still require a pre-hybridisation PCR amplification because of their insufficient sensitivity to directly detect viral nucleic acids from clinical specimens. Arrays are still low-throughput, high-turnaround time diagnostic options. At their most robust, microarrays, like PCR, rely on the existence of conserved regions of sequence to detect unknown viruses and they too can detect previously unknown HRV strains [126], although nothing vastly different from what is already known. Rapid protein- or virion-based assays are not (yet) adequately sensitive [127, 128].

PCR does have some downsides, some of which have been mentioned already. Detection of microbial genomic nucleic acids cannot yield the same information about infectivity as cell culture, but there have been good correlations reported between infectivity and viral genome detection for yellow fever virus [129] and in a comprehensive birth cohort study characterising frequent respiratory infections in which PCR data were found to correlate very well with symptomatic respiratory illness [130]. Despite the 'closed' nature of the modern generation of rtPCR techniques, they are PCR-based and as such still subject to contamination by amplicon from previous runs and template from extraction areas or infected technologists. Efficient PCR relies entirely on conserved sequence targets and thus an extensive foreknowledge of each virus is being sought. If the region targeted by oligonucleotides is subject to genetic variation, PCR will continue the diagnostic trend towards underestimating viruses in CFLIs. Even for conserved targets, PCR primer pair designs that yield a single specific amplicon from clinical specimen extracts can be extremely difficult to achieve when faced with the highly variable cellular and microbial content of respiratory tract specimens and the sequence similarities between viruses and humans for some targets. Non-specificity can render quantification methods useless [131] as can the absence of suitable housekeeping gene targets to permit normalisation of viral nucleic acid input. Because the success of PCR has led to an increase in the number of virus detections and a reduction in the number of virions required for a positive result, positive PCR methods are sometimes greeted with scepticism due to them being perceived as too sensitive. Such concerns must be addressed by careful epidemiology.

Questions raised by the co-detection of viruses among CFLIs

When thorough screening is conducted for all relevant viruses in each specimen, multiple virus detections are a frequent result. In particular, this has been the case since the more widespread adoption of PCR as the diagnostic method of choice because it is significantly more sensitive than the traditional methods of culture and direct or indirect fluorescent antibody assays. PCR is also better than other diagnostic methods at rapidly and specifically discriminating multiple targets representing different viral genes or strains, fuelling an increasing number of reports of microbial co-detections in 20% or more of specimens [114, 132–137]. For viral co-detections that include HRSV, interferon gamma (IFN-γ) levels are reduced [100]. This suggests a mechanism of immune intervention that creates a beachhead in the host's innate immune response, which subsequently permits additional viruses to gain a foothold, thereby increasing the frequency of co-detections. Although a description of all of a patient's viruses is necessary before the significance of co-detections can be determined, it does complicate the interpretation of results and the traditional assignation of a "causal" virus. Historically, to save labour and costs, causality has been associated with a "first-past-the-post" approach in which the initial virus to be detected is assigned the causal role [122]. Many laboratories have yet to completely adopt PCR, and so the occurrence of co-detections is not globally acknowledged, further complicating their impact compared to single detections.

What the detection of more than one virus, as well as the particular mix of viruses involved, means to the clinical outcome is controversial, with studies describing illness severity that is worsened [138–140] or unchanged [137, 141] by multiple detections. Among infants hospitalised with bronchiolitis, there was a 2.7-fold increased likelihood of infants with viral co-detections being admitted to a paediatric intensive care unit than those with single detections [114]. Considering their ubiquity, it is interesting that relatively low numbers of concurrent detections of other respiratory viruses occur with HRV strains [47, 142]. In fact, HRV strains are co-detected with other pathogens in reproducible, but clinically undefined, patterns [111]. Nonetheless, there is an increasing number of single HRV detections being made from patients with significant LRTIs and with acute otitis media [143]: it is becoming clearer that the HRV infection process can directly cause illness and that HRVs are not merely passengers in the clinical outcome of the infection [44].

The increasing proportion of viruses found in the company of other viruses, and also with bacteria, raises some interesting questions. Is it possible that a certain number, or certain mix, of viruses, or both, is necessary to tip the host into a state of symptomatic illness? This question may be especially relevant for viruses traditionally thought of as causing more mild respiratory illness, such as the HAdVs and perhaps HBoV. It is noteworthy that the proportion of asymptomatic episodes decreases with the number of micro-organisms detected and increases with age in children [138]. If not the nature then perhaps it is the order of infection that is important as has been suggested for some viral and bacterial pairings. This is poorly addressed by examining data from the clinical microbiology laboratory since such testing is only a cross-sectional snapshot of the host's condition. To address this question accurately, carefully planned, longitudinal cohort studies are required. In a study of 27 children during the first year of life who contracted five or more moderate-to-severe respiratory illnesses, it was apparent that the same viral species or strain did not usually recur during a 12-month period [130]. Another question is whether infection by one virus or bacterium predisposes the host to infection by one or more others.

The proportion of asymptomatic PCR positives is virus specific and occurs in more than a third of children during a CFLI season [144]. A particularly confounding and relevant issue for viral epidemiology is that raised by the criteria used to define an illness in some studies. Some criteria are so stringent that they may miss mild, but nonetheless common and virally induced CFLI symptoms such as headaches [144]. Such omissions are likely to contribute to the number of 'asymptomatic' cases reported by some investigations [114] and to the severity scores used for studies linking single and multiple detections to clinical outcome. It might be simple coincidence that two or more viruses can be detected in the same specimen, reflecting an overlap of their seasonal peaks [114] when it is more likely that hosts will come into contact with more than one virus in the community. However, we believe this is not the case for two reasons. We have not seen a

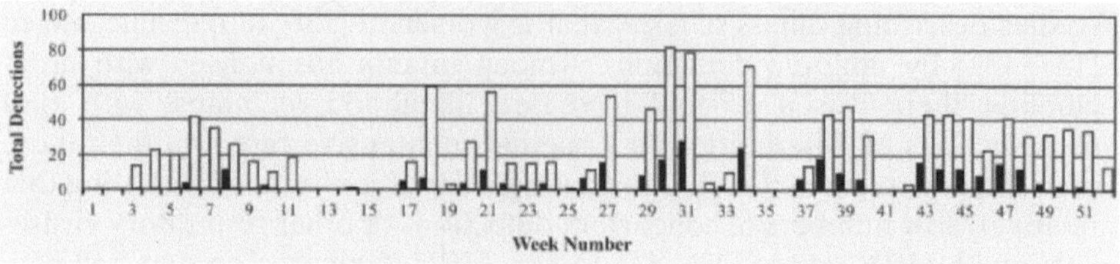

Figure 2. The total number of virus detections (open bars) and co-detections (filled bars) during each week of 2003. Viruses tested included, HRSV, HMPV, IFAV, IFBV, HAdV, HBoV, HPIVs, non-SARS HCoVs and respiratory picornaviruses. Data are derived from [8] and [32].

seasonal trend towards more co-detections in certain seasons (Fig. 2) but we have seen patterns that indicate virus-specific factors drive the association between co-detected viruses.

When we statistically analysed co-detections from earlier studies of HRV-QPM [32], which also included screening for traditional respiratory viruses and NIVs, we identified that patterns existed that particularly involved the association of certain viruses. Specifically, HRVs were the virus or virus group with the lowest statistically significant proportion of co-detections. We believe that this may be an example of a strong HRV interference effect. Others have shown that epidemics of HRSV may be interrupted or apparently staved off by an epidemic of IFV [33, 145]. A possible mechanism for the separation often seen between an epidemic peak due to one virus and that from another could be competition between different viruses for replication in the same host cells or tissues or for use of the same, or very similar, receptor molecules required for infection. Interference may also be due to the nature of the immune response elicited by the infected host in response to infection by the first virus [73, 146]. Seasonal variation in the prevalence of any virus may be influenced by interference, whereby the peak prevalence of one respiratory virus impedes or prevents the processes that let other viruses establish themselves at the same time, in the same host population [145].

Despite extensive investigation of respiratory specimens taken from patients requiring hospitalisation, oxygen therapy and/or drug treatment, we noted the retention of a large proportion (34%) of specimens from which no virus could be detected [8]. Other studies have found similar frequencies of negative specimens and such findings indicate the likely existence of yet-to-be characterised viral causes of respiratory illness. Extrapolating from all the known respiratory viruses and recent research findings, it is reasonable to assume that any new agents of respiratory disease will be associated with CFLIs as well as possibly more severe disease in some populations and also both as sole agents and in the company of other viruses and bacteria.

Associations between acute virus infections and chronic respiratory disease

CFLI is linked with a number of more serious clinical conditions that may require hospitalisation, invasive testing procedures and the use of drugs and other supportive measures. An URTI may develop into a LRTI or it may acutely exacerbate pre-existing chronic conditions including asthma and COPD. Such exacerbations mask CFLI epidemiology by favouring the clinical diagnosis of the LRTI. Acute LRTIs contribute to more morbidity and mortality than HIV infection, malaria, cancer or heart attack [147] worldwide. Because of equivalent isolation frequencies from well and ill children, the presence of potential bacterial pathogens cannot reliably be correlated with LRT symptoms [145].

As we stated earlier in the chapter, many respiratory viruses that are associated with serious disease are also associated with milder common cold-like illnesses; the converse is also true. Viruses, especially the HRVs, that were previously deemed to be capable of causing only mild illness [138] are now being frequently associated with costly and distressing illnesses and CFLI complications. In particular, respiratory viruses often cause more severe LRT symptoms in neonates and infants, because of airway swelling, excessive secretions and smooth muscle contraction in their narrow immature airways resulting from infection [148].

The importance of HRV infection associated with LRT morbidity during the first year of life is both significant [13] and underappreciated [149]. HRVs replicate in non-nasal tissues including smooth muscle [150] and bronchial epithelial cells [151, 152]. In addition, the immunopathological effect of viral replication in the upper airways may be transmitted systemically [148]. If HRVs naturally replicate in the LRT, as has been reported [83], then a local host inflammatory effect is a likely pathogenic mechanism.

In one example, a German birth cohort study found a positive association between repeated LRTI (pneumonia, bronchitis, pertussis, tracheobronchitis, 'flu', croup and bronchitis) before the age of 3 and wheeze at the age of 7 [13]. Nonetheless, the impact of LRTIs on immune development and the contribution of genetic predisposition to LRTIs remain unclear [14, 153, 154]. This study also found a significant inverse relationship between recurrent "runny nose" episodes and subsequent atopic sensitisation, and these repeated infections imparted most of their protective effect during the first year of life [13]. A study of infants found that a sixth of HRV isolate-positive patients exhibited symptoms of LRTIs (mostly wheezing) [155]. In adults ≥40 years of age, the duration of symptoms and frequency of LRTIs associated with HRV isolation starts to increase with age [156].

Although HRVs have been associated with threefold more LRT and wheezy LRT illnesses than HRSV [149], the risk of obstructive airway disease is similar whether an HRV or HRV and HRSV are detected [100].

Studies of children in hospital-based populations usually report more significant clinical outcomes, especially those relating to the LRT [157]. These data can be considered a condensed sampling of illness among community-based populations but conclusions should be interpreted cautiously. LRT illness has also been identified in other age and patient groups [74, 91, 99, 100, 155, 158–161]; nonetheless, hospital-based populations retain importance for probing the potential of a virus to cause severe clinical outcomes, especially due to a first infection. This environment provides cases with the strongest influence on future prioritisation of therapeutic developments [145].

HRVs and expiratory wheezing exacerbations

Acute wheezing episodes (including bronchiolitis and acute asthma, which share similar pathologies) are a common epidemic and seasonal LRT manifestation of respiratory virus infection of the URT and LRT of children from all ages, but especially among males and during the first year of life [145, 158, 162, 163]. The mechanisms underlying the induction or exacerbation of asthma are not yet fully understood [148, 164] but wheezing is blamed for excessive use of antibiotics, for being the primary cause of hospitalisation among children and, rarely, for death [48, 165, 166]. Exacerbations of asthma and COPD are often preceded by a symptomatic rather than asymptomatic HRV episode [166–171], although, in some instances, an exacerbation is the only evidence of symptoms [172]. Reduced peak expiratory volume in children is especially associated with detection of respiratory picornaviruses [170].

Traditionally, it is HRSV infection that is causally associated with expiratory wheezing because of the virus's well-known ability to infect the LRT, but periods of epidemic wheezing unaccompanied by high rates of HRSV detection are common [163, 173]. The Childhood Origins of Asthma Study (COAST) used sampling criteria that were designed to intentionally investigate the role of HRSV in illness, but instead of HRSV, the data indicated that HRVs were the most important predictor of subsequent wheezing in early childhood [174, 175]. Although the total number of symptomatic respiratory illnesses did not differ significantly, asthmatics had more HRV infections, while their siblings had more bacterial infections. Since asthmatics are more often treated with antibiotics, bacterial detection rates may be falsely lowered in some reports [176]. Significantly higher rates of HRV detection with more obvious LRT symptoms are more common in asthmatic children than in non-asthmatic populations [166, 176–178]. History of asthma in children also appears to be a risk factor for more frequent symptomatic viral infections. However, the presence of atopy or allergy does not appear to be a common feature [162, 166] since only a small proportion of allergic children have asthma [179].

Impact and cost of the common cold

For any illness or syndrome, mapping the epidemiology and burden of disease is needed for a number of reasons, but key amongst them is prioritising the need for prevention, treatment, and further research efforts. There are three pieces of evidence required by those developing health policies in assessing whether to recommend or implement a publicly funded prevention or treatment program: epidemiology of the targeted illness, the efficacy of the intervention, and the cost effectiveness of the intervention [180]. Evaluations of cost effectiveness consist of a number of key components, including how common the illness is, the cost associated with illness, and the cost of any intervention, either prevention or treatment [181]. Given the ubiquitous nature of the common cold syndrome, there has been little attention paid to documenting impact. This is a feature colds have in common with the less frequent, but more severe end of the respiratory infection spectrum. Based on estimates from the Global Burden of Disease study, acute respiratory diseases, despite being one of the largest contributors to disability-adjusted life-years (DALYs), receive a discouragingly low proportion of health-related research funds [182].

The value used in cost-effectiveness evaluations is a product of counts of illness and impact of individual illness, often presented as DALYs [181]. Even though CFLIs have lower severity compared with complicated URTIs and LRTIs, due to the frequency their burden cannot be ignored. Acute respiratory infection incidence is highest in the first 2 years of life, with up to 13 episodes per year, and it is not uncommon to average close to one infection per child-month [130, 183]. Whereas illnesses can often be managed in the community with supportive care from parents, complications requiring a medical visit in which antibiotic therapy is prescribed, such as otitis media (30%) and sinusitis (8%), are common [184]. In pre-school aged children, nearly 50% of general practitioner visits are for acute respiratory infections [185], many of which will only involve self-limiting URT symptoms.

The availability of preventive vaccines and therapeutic antivirals means that interpandemic influenza is the most studied of respiratory viruses associated with the cold. Estimates around the cost impact of other respiratory viruses are rare – particularly compared to their relative frequency. Some estimates about the cost impact of non-influenza viruses are available from the US. Using a telephone survey of over 4000 households, researchers collected self-reported incidence and resource use during non-influenza, viral respiratory infections [186]. These figures were extrapolated to the US population and costs attached to resource use. The direct costs associated with viral respiratory infections were US$17 billion annually, with these being outweighed by the indirect cost burden of US$22.5 billion. The indirect cost component was made up of missed workdays due to illness, totalling 70 million days, and missed workdays while caring for a household member, totalling 189 million days [186]. The annual cost burden of antibiotic use for acute respiratory tract illness in the US is over US$1.3 billion alone [187]. This compares with a recent modelling assessment of seasonal influenza suggesting annual costs US$87.1 billion, with 83% of this cost due to annual deaths [188]. Information about HRSV impact is more common than other non-influenza viruses, but pertains mainly to those groups of children who are currently eligible for preventive interventions: those born prematurely with associated lung disease, or with specific congenital cardiopulmonary malformations [189–191]. A US study using three national databases and an assumption that 15% of all acute otitis media was due to HRSV calculated direct medical costs from HRSV to be over US$1.3 billion (2002 dollars) per annum, with 98% of these costs associated with illness in the less than 5-year age group [192].

Although national data are rare, community-level impact is even less commonly measured. Two recent community-level studies have included an assessment of acute respiratory illness in children using a sensitive definition for influenza-like illness [47, 110, 193–195]. The threshold for burden data collection for study children could be met with a combination of two non-specific symptoms, such as nasal stuffiness and decreased activity [47, 194]. Standard costs were applied to burden data to derive a syndrome cost [193] and a virus-specific cost of illness [195]. A mean cost for community-managed illness from each study was AUD$241 from the 2001 pilot study [193], and AUD$309 from the 2003/2004 main study [195] (average exchange rates during study period: United Kingdom pound £1 = AUD$2.49, Euro €1 = AUD$1.73, and US$1 = AUD$1.50) [196]. The main study included an influenza season of higher than normal activity with H3N2 influenza A (drifted strain subtype A/Fujian/411/2002-like) being the predominant circulating type [197].Virus-specific cost of illness for all viruses other than influenza fell within a relatively narrow band, and picornaviruses (not further differentiated) had an mean cost of AUD$267 per illness [195]. A recent UK study looking at the cost impact of individual cough illnesses in children aged 3–59 months, without detailed recording of indirect costs, reported a mean cost per episode to the National Health Service (NHS) of £27, a mean cost for the family of £15, and an annual cost to the NHS £31.5 million [198].

These findings show that, although there are some data on illnesses associated with more serious outcomes and specific viruses, there continues to be little in the way of targeted research at the national or community level documenting the simple burden associated with the common cold. Future community-based studies into the common cold and associated respiratory tract illness, integrating epidemiology and economic methods, are required [199].

Conclusions

The common cold is the syndromic child of many parents. The nature of the child, its epidemiology, severity, and impact, is determined by interaction of host, pathogen, and environmental effects. HRVs are the agents most commonly associated with CFLIs, but other respiratory viruses, including influenza viruses and HRSV, can be associated with the syndrome. The recent expansion in the use of PCR has brought improved detection of known viruses, but also detection of NIVs. Through these means, the diagnostic gap in all respiratory illnesses is reduced. The contribution of HRV Cs in respiratory illness appears to overshadow that of other known RVs; however, it is difficult to judge given the paucity of data from the other species, and further documentation of HRV epidemiology and impact are research priorities for the coming years. Although our knowledge of the causes of CFLIs has improved in past few years, the collation of impact data is some way behind. Documenting burden is an important step in the progress towards improved control and management of these illnesses.

Acknowledgements.

This work was possible because of funding from NH&RMC project grant 455905 and RCHF Project Seeding grant 10281.

References

1 Wat D (2004) The common cold: A review of the literature. *Eur J Intern Med* 15: 79–88
2 Mäkelä MJ, Puhakka T, Ruuskanen O, Leinonen M, Saikku P, Kimpimäki M, Blomqvist S, Hyypiä T, Arstila P (1998) Viruses and bacteria in the etiology of the common cold. *J Clin Microbiol* 36: 539–542
3 Arruda E, Pitkäranta A, Witek TJ, Doyle CA, Hayden FG (1997) Frequency and natural history of rhinovirus infections in adults during autumn. *J Clin Microbiol* 35: 2864–2868
4 van den Hoogen BG, de Jong JC, Groen J, Kuiken T, de Groot R, Fouchier RAM, Osterhaus ADME (2001) A newly discovered human pneumovirus isolated from young children with respiratory tract disease. *Nat Med* 7: 19–24
5 van der Hoek L, Pyrc K, Jebbink MF, Vermeulen-Oost W, Berkhout RJM, Wolthers KC, Wertheim-van Dillen PME, Kaandorp J, Spaargaren J, Berkhout B (2004) Identification of a new human coronavirus. *Nat Med* 10: 368–373
6 Woo PCY, Lau SKP, Chu C-M, Chan K-H, Tsoi H-W, Huang Y, Wong BHL, Poon RWS, Cai JJ, Luk W-K et al. (2005) Characterization and complete genome sequence of a novel coronavirus, coronavirus HKU1, from patients with pneumonia. *J Virol* 79: 884–895
7 Allander T, Tammi MT, Eriksson M, Bjerkner A, Tiveljung-Lindell A, Andersson

B (2005) Cloning of a human parvovirus by molecular screening of respiratory tract samples. *Proc Nat Acad Sci USA* 102: 12891–12896
8 Arden KE, McErlean P, Nissen MD, Sloots TP, Mackay IM (2006) Frequent detection of human rhinoviruses, paramyxoviruses, coronaviruses, and bocavirus during acute respiratory tract infections. *J Med Virol* 78: 1232–1240
9 Lamson D, Renwick N, Kapoor V, Liu Z, Palacios G, Ju J, Dean A, St GK, Briese T, Lipkin WI (2006) MassTag polymerase-chain-reaction detection of respiratory pathogens, including a new rhinovirus genotype, that caused influenza-like illness in New York State during 2004–2005. *J Infect Dis* 194: 1398–1402
10 Lau SKP, Yip CCY, Tsoi H-W, Lee RA, So L-Y, Lau Y-L, Chan K-H, Woo PCY, Yuen K-Y (2007) Clinical features and complete genome characterization of a distinct human rhinovirus genetic cluster, probably representing a previously undetected HRV species, HRV-C, associated with acute respiratory illness in children. *J Clin Microbiol* 45: 3655–3664
11 McErlean P, Shackleton LA, Andrewes E, Webster DR, Lambert SB, Nissen MD, Sloots TP, Mackay IM (2008) Distinguishing molecular features and clinical characteristics of a putative new rhinovirus species, human rhinovirus C (HRV C). *PLoS One* 3: e1847
12 Esposito S, Bosis S, Niesters HG, Tremolati E, Sabatini C, Porta A, Fossali E, Osterhaus AD, Principi N (2008) Impact of human bocavirus on children and their families. *J Clin Microbiol* 46: 1337–1342
13 Illi S, von ME, Lau S, Bergmann R, Niggemann B, Sommerfeld C, Wahn U (2001) Early childhood infectious diseases and the development of asthma up to school age: A birth cohort study. *BMJ* 322: 390–395
14 Hershenson MB, Johnston SL (2006) Rhinovirus infections: More than a common cold. *Am J Respir Crit Care Med* 174: 1284–1285
15 Heikkinen T, Järvinen A (2003) The common cold. *Lancet* 361: 51–59
16 Johnston SL, Sanderson G, Pattemore PK, Smith S, Bardin PG, Bruce CB, Lambden PR, Tyrrell DAJ, Holgate ST (1993) Use of polymerase chain reaction for diagnosis of picornavirus infection in subjects with and without respiratory symptoms. *J Clin Microbiol* 31: 111–117
17 Turner RB (1998) The common cold. *Pediatr Ann* 27: 790–795
18 Pappas DE, Hendley JO, Hayden FG, Winther B (2008) Symptom profile of common colds in school-aged children. *Pediatr Infect Dis J* 27: 8–11
19 Eccles R (2007) Mechanisms of symptoms of the common cold and influenza. *Br J Hosp Med* 68: 578–582
20 Pizzichini MMM, Pizzichini E, Efthimiadis A, Chauhan AJ, Johnston SL, Hussack P, Mahony J, Dolovich J, Hargreave FE (1998) Asthma and natural colds. *Am J Respir Crit Care Med* 158: 1178–1184
21 Lemanske RF, Gern JE, Gangnon RE (2006) Viral specimen collection by parents increases response rate in population-based virus studies. *J Allergy Clin Immunol* 117: 956–957
22 Phillips CA, Melnick JL, Grim CA (1968) Rhinovirus infections in a student population: Isolation of the five new serotypes. *Am J Epidemiol* 87: 447–456
23 Minor TE, Dick EC, Peterson JA, Docherty DE (1974) Failure of naturally acquired rhinovirus infections to produce temporal immunity to heterologous serotypes. *Infect Immun* 10: 1192–1193

24 Cooney MK, Kenny GE (1977) Demonstration of dual rhinovirus infection in humans by isolation of different serotypes in human heteroploid (HeLa) and human diploid fibroblast cell cultures. *J Clin Microbiol* 5: 202–207
25 Cooney MK, Hall CB, Fox JP (1972) The Seattle virus Watch. III. Evaluation of isolation methods and summary of infections detected by virus isolations. *Am J Epidemiol* 96: 286–305
26 Renwick N, Schweiger B, Kapoor V, Liu Z, Villari J, Bullmann R, Miething R, Briese T, Lipkin WI (2007) A recently identified rhinovirus genotype is associated with severe respiratory-tract infection in children in Germany. *J Infect Dis* 196: 1754–1760
27 Lee W-M, Kiesner C, Pappas T, Lee I, Grindle K, Jartti T, Jakiela B, Lemanske RF, Shult PA, Gern JE (2007) A diverse group of previously unrecognized human rhinoviruses are common causes of respiratory illness in infants. *PLoS One* 2: e966
28 Peltola V, Waris M, Österback R, Susi P, Ruuskanen O, Hyypiä T (2008) Rhinovirus transmission within families with children: Incidence of symptomatic and asymptomatic infections. *J Infect Dis* 197: 382–389
29 Yusuf S, Piedimonte G, Auais A, Demmler G, Krishnan S, van Caseele P, Singleton R, Broor S, Parveen S, Avendano L et al. (2007) The relationship of meteorological conditions to the epidemic activity of respiratory syncytial virus. *Epidemiol Infect* 135: 1077–1090
30 Mackay IM, Waliuzzaman Z, Chidlow GR, Fegredo DC, Laingam S, Adamson P, Harnett GB, Rawlinson W, Nissen MD, Sloots TP (2004) Use of the P gene to genotype human metapneumovirus identifies 4 viral subtypes. *J Infect Dis* 190: 1913–1918
31 Mackay IM, Bialasiewicz S, Jacob KC, McQueen E, Arden KE, Nissen MD, Sloots TP (2006) Genetic diversity of human metapneumovirus over 4 consecutive years in Australia. *J Infect Dis* 193: 1630–1633
32 McErlean P, Shackleton LA, Lambert SB, Nissen MD, Sloots TP, Mackay IM (2007) Characterisation of a newly identified human rhinovirus, HRV-QPM, discovered in infants with bronchiolitis. *J Clin Virol* 39: 67–75
33 Glezen WP, Paredes A, Taber LH (1980) Influenza in children relationship to other respiratory agents. *JAMA* 243: 1345–1349
34 Chew FT, Doraisingham S, Ling AE, Kumarasinghe G, Lee BW (1998) Seasonal trends of viral respiratory tract infections in the tropics. *Epidemiol Infect* 121: 121–128
35 Jansen AG, Sanders EA, Van der Ende A, van Loon AM, Hoes AW, Hak E (2008) Invasive pneumococcal and meningococcal disease: Association with influenza virus and respiratory syncytial virus activity? *Epidemiol Infect* 136: 1448–1454
36 Johnson HE, Altman R, Hamre D, Ward T (1964) Viral infections and the common cold. *Chest* 45: 46–53
37 Al-Sunaidi M, Williams CH, Hughes PJ, Schnurr DP, Stanway G (2007) Analysis of a new human parechovirus allows the definition of parechovirus types and the identification of RNA structural domains. *J Virol* 81: 1013–1021
38 Hamre D, Connelly AP, Procknow JJ (1966) Virologic studies of acute respira-

tory disease in young adults. IV. Virus isolations during four years of surveillance. *Am J Epidemiol* 83: 238–249
39 Johnston NW, Johnston SL, Norman GR, Dai J, Sears MR (2006) The September epidemic of asthma hospitalization: School children as disease vectors. *J Allergy Clin Immunol* 117: 557–562
40 Deal EC Jr, McFadden ER Jr, Ingram RH Jr, Breslin FJ, Jaeger JJ (1980) Airway responsiveness to cold air and hyperpnea in normal subjects and in those with hay fever and asthma. *Am Rev Respir Dis* 121: 621–628
41 Winther B, Hayden FG, Hendley JO (2006) Picornavirus infections in children diagnosed by RT-PCR during longitudinal surveillance with weekly sampling: Association with symptomatic illness and effect of season. *J Med Virol* 78: 644–650
42 Vesa S, Kleemola M, Blomqvist S, Takala A, Kilpi T, Hovi T (2001) Epidemiology of documented viral respiratory infections and acute otitis media in a cohort of children followed from two to twenty-four months of age. *Pediatr Infect Dis J* 20: 574–581
43 Silva MJ, Ferraz C, Pissarra S, Cardoso MJ, Simões J, Vitór AB (2007) Role of viruses and atypical bacteria in asthma exacerbations among children in Oporto (Portugal). *Allergol Immunopathol* 35: 4–9
44 Miller EK, Lu X, Erdman DD, Poehling KA, Zhu Y, Griffin MR, Hartvert TV, Anderson LJ, Weinberg GA, Hall CB et al. (2007) Rhinovirus-associated hospitalizations in young children. *J Infect Dis* 195: 773–781
45 Gwaltney JM Jr, Hendley JO, Simon G, Jordan WS Jr (1966) Rhinovirus infections in an industrial population. I. The occurrence of illness. *N Engl J Med* 275: 1261–1268
46 Fox JP, Cooney MK, Hall CE (1975) The Seattle virus watch. V. Epidemiologic observation of rhinovirus infections, 1965–1969 in families with young children. *Am J Epidemiol* 101: 122–143
47 Lambert SB, Allen KM, Druce JD, Birch CJ, Mackay IM, Carlin JB, Carapetis JP, Sloots TP, Nissen MD, Nolan TM (2007) Community epidemiology of human metapneumovirus, human coronavirus NL63, and other respiratory viruses in healthy preschool-aged children using parent-collected specimens. *Pediatrics* 120: e929–e937
48 Jartti T, Lehtinen P, Vuorinen T, Österback R, van den Hoogen B, Osterhaus ADME, Ruuskanen O (2004) Respiratory picornaviruses and respiratory syncytial virus as causative agents of acute expiratory wheezing in children. *Emerg Infect Dis* 10: 1095–1101
49 Wald TG, Shult P, Krause P, Miller BA, Drinka P, Gravenstein S (1995) A rhinovirus outbreak among residents of a long-term care facility. *Ann Intern Med* 123: 588–593
50 Dick EC, Blumer CR, Evans AS (1967) Epidemiology of infections with rhinovirus types 43 and 55 in a group of university of Wisconsin student families. *Am J Epidemiol* 86: 386–400
51 Hament JM, Kimpen JL, Fleer A, Wolfs TF (1999) Respiratory viral infection predisposing for bacterial disease: A concise review. *FEMS Immunol Med Microbiol* 26: 189–195

52 Peltola VT, McCullers JA (2004) Respiratory viruses predisposing to bacterial infections: Role of neuraminidase. *Pediatr Infect Dis J* 23: S87–S97
53 Selinger DS, Reed WP, McLaren LC (1981) Model for studying bacterial adherence to epithelial cells infected with viruses. *Infect Immun* 32: 941–944
54 McCullers JA, Bartmess KC (2003) Role of neuraminidase in lethal synergism between influenza virus and *Streptococcus pneumoniae*. *J Infect Dis* 187: 1000–1009
55 Okamoto S, Kawabata S, Nakagawa I, Okuno Y, Goto T, Sano K, Hamada S (2003) Influenza A virus-infected hosts boost an invasive type of *Streptococcus pyogenes* infection in mice. *J Virol* 77: 4104–4112
56 Ishizuka S, Yamaya M, Suzuki T, Takahashi H, Ida S, Sasaki T, Inoue D, Sekizawa K, Nishimura H, Sasaki H (2003) Effects of rhinovirus infection on the adherence of *Streptococcus pneumoniae* to cultured human airway epithelial cells. *J Infect Dis* 188: 1928–1939
57 Oliver BG, Lim S, Wark P, Laza-Stanca V, King N, Black JL, Burgess JK, Roth M, Johnston SL (2008) Rhinovirus exposure impairs immune responses to bacterial products in human alveolar macrophages. *Thorax* 63: 519–525
58 Watson M, Gilmour R, Menzies R, Ferson M, McIntyre P (2006) The association of respiratory viruses, temperature, and other climatic parameters with the incidence of invasive pneumococcal disease in Sydney, Australia. *Clin Infect Dis* 42: 211–215
59 Murdoch DR, Jennings LC (2009) Association of respiratory virus activity and environmental factors with the incidence of invasive pneumococcal disease. *J Infect* 58: 37–46
60 Madhi SA, Klugman KP (2004) A role for *Streptococcus pneumoniae* in virus-associated pneumonia. *Nat Med* 10: 811–813
61 Kaiser L, Aubert J-D, Pache J-C, Deffernez C, Rochat T, Garbino J, Wunderli W, Meylan P, Yerly S, Perrin L et al. (2006) Chronic rhinoviral infection in lung transplant recipients. *Am J Respir Crit Care Med* 174: 1392–1399
62 Larson HE, Reed SE, Tyrrell DAJ (1980) Isolation of rhinoviruses and coronaviruses from 38 colds in adults. *J Med Virol* 5: 221–229
63 Denny FW, Clyde WA Jr (1986) Acute lower respiratory tract infections in nonhospitalized children. *J Pediatr* 108: 635–646
64 Whelen AC, Persing DH (1996) The role of nucleic acid amplification and detection in the clinical microbiology laboratory. *Annu Rev Microbiol* 50: 349–373
65 Carman WF, Wallace LA, Walker J, McIntyre S, Noone A, Christie P, Millar J, Douglas JD (2000) Rapid virological surveillance of community influenza infection in general practice. *Br Med J* 321: 736–737
66 Ogilvie M (2001) Molecular techniques should not now replace cell culture in diagnostic virology laboratories. *Rev Med Virol* 11: 351–354
67 Leland DS, Ginocchio CC (2007) Role of cell culture for virus detection in the age of technology. Clin *Microbiol Rev* 20: 49–78
68 Mahony JB (2008) Detection of respiratory viruses by molecular methods. Clin *Microbiol Rev* 21: 716–747
69 Andrewes CH, Chaproniere DM, Gompels AEH, Pereira HG, Roden AT

(1953) Propagation of common-cold virus in tissue cultures. *Lancet* 265: 546–547
70 Andrewes CH (1966) Rhinoviruses and common colds. *Annu Rev Med* 17: 361–370
71 Pelon W, Mogabgab WJ, Phillips LA, Pierce WE (1957) A cytopathogenic agent isolated from naval recruits with mild respiratory illnesses. *Proc Soc Exp Biol Med* 94: 262–267
72 Price WH (1956) The isolation of a new virus associated with respiratory clinical disease in humans. *Proc Natl Acad Sci USA* 42: 892–896
73 Olson LC, Willhight M, Buescher EL (1972) Recovery and characterization of non-cytopathogenic rhinoviruses. *J Gen Virol* 17: 237–240
74 Douglas RG Jr, Cate TR, Gerone PJ, Couch RB (1966) Quantitative rhinovirus shedding patterns in volunteers. *Am Rev Respir Dis* 94: 159–167
75 D'Alessio DJ, Meschievitz CK, Peterson JA, Dick CR, Dick EC (1984) Short-duration exposure and the transmission of rhinoviral colds. *J Infect Dis* 150: 189–194
76 Cate TR, Couch RB, Fleet WF, Griffith WR, Gerone PJ, Knight V (1965) Production of tracheobronchitis in volunteers with rhinovirus in a small-particle aerosol. *Am J Epidemiol* 81: 95–105
77 Hendley JO, Wenzel RP, Gwaltney JM Jr (1973) Transmission of rhinovirus colds by self-inoculation. *N Engl J Med* 288: 1361–1364
78 Sethi SK (1978) Reproducible plaquing system for rhinovirus serotypes in HeLa cells – Agarose suspension. *Acta Virol* 22: 60–65
79 Gwaltney JM Jr (1966) Micro-neutralization test for identification of rhinovirus serotypes. *Proc Soc Exp Biol Med* 122: 1137–1141
80 Behbehani AM, Lee LH (1964) Growth, plaque production and cationic stabilization of rhinovirus type 1 (Echovirus 28). *J Bacteriol* 88: 1608–1611
81 Fiala M, Kenny GE (1966) Enhancement of rhinovirus plaque formation in human heteroploid cell cultures by magnesium and calcium. *J Bacteriol* 92: 1717–1715
82 Parsons R, Tyrrell DAJ (1961) A plaque method for assaying some viruses isolated from common colds. *Nature* 189: 640–642
83 Papadopoulos NG, Sanderson G, Hunter J, Johnston SL (1999) Rhinoviruses replicate effectively at lower airway temperatures. *J Med Virol* 58: 100–104
84 Rosenbaum MJ, De Berry P, Sullivan EJ, Pierce WE, Mueller RE, Peckinpaugh RO (1971) Epidemiology of the common cold in military recruits with emphasis on infections by rhinovirus types 1A, 2, and two unclassified rhinoviruses. *Am J Epidemiol* 93: 183–193
85 Mogabgab WJ, Pelon W (1957) Problems in characterizing and identifying an apparently new virus found in association with mild respiratory disease in recruits. *Ann N Y Acad Sci* 67: 403–412
86 Hendley JO, Edmondson WP Jr, Gwaltney JM Jr (1972) Relation between naturally acquired immunity and infectivity of two rhinoviruses in volunteers. *J Infect Dis* 125: 243–248
87 Relman DA (2003) Shedding light on microbial detection. *N Engl J Med* 349: 2162–2163
88 Kuypers J, Wright N, Ferrenberg J, Huang M-L, Cent A, Corey L, Morrow R

(2006) Comparison of real-time PCR assays with fluorescent-antibody assays for diagnosis of respiratory virus infections in children. *J Clin Microbiol* 44: 2382–2388
89 Falsey AR, Walsh EE (2006) Viral pneumonia in older adults. *Clin Infect Dis* 42
90 Johnston SL, Bardin PG, Pattemore PK (1993) Viruses as precipitants of asthma symptoms. III. Rhinoviruses: Molecular biology and prospects for future intervention. *Clin Exp Allergy* 23: 237–246
91 Ketler A, Hamparian VV, Hilleman MR (1962) Characterization and classification of ECHO 28-rhinovirus-coryzavirus agents. *Proc Soc Exp Biol Med* 110: 821–831
92 Conant RM, Hamparian VV (1968) Rhinoviruses: Basis for a numbering system. II. Serologic characterization of prototype strains. *J Immunol* 100: 107–113
93 Gwaltney JM Jr, Hendley JO (1978) Rhinovirus transmission: One if by air, two if by hand. *Am J Epidemiol* 107: 357–361
94 Ledford RM, Patel NR, Demenczuk TM, Watanyar A, Herbertz T, Collett MS, Pevear DC (2004) VP1 sequencing of all human rhinovirus serotypes: Insights into genus phylogeny and susceptibility to antiviral capsid-binding compounds. *J Virol* 78: 3663–3674
95 Oberste MS, Maher K, Kilpatrick DR, Pallansch LA (1999) Molecular evolution of the human enteroviruses: Correlation of serotype with VP1 sequence and application to picornavirus classification. *J Virol* 73: 1941–1948
96 van de Pol AC, van Loon AM, Wolfs TF, Jansen NJ, Nijhuis M, Breteler EK, Schuurman R, Rossen JW (2007) Increased detection of respiratory syncytial virus, influenza viruses, parainfluenza viruses, and adenoviruses with real-time PCR in samples from patients with respiratory symptoms. *J Clin Microbiol* 45: 2260–2262
97 Pitkäranta A, Arruda E, Malmberg H, Hayden FG (1997) Detection of rhinovirus in sinus brushings of patients with acute community-acquired sinusitis by reverse transcription-PCR. *J Clin Microbiol* 35: 1791–1793
98 Kämmerer U, Kunkel B, Korn K (1994) Nested PCR for specific detection and rapid identification of human picornaviruses. *J Clin Microbiol* 32: 285–291
99 Andeweg AC, Bestebroer TM, Huybreghs M, Kimman TG, de Jong JC (1999) Improved detection of rhinoviruses in clinical samples by using a newly developed nested reverse transcription-PCR assay. *J Clin Microbiol* 37: 524–530
100 Aberle JH, Aberle SW, Pracher E, Hutter H-P, Kundi M, Popw-Kraupp T (2005) Impact on clinical course of disease and interferon-γ response. *Pediatr Infect Dis J* 24: 605–610
101 Versteegh FGA, Weverling GJ, Peeters MF, Wilbrink B, Veenstra-van Schie MTM, van Leewen-Gerritsen JM, Mooi-Kokenberg EANM, Schellekens JFP, Roord JJ (2005) Community-acquired pathogens associated with prolonged coughing in children: A prospective cohort study. *Clin Microbiol Infect* 11: 801–807
102 Hutchinson AF, Ghimire AK, Thompson MA, Black JF, Brand CA, Lowe AJ, Smallwood DM, Vlahos R, Bozinovski S, Brown GV et al. (2007) A communi-

ty-based, time-matched, case-control study of respiratory viruses and exacerbations of COPD. *Respir Med* 101: 2472–2481

103 Arruda E, Hayden FG (1993) Detection of human rhinovirus RNA in nasal washings by PCR. *Mol Cell Probe* 7: 373–379

104 Lu X, Holloway B, Dare RK, Kuypers J, Yagi S, Williams JV, Hall CB, Erdman DD (2008) Real-time reverse transcription-PCR assay for comprehensive detection of human rhinoviruses. *J Clin Microbiol* 46: 533–539

105 Suvilehto J, Roivainen M, Seppänen M, Meri S, Hovi T, Carpén O, Pitkäranta A (2006) Rhinovirus/enterovirus RNA in tonsillar tissue of children with tonsillar disease. *J Clin Virol* 35: 292–297

106 Mackay IM, Bustin S, Andrade JM, Nissen MD, Sloots TP (2007) Quantification of microorganimsms: Not human, not dimple, not quick. In: IM Mackay (ed): *Real-time PCR in microbiology.* Caister Academic Press, Norfolk, 133–182

107 Stensballe LG, Trautner S, Kofoed PE, Nante E, Hedegaard K, Jensen IP, Aaby P (2002) Comparison of nasopharyngeal aspirate and nasal swab specimens for detection of respiratory syncytial virus in different settings in a developing country. *Trop Med Int Health* 7: 317–321

108 Macfarlane P, Denham J, Assous J, Hughes C (2005) RSV testing in bronchiolitis: Which nasal sampling method is best? *Arch Dis Child* 90: 634–635

109 Lambert SB, Whiley DM, O'Neill NT, Andrews EC, Canavan FM, Bletchly C, Siebert DJ, Sloots TP, Nissen MD (2008) Comparing nose-throat swabs and nasopharyngeal aspirates collected from children with symptoms for respiratory virus identification using real-time polymerase chain reaction. *Pediatrics* 122: e615-e620

110 Lambert SB, Allen KM, Nolan TM (2008) Parent-collected respiratory specimens – A novel method for respiratory virus and vaccine efficacy research. *Vaccine* 26: 1826–1831

111 Brunstein JD, Cline CL, McKinney S, Thomas E (2008) Evidence from multiplex molecular assays for complex multipathogen interactions in acute respiratory infections. *J Clin Microbiol* 46: 97–102

112 Stott EJ, Eadie MB, Grist NR (1969) Rhinovirus infections of children in hospital: Isolation of three possibly new rhinovirus serotypes. *Am J Epidemiol* 90: 45–52

113 Tiveljung-Lindell A, Rotzen-Ostlund M, Gupta S, Ullstrand R, Grillner L, Zweygberg-Wirgart B, Allander T (2009) Development and implementation of a molecular diagnostic platform for daily rapid detection of 15 respiratory viruses. *J Med Virol* 81: 167–175

114 Richard N, Komurian-Pradel F, Javouhey E, Perret M, Rajoharison A, Bagnaud A, Billaud G, Vernet G, Lina B, Floret D et al. (2008) The impact of dual viral infection in infants admitted to a pediatric intensive care unit associated with severe bronchiolitis. *Pediatr Infect Dis J* 27: 1–5

115 Gunson RN, Collins TC, Carman WF (2005) Real-time RT-PCR detection of 12 respiratory viral infections in four triplex reactions. *J Clin Virol* 33: 341–344

116 Nolte FS, Marshall DJ, Rasberry C, Schievelbein S, Banks GG, Storch GA, Arens MQ, Buller RS, Prudent JR (2007) MultiCode-PLx system for multiplexed detection of seventeen respiratory viruses. *J Clin Microbiol* 45: 2779–2786

117 Mahony J, Chong S, Merante F, Yaghoubian S, Sinha T, Lisle C, Janeczko R (2007) Development of a respiratory virus panel test for detection of twenty human respiratory viruses by use of multiplex PCR and a fluid microbead-based assay. *J Clin Microbiol* 45: 2965–2970
118 Drews SJ, Blair J, Lombos E, DeLima C, Burton L, Mazzulli T, Low DE (2008) Use of the Seeplex RV Detection kit for surveillance of respiratory viral outbreaks in Toronto, Ontario, Canada. *Ann Clin Lab Sci* 38: 376–379
119 Yoo SJ, Kuak EY, Shin BM (2007) Detection of 12 respiratory viruses with two-set multiplex reverse transcriptase-PCR assay using a dual priming oligonucleotide system. *Korean J Lab Med* 27: 420–427
120 Roh KH, Kim J, Nam MH, Yoon S, Lee CK, Lee K, Yoo Y, Kim MJ, Cho Y (2008) Comparison of the Seeplex reverse transcription PCR assay with the R-mix viral culture and immunofluorescence techniques for detection of eight respiratory viruses. *Ann Clin Lab Sci* 38: 41–46
121 Han J, Swan DC, Smith SJ, Lum SH, Sefers SE, Unger ER, Tang YW (2006) Simultaneous amplification and identification of 25 human papillomavirus types with Templex technology. *J Clin Microbiol* 44: 4157–4162
122 Brunstein J, Thomas E (2006) Direct screening of clinical specimens for multiple respiratory pathogens using the Genaco Respiratory Panels 1 and 2. *Diagn Mol Pathol* 15: 169–173
123 Li H, McCormac MA, Estes RW, Sefers SE, Dare RK, Chappell JD, Erdman DD, Wright PF, Tang Y-W (2007) Simultaneous detection and high-throughput identification of a panel of RNA viruses causing respiratory tract infections. *J Clin Microbiol* 45: 2105–2109
124 Briese T, Palacios G, Kokoris M, Jabado O, Liu Z, Renwick N, Kapoor V, Casas I, Pozo F, Limberger R et al. (2005) Diagnostic system for rapid and sensitive differential detection of pathogens. *Emerg Infect Dis* 11: 310–313
125 Dominguez SR, Briese T, Palacios G, Hui J, Villari J, Kapoor V, Tokarz R, Glode MP, Anderson MS, Robinson CC et al. (2008) Multiplex MassTag-PCR for respiratory pathogens in pediatric nasopharyngeal washes negative by conventional diagnostic testing shows a high prevalence of viruses belonging to a newly recognized rhinovirus clade. *J Clin Virol* 43: 219–222
126 Wang D, Coscoy L, Zylberberg M, Avila PC, Boushey HA, Ganem D, DeRisi JL (2002) Microarray-based detection and genotyping of viral pathogens. *Proc Natl Acad Sci USA* 99: 15687–15692
127 Ostroff R, Ettinger A, La H, Rihanek M, Zalman L, Meador III J, Patick AK, Worland S, Polisky B (2001) Rapid multiserotype detection of human rhinoviruses on optically coated silicon surfaces. *J Clin Virol* 21: 105–117
128 Shanmukh S, Jones L, Driskell J, Zhao Y, Dluhy R, Tripp RA (2006) Rapid and sensitive detection of respiratory virus molecular signatures using a silver nanorod array SERS substrate. *Nano Lett* 6: 2630–2636
129 Bae HG, Nitsche A, Teichmann A, Biel SS, Niedrig M (2003) Detection of yellow fever virus: A comparison of quantitative real-time PCR and plaque assay. *J Virol Methods* 110: 185–191
130 Jartti T, Lee W-M, Pappas T, Evans M, Lemanske RF, Gern JE (2008) Serial viral infections in infants with recurrent respiratory illnesses. *Eur Respir J* 32: 314–320

131 Mackay IM, Arden KE, Nissen MD, Sloots TP (2007) Challenges facing real-time PCR characterization of acute respiratory tract infections. In: IM Mackay (ed): *Real-Time PCR in Microbiology: From Diagnosis to Characterization*. Caister Academic Press, Norfolk, 269–318

132 Brouard J, Freymuth F, Vabret A, Jokic M, Guillois B, Duhamel JF (2000) Viral co-infections in immunocompetent infants with bronchiolitis: Prospective epidemiologic study (in French). *Arch Pediatr* 7 (Suppl 3): 531s–535s

133 Papadopoulos NG, Moustaki M, Tsolia M, Bossios A, Astra E, Prezerakou A, Gourgiotis D, Kafetzis D (2002) Association of rhinovirus infection with increased disease severity in acute bronchiolitis. *Am J Respir Crit Care Med* 165: 1285–1289

134 Maggi F, Pifferi M, Vatteroni M, Fornai C, Tempestini E, Anzilotti S, Lanini L, Andreoli E, Ragazzo V, Pistello M et al. (2003) Human metapneumovirus associated with respiratory tract infections in a 3-year study of nasal swabs from infants in Italy. *J Clin Microbiol* 41: 2987–2991

135 Peltola J, Waris M, Hyypiä T, Ruuskanen O (2006) Respiratory viruses in children with invasive pneumococcal disease. *Clin Infect Dis* 43: 266–268

136 Juvén T, Mertsola J, Waris M, Leinonen M, Meurman O, Roivainen M, Eskola J, Saikku P, Ruuskanen O (2000) Etiology of community-acquired pneumonia in 254 hospitalized children. *Pediatr Infect Dis J* 19: 293–298

137 Garcia-Garcia ML, Calvo C, Perez-Brena P, De Cea JM, Acosta B, Casas I (2006) Prevalence and clinical characteristics of human metapneumovirus infections in hospitalized infants in Spain. *Pediatr Pulmonol* 41: 863–871

138 van der Zalm MM, van Ewijk BE, Wilbrink B, Uiterwaal CSPM, Wolfs TFW, van der Ent CK (2009) Respiratory pathogens in children with and without respiratory symptoms. *J Pediatr* 154: 396–400

139 Aberle JH, Aberle SW, Pracher E, Hutter H-P, Kundi M, Popw-Kraupp T (2005) Single *versus* dual respiratory virus infections in hospitalized infants: Impact on clinical course of disease and interferon-gamma response. *Pediatr Infect Dis J* 24: 605–610

140 Greensill J, McNamara PS, Dove W, Flanagan B, Smyth RL, Hart CA (2003) Human metapneumovirus in severe respiratory syncytial virus bronchiolitis. *Emerg Infect Dis* 9: 372–375

141 Simon A, Wilkesmann A, Muller A, Schildgen O (2007) HMPV infections are frequently accompanied by co-infections. *Pediatr Pulmonol* 42: 98

142 Mackay IM (2007) Human bocavirus: Multisystem detection raises questions about infection. *J Infect Dis* 196: 968–970

143 Winther B, Alper CM, Mandel EM, Doyle WJ, Hendley JO (2007) Temporal relationships between colds, upper respiratory viruses detected by polymerase chain reaction, and otitis media in young children followed through a typical cold season. *Pediatrics* 119: 1069–1075

144 Alper CM, Doyle WJ, Winther B, Hendley JO (2008) Upper respiratory virus detection without parent-reported illness in children is virus-specific. *J Clin Virol* 43: 120–122

145 Glezen WP, Denny FW (1973) Epidemiology of acute lower respiratory disease in children. *N Engl J Med* 288: 498–505

146 Hitchcock G, Tyrrell DA (1960) Some virus isolations from common colds. II. Virus interference in tissue cultures. *Lancet* 1: 237–239
147 Mizgerd JP (2006) Lung infection-a public health priority. PloS Medicine 3: e76
148 Bardin PG, Johnston SL, Pattemore PK (1992) Viruses as precipitants of asthma symptoms. II. Physiology and mechanisms. *Clin Exp Allergy* 22: 809–822
149 Kusel MMH, de Klerk NH, Holt PG, Kebadze T, Johnston SL, Sly PD (2006) Role of respiratory viruses in acute upper and lower respiratory tract illness in the first year of life. *Pediatr Infect Dis J* 25: 680–686
150 Hakonarson H, Maskeri N, Carter C, Hodinka RL, Campbell D, Grunstein MM (1998) Mechanism of rhinovirus-induced changes in airway smooth muscle responsiveness. *J Clin Invest* 102: 1732–1741
151 Gern JE, Galagan DM, Jarjour NN, Dick EC, Busse WW (2008) Detection of rhinovirus RNA in lower airway cells during experimentally induced infection. *Am J Respir Crit Care Med* 155: 1159–1161
152 Jakiela B, Brockman-Schneider R, Amineva S, Lee W-M, Gern JE (2008) Basal cells of differentiated bronchial epithelium are more susceptible to rhinovirus infection. *Am J Respir Cell Mol Biol* 38: 517–523
153 Gern JE, Busse WW (2002) Relationship of viral infections to wheezing illnesses and asthma. *Nat Rev Immunol* 2: 132–138
154 Martin JG, Siddiqui S, Hassan M (2006) Immune responses to viral infections: Relevance for asthma. *Paediatr Respir Rev* 7S: S125-S127
155 Krilov L, Pierik L, Keller E, Mahan K, Watson D, Hirsch M, Hamparian V, McIntosh K (1986) The association of rhinoviruses with lower respiratory tract disease in hospitalized patients. *J Med Virol* 19: 345–352
156 Monto AS, Bryan ER, Ohmit S (1987) Rhinovirus infections in Tecumseh, Michigan: Frequency of illness and number of serotypes. *J Infect Dis* 156: 43–49
157 El-Sahly HM, Atmar RL, Glezen WP, Greenberg SB (2000) Spectrum of clinical illness in hospitalized patients with "Common cold" virus infections. *Clin Infect Dis* 31: 96–100
158 Glezen WP, Loda FA, Clyde WA, Senior RJ, Sheaffer CI, Conley WG, Denny FW (1971) Epidemiologic patterns of acute lower respiratory disease of children in a pediatric group practice. *J Pediatr* 78: 397–406
159 Bloom HH, Forsyth BR, Johnson KM, Chanock RM (1963) Relationship of rhinovirus infection to mild upper respiratory disease. *JAMA* 186: 38–45
160 Collinson J, Nicholson KG, Cancio E, Ashman J, Ireland DC, Hammersley V, Kent J, O'Callaghan C (1996) Effects of upper respiratory tract infections in patients with cystic fibrosis. *Thorax* 51: 1115–1122
161 Andréoletti L, Lesay M, Deschildre A, Lambert V, Dewilde A, Wattré P (2000) Differential detection of rhinoviruses and enteroviruses RNA sequences associated with classical immunofluorescence assay detection of respiratory virus antigens in nasopharyngeal swabs from infants with bronchiolitis. *J Med Virol* 61: 341–346
162 Rakes GP, Arruda E, Ingram JM, Hoover GE, Zambrano JC, Hayden FG, Platts-Mills TAE, Heymann PW (1999) Rhinovirus and respiratory syncytial

virus in wheezing children requiring emergency care. *Am J Respir Crit Care Med* 159: 785–790

163 Henderson FW, Clyde WA, Collier AM, Denny FW, Senior RJ, Sheaffer CI, Conley WG, Christian RM (1979) The etiologic and epidemiologic spectrum of bronchiolitis in pediatric practice. *J Pediatr* 95: 183–190

164 Martinez FD (2007) Gene-environment interactions in asthma. *Proc Am Thorac Soc* 4: 26–31

165 Mallia P, Johnston SL (2006) How viral infections cause exacerbation of airway diseases. *Chest* 130: 1203–1210

166 Pattemore PK, Johnston SL, Bardin PG (1992) Viruses as precipitants of asthma symptoms. I. Epidemiology. *Clin Exp Allergy* 22: 325–336

167 Heymann PW, Platts-Mills TAE, Johnston SL (2005) Role of viral infections, atopy and antiviral immunity in the etiology of wheezing exacerbations among children and young adults. *Pediatr Infect Dis J* 24: S217-S222

168 Lidwell OM, Sommerville T (1951) Observations on the incidence and distribution of the common cold in a rural community during 1948 and 1949. *J Hyg (Lond)* 49: 365–381

169 Green RM, Custovic A, Sanderson G, Hunter J, Johnston SL, Woodcock A (2007) Synergism between allergens and viruses and risk of hospital admission with asthma: Case-control study. *Br Med J* 324: 1–5

170 Johnston SL, Pattemore PK, Sanderson G, Smith S, Lampe F, Josephs L, Symington P, O'Toole S, Myint SH, Tyrrell DAJ et al. (1995) Community study of role of viral infections in exacerbations of asthma in 9–11 year old children. *Br Med J* 310: 1225–1229

171 Minor TE, Dick EC, DeMeo AN, Ouellette JJ, Cohen M, Reed CE (1974) Viruses as precipitants of asthmatic attacks in children. *JAMA* 227: 292–298

172 Roldaan AC, Masural N (1982) Viral respiratory infections in asthmatic children staying in a mountain resort. *Eur J Respir Dis* 63: 140–150

173 Lemanske RF (2002) The childhood origins of asthma (COAST) study. Pediatr Allergy Immunol 15: 1–6

174 van der Zalm MM, Uiterwaal CSPM, de Jong BM, Wilbrink B, van der Ent CK (2006) Viral specimen collection by parents increases response rate in population-based virus studies. *J Allergy Clin Immunol* 117: 955–957

175 Lemanske RF, Jackson DJ, Gangnon RE, Evans MD, Li Z, Shult PA, Kirk CJ, Reisdorf E, Roberg KA, Anderson EL et al. (2005) Rhinovirus illnesses during infancy predict subsequent childhood wheezing. *J Allergy Clin Immunol* 116: 571–577

176 Minor TE, Baker JW, Dick EC, DeMeo AN, Ouellette JJ, Cohen M, Reed CE (1974) Greater frequency of viral; respiratory infections in asthmatic children as compared with their nonasthmatic siblings. *J Pediatr* 85: 472–477

177 Nicholson KG, Kent J, Ireland DC (1993) Respiratory viruses and exacerbations of asthma in adults. *Br Med J* 307: 982–986

178 Rawlinson WD, Waliuzzaman Z, Carter IW, Belessis YC, Gilbert KM, Morton JR (2003) Asthma exacerbations in children are associated with rhinovirus but not human metapneumovirus infection. *J Infect Dis* 187: 1314–1318

179 Yoo J, Tcheurekdjian H, Lynch SV, Cabana M, Boushey HA (2007) Microbial

manipulation of immune function for asthma prevention. Inferences from clinical trials. *Proc Am Thorac Soc* 4: 277–282
180 Fedson DS, Nichol KL (2006) Influenza vaccination: Policy *versus* evidence: No gap between policy and evidence. *BMJ* 333: 1020
181 Drummond M, Sculpher M, Torrance G (2005) *Methods for the economic evaluation of health care programmes.* Oxford University Press: Oxford
182 Michaud CM, Murray CJ, Bloom BR (2001) Burden of disease – implications for future research. *JAMA* 285: 535–539
183 Monto AS (2002) Epidemiology of viral respiratory infections. *Am J Med* 112: 4S–12S
184 Revai K, Dobbs LA, Nair S (2007) Incidence of acute otitis media and sinusitis complicating upper respiratory tract infection: The effect of age. *Pediatrics* 119: e1408–1412
185 Bridges-Webb C, Britt H, Miles DA, Neary S, Charles J, Traynor V (1993) Morbidity and treatment in general practice in Australia. *Aust Fam Physician* 22: 336–339–342–346
186 Fendrick AM, Monto AS, Nightengale B (2003) The economic burden of non-influenza-related viral respiratory tract infection in the United States. *Arch Intern Med* 163: 487–494
187 Bertino JS (2002) Cost burden of viral respiratory infections: Issues for formulary decision makers. *Am J Med* 112: 42S–49S
188 Molinari NA, Ortega-Sanchez IR, Messonnier ML (2007) The annual impact of seasonal influenza in the US: Measuring disease burden and costs. *Vaccine* 25: 5086–5096
189 O'Shea TM, Sevick MA, Givner LB (1998) Costs and benefits of respiratory syncytial virus immunoglobulin to prevent hospitalization for lower respiratory tract illness in very low birth weight infants. *Pediatr Infect Dis J* 17: 587–593
190 Numa A (2000) Outcome of respiratory syncytial virus infection and a cost-benefit analysis of prophylaxis. *J Paediatr Child Health* 36: 422–427
191 Rietveld E, DeJonge HC, Polder JJ (2004) Anticipated costs of hospitalization for respiratory syncytial virus infection in young children at risk. *Pediatr Infect Dis J* 23: 523–529
192 Paramore LC, Ciuryla V, Ciesla G (2004) Economic impact of respiratory syncytial virus-related illness in the US: An analysis of national databases. *Pharmacoeconomics* 22: 275–284
193 Lambert S, O'Grady K-A, Gabriel S, Carter R, Nolan T (2004) The cost of seasonal respiratory illnesses in Australian children: The dominance of patient and family costs and implications for vaccine use. *Commun Dis Intell* 28: 510–516
194 Lambert SB, Allen KM, Druce JD (2005) Respiratory illness during winter: A cohort study of urban children from temperate Australia. *J Paediatr Child Health* 41: 125–129
195 Lambert SB, Allen KM, Carter RC, Nolan TM (2008) The cost of community-managed viral respiratory illnesses in a cohort of healthy preschool-aged children. *Respir Res* 9: 1–11
196 Australian Bureau of Statistics (2007) Australian Bureau of Statistics: Australian Economic Indicators: May 2004

197 Turner J, Tran T, Birch C (2004) Higher than normal seasonal influenza activity in Victoria, 2003. *Commun Dis Intell* 28: 175–180
198 Hollinghurst S, Gorst C, Fahey T (2008) Measuring the financial burden of acute cough in pre-school children: A cost of illness study. BMC *Fam Pract* 9: 10
199 Coleman MS, Washington ML, Orenstein WA (2006) Interdisciplinary epidemiologic and economic research needed to support a universal childhood influenza vaccination policy. *Epidemiol Rev* 28: 41–46

Common Cold
ed. by R. Eccles and O. Weber

The role of viruses in the etiology and pathogenesis of common cold

Olaf Weber

Rheinische Friedrich-Wilhelms-Universität, Institute of Molecular Medicine and Experimental Immunology, Sigmund-Freud-Straße 25, 53105 Bonn, Germany

Abstract

Numerous viruses are able to cause respiratory tract infections. With the availability of new molecular techniques, the number of pathogens detected in specimens from the human respiratory tract has increased. Some of these viral infections have the potential to lead to severe systemic disease. Other viruses are limited to playing a role in the pathogenesis of the common cold syndrome. This chapter focuses on the viral pathogens that are linked to common cold. It is not the intention to comprehensively review all the viruses that are able to cause respiratory tract infections – this would go beyond the scope of this book. The list of viruses that are briefly reviewed here includes rhinoviruses, respiratory syncytial virus, parainfluenza virus, adenovirus, metapneumovirus and coronavirus. Bocavirus is discussed as one example of a newly identified pathogen with a less established role in the etiology and pathogenesis of common cold. Influenza virus does not cause what is defined as common cold. However, influenza viruses are associated with respiratory disease and the clinical picture of mild influenza and common cold frequently overlaps. Therefore, influenza virus has been included in this chapter. It is important to note that a number of viruses are frequently co-detected with other viruses in humans with respiratory diseases. Therefore, the viral etiology and the role of viruses in the pathogenesis of common cold is complex, and numerous questions remain to be answered.

Introduction: The role of viruses in the etiology and pathogenesis of common cold

Numerous viruses are able to cause respiratory tract infections. Some of these may also cause severe diseases. Others are limited to a role in the pathogenesis of the common cold syndrome. With the availability of new molecular techniques, the number of pathogens detected in specimens from the human respiratory tract has increased. The association of some of these agents with human respiratory disease is not always clear. It is not the intention of this chapter to comprehensively review the virology of all the viruses that cause or potentially cause respiratory tract infections. The chapter focuses on some pathogens that are linked to common cold. The list of viruses described includes rhinovirus, respiratory syncytial virus, parainfluenza virus, adenovirus, metapneumovirus and coronavirus. Bocavirus is discussed as an example of a newly identified pathogen with a less established role in the etiology and pathogenesis of common cold. Influenza virus does not cause what is defined as common cold, but is associated with respiratory disease and the clinical picture of mild influenza frequently overlaps with that of the common cold. Therefore, influenza viruses are briefly described in this chapter.

For details on the biology of the individual viruses and their role in pathogenesis of respiratory diseases further reading of standard literature and text books of virology is recommended.

Viruses with an established role in common cold are rhinoviruses, adenoviruses, parainfluenza viruses, coronaviruses and the respiratory syncytial virus, and these are reviewed in greater detail here. Their structure and replication, the transmission and epidemiology and the clinical symptoms are described. In addition, some brief comments about current models of pathogenesis and animal models, respectively, complete the respective subchapters.

Table 1 provides an overview of the viruses that cause respiratory tract infections and that do, or may, play a role as a cause or in the pathogenesis of common cold.

A number of viruses are frequently co-detected with other viruses in humans with respiratory diseases. Therefore, the viral etiology and the role of viruses in the pathogenesis of common cold is complex and it is safe to say, not fully understood for each and every virus that is linked to respiratory tract infection.

Recent developments in the field of antivirals are described in the chapter by Tom Jefferson in this book.

Rhinoviruses

Rhinoviruses cause the vast majority of the common colds in humans. Although the infection usually is self limiting and the symptoms of the disease are mild in healthy adults, rhinovirus infections may cause serious illness in children or patients with pre-existing medical problems [1].

Taxonomy, structure and replication

Rhinoviruses (RV) are members of the order *Picornavirales*, family *Picornaviridae*, genus: Enterovirus [2]. (In the virus taxonomy list of the year 2007 of the International Committee on the Taxonomy of Viruses the rhinoviruses still constituted a separate genus: Rhinovirus.)

Table 1. Viruses that cause illness of the respiratory tract (for references see text)

Agents	Taxonomy	Disease/symptoms	Epidemiology	Transmission	Treatment	Prophylaxis
Rhinovirus (RV)	**Order**: Picornavirales **Family**: Picornaviridae **Genus**: Enterovirus **Species**: Human rhinovirus A / B	Rhinitis, pharyngitis, cough, fever, otitis media, sinusitis, acute disease or exacerbation of chronic pulmonary diseases	~60–80% of the patients with a common cold syndrome, between August and November	Direct contact human-to-human, aerosols	Symptomatic	Hygiene, disinfection, chemoprophylaxis
Respiratory Syncytial Virus (RSV)	**Order**: Mononegavirales **Family**: Paramyxoviridae **Subfamily**: Pneumovirinae **Genus**: Pneumovirus **Species**: Human respiratory syncytial virus	Rhinitis, pharyngitis, cough, bronchiolitis, pneumonia, complications in patients with immunodeficiency or underlying conditions like cystic fibrosis, chronic heart disease etc.	WHO: RSV causes 64 million infections and 160 000 deaths annually, seasonal: winter/ early spring	Epidemic, mostly saliva/respiratory droplets, human-human, hand-to-mouth or hand-to-eye, contaminated surfaces	Immunoglobulins, antibodies, ribavirin; symptomatic	Vaccines in development
Parainfluenza virus (PIV) 1 / 3	**Order**: Mononegavirales **Family**: Paramyxoviridae **Subfamily**: Paramyxovirinae **Genus**: Respirovirus **Species**: Human parainfluenza virus1/ 3	Rhinitis, pharyngitis, cough, hoarseness, fever, croup, bronchiolitits, pneumonia	Children, infants, most children infected by 5 years of age, PIV 1: epidemics in fall PIV 3: epidemics in early spring	Human-to-human, aerosols	Symptomatic	Hygiene, disinfection, no effective vaccines available

Table 1 (continued)

Agents	Taxonomy	Disease/symptoms	Epidemiology	Transmission	Treatment	Prophylaxis
Parainfluenza virus (PIV)	**Order**: Mononegavirales **Family**: Paramyxoviridae **Subfamily**: Paramyxovirinae **Genus**: Rubulavirus **Species**: Human parainfluenza virus 2/ 4	Rhinitis, pharyngitis, cough PIV 2: croup, bronchiolitits, pneumonia PIV 4: mild upper respiratory tract disease	PIV 2 epidemics mainly in autumn	Human-to-human, aerosols	Symptomatic	Hygiene, disinfection, no effective vaccines available
Adenovirus (AV)	**Order**: not assigned **Family**: Adenoviridae **Genus**: Mastadenovirus Species: Human adenovirus C (B) (A-F)	URTI, rhinitis, conjunctivitis, tonsillitis, (gastroenteritis)	5% of URTI in children, institutional infections, AV account for 10% of pneumonia in children; respir. infections seasonal (mainly late winter to early summer)	Aerosols, human-human	Symptomatic, cidofovir in immuno-suppressed patients	Hygiene
Metapneumovirus (hMPV)	**Order**: Mononegavirales **Family**: Paramyxoviridae **Subfamily**: Pneumovirinae **Genus**: Metapneumovirus **Species**: Human metapneumovirus virus	Cough, wheezing, coryza, fever, diarrhea, vomiting bronchiolitis, pneumonia, complications in patients with immunodeficiency or underlying conditions such as asthma, COPD	Seasonal distribution in temperate regions (i.e., late winter, spring) third leading cause of ARTI in humans	Epidemic, mostly saliva/respiratory droplets (not aerosols), human-human, hand-to-mouth or hand-to-eye, contaminated surfaces	Symptomatic, ribavirin	Hygiene

Boca Virus (HBoV)	**Order**: not assigned **Family**: Parvoviridae **Subfamily**: Parvovirinae **Genus**: Bocavirus **Species**: Human Bocavirus (not listed in the 2008 ICTV database)	Rhinitis, pharyngitis, cough, LRTI	Role to be established, frequent co-infections			
Coronavirus (hCoV)	**Order**: Nidovirales **Family**: Coronaviridae **Genus**: Coronavirus **Species**: Human coronavirus (several species: 229E, HKU1, NL 63, OC43)	Rhinitis, pharyngitis, cough, otitis media	Up to 25% of common cold cases are estimated to be caused by HCoV	Aerosols, human-human, winter season	Symptomatic	Hygiene
Influenza A/B Virus (IAV, IBV)	**Order**: not assigned **Family**: Orthomyxoviridae **Genus**: Influenza virus **Species**: Influenza virus A, B	Influenza, URTI, manifestations possible in the central nervous system, muscle (myositis/rhabdomyositis), heart (myocarditis), toxic/septic shock	- WHO: 5–15% of the population are affected with URTI/year - 3–5 million cases of severe illness - 250 000–500 000 deaths/year worldwide - most deaths >65 years of age - seasonal distribution in temperate regions (i.e., winter)	Epidemic, pandemic (not IB), aerosols, human-human, seabirds, poultry, animals	Symptomatic, neuraminidase-inhibitors	Vaccination, hygiene

ARTI: acute respiratory tract infection

More than 100 serotypes, strains and isolates of RV have been isolated from humans. Two human RV species have been described: Human rhinovirus (HRV) A and B. Eighteen serotypes and 2 subtypes (HRV 1A and 1B) belong to HRV A. Five serotypes are assigned to HRV B and 82 serotypes are not yet assigned to a species including bovine rhinoviruses (BRV) 1–3.

RV are non-enveloped viruses with an icosahedral symmetry. The virus is small and has a diameter of approximately 30 nm. Four capsid proteins, VP1–4 have been described. A protomer is composed of one copy of VP1, VP3 and VP0 (a precursor where VP4 and VP2 are covalently linked). Cleavage of VP0 is the final step of the assembly process [3]. One or two copies of VP0 will remain uncleaved; no role for this uncleaved VP0 has been established yet. Five protomers are arranged symmetrically about a fivefold axis, forming a pentamer that represents a corner of the icosahedron. The capsid is formed by 12 pentamers. RV have, similar to human enteroviruses, the same comparatively uneven surface with its characteristic canyon around the fivefold axis [4]. The canyon serves as an attachment site for the cell receptor [5]. In CsCl, RV have a buoyant density of 1.38–1.42 g/cm^3. Virions are unstable at a pH below 5–6, a feature, which distinguishes RV from other enteroviruses. However, as they are non-enveloped viruses, RV are stable against detergents and most organic solvents. On the other hand, alcohol and phenol are effective virucidal agents.

The RV genome is organized as a single-stranded positive-sense RNA of approximately 7100–7200 nucleotides in length with its 5' terminus covalently linked to a small protein, VPg. The 5'-untranslated region (UTR) of approximately 0.65 kb is shorter than that of other enteroviruses, owing to a deletion of approximately 100 nucleotides between the internal ribosomal entry site (IRES) and the translation start site. One open reading frame (ORF) of about 2150 codons, a 3'-UTR of approximately 40 nucleotides and a 3' poly(A) tail complete the structure of the genome. RV have a characteristic nucleotide composition with a preponderance of A and U, particularly in the third position of the codons. The genome is fully sequenced and has the accession number [K02121]; [K02021] [2].

Replication is initiated through attachment to the cell receptor. For most RV serotypes this is intercellular adhesion molecule-1 (ICAM-1) [6, 7]. It is hypothesized that the viral canyon structure releases a lipid moiety upon ICAM-1 binding, which, in turn, leads to a change in conformation, destabilization and the release of the viral RNA into the cytoplasm [8]. RV shut off host cell protein synthesis by inactivating the cap binding complex. Their IRES allows them to replicate despite this inactivation.

The RNA serves as a messenger RNA encoding a single polyprotein which is cleaved post-translationally by virus-encoded proteases. Once the first round of translation and subsequent processing is complete a $3D^{pol}$ RNA-dependent RNA polymerase produces negative-sense RNA from the genomic template, which in turn serve as template for the production of positive-sense genomic RNA. The synthesis of a single virus polyprotein requires post-translational processing to facilitate subsequent steps in viral replication. At least two proteolytic activities are encoded by the virus: $2A^{pro}$ performs the first cleavage releasing capsid precursors and $3C^{pro}$ catalyzes most other cleavage reactions. The protease has a trypsin-like structure but the active site of the enzyme is a cysteine sulfydryl [9].

Pathogenesis, immunology and clinical symptoms

RV are transmitted mainly by direct contact and less frequently through aerosols (for details see the chapter by Diane Pappas and Owen Hendley). Virus can frequently be isolated from the hands of an infected individual and is transmitted to other individuals or to objects in the environment. During RV infection virus titers in nasal secretions are as high as 10^2–10^3 $TCID_{50}$/ml of nasal lavage fluid [10, 11].

Infection of humans is very effective and less RV may be needed for infection of seronegative volunteers by nasal drops than needed for infection of a human embryonic fibroblast tissue culture [12]. In contrast, when the same virus was used for inhalation of aerosols a 20-fold disparity in infectious dose has been described [13], suggesting that the lower respiratory tract is less susceptible for infection than the nasopharynx.

After a short incubation period of 1–4 days virus is shed, peaks after another 2–3 days, and declines thereafter [13, 14]. The primary site of viral replication is ciliated epithelial cells as detected by *in situ* hybridization [15].

The histopathology of RV infection is not as yet very detailed. Nasal mucosa biopsies reveal only few or no histopathological abnormalities despite active virus shedding. Explant cultures inoculated with rhinovirus failed to develop cytopathic effects (CPE) [16]. Biopsies showed marked edema of connective tissue, sparse infiltration of inflammatory cells, hyperemia and exudation of seromucous fluids [17–19]. Infection of bovine tracheal organ cultures with BRV leads to shedding of ciliated cells.

It has been suggested that the immune response of the host contributes to the symptom complex. Increased concentrations of the pro-inflammatory cytokines IL-8, IL-1 and IL-6 [20–22] have been found in nasal secretions of subjects with symptomatic RV infection. A direct correlation between concentration in nasal fluids and symptom severity has been described for IL-6 [22].

RV infection is usually accompanied by the typical common cold symptoms: nasal discharge and obstruction, sneezing, coughing, sore throat and, less frequently, fever. Gastrointestinal symptoms are sometimes observed in children. The infection is usually limited to the upper respiratory tract. It is commonly believed that RV infection increases the risk for subsequent or secondary bacterial infections. In patients predisposed with existing underlying diseases, like cystic fibrosis or chronic bronchitis, and in immunocompromised patients, elderly and infants, RV can cause serious infections of the lower respiratory tract. RV infection of the lower respiratory tract (LRTI) was demonstrated by Papadopoulos and co-workers [23] using *in situ* hybridization techniques. These authors demonstrated RV infection not only in epithelial cells but also in underlying submucosal cells. Exacerbation of chronic bronchitis or asthma may be a consequence in these patients [24, 25]. Indeed, approximately 80% of asthma exacerbations in children [26] and about 70% in adults [27] are associated with respiratory virus infections, and the vast majority of these are RV infections [28]. Examination of the early innate immune responses to RV infection in asthmatic bronchial epithelia revealed profound impairment of virus-induced interferon (IFN)-β expression leading to impaired apoptotic responses and enhanced RV replication [29].

RV infections lead to the production of type-specific IgA, IgG and IgM antibodies. However, frequencies of response to natural infection have been reported to vary between 37% and 92% [30]. Infected patients usually develop neutralizing antibodies to the infecting virus within 1–3 weeks after infection. IgA is the dominant immunoglobulin in nasal secretions, has a protective role and may prevent re-infections with homotypic viruses or reduce the symptoms upon reinfection. The involvement in the viral clearance process is less clear and other mechanisms like the induction of an innate immune response are being discussed. Both serum and secretory antibodies persist for several years after infection.

Epidemiology, diagnosis and treatment

In the absence of effective antiviral treatments, the diagnosis of RV infection for guiding an anti-RV therapy is not useful. The diagnosis of RV infection largely relies on the clinical symptoms. Approximately 60–80% of the patients with a common cold syndrome of afebrile prominent nasal symptoms but minimal systemic disease that occurs between August and early November have RV infection [31]. However, the general method for identifying the etiological agent is the isolation and propagation in cell culture. In addition, polymerase chain reaction (PCR) can be used for rapid identification of RV in specimens. Point-of-care diagnostics are under development.

Experimental models

A major obstacle to understanding disease pathogenesis has been the lack of a small-animal model for RV infection. RV have shown a high degree of species specificity, limiting the use of experimental animal systems.

Therefore, aspects of pathogenesis have been studied in experimentally induced colds in human volunteers.

Infection of rabbits, guinea pigs or weanling mice by parenteral routes was not successful with certain strains of the virus [32–34], but infection of mice was possible using a tissue-culture adapted HRV-2 [35]. Chimpanzees or gibbons has been experimentally infected using specific strains of HRV [36, 37].

Approximately 90% of the RV use human ICAM-1 as their cell receptor and do not bind mouse ICAM-1; the remaining 10% use a member of the low-density lipoprotein receptor family and can bind the mouse counterpart. Recently, three novel mouse models of RV infection: minor-group RV infection of BALB/c mice, major-group RV infection of transgenic BALB/c mice expressing a mouse-human ICAM-1 chimera and RV-induced exacerbation of allergic airway inflammation were described by Bartlett et al. [38]. These models have features similar to those observed in RV infection in humans, including augmentation of allergic airway inflammation, and may be useful in the development of future therapies for colds and asthma exacerbations. Association between common cold symptoms and inflammatory mediators is an important aspect of understanding common cold and RV infection. Although this association seems obvious, the exact mechanisms are less clear and one might expect a better understanding of the detailed mechanism(s) once inhibitors of viral replication are available for studies in humans. In addition, the new animal models developed by Bartlett et al. [38] can be expected to support efforts to study pathogenesis of RV infection *in vivo* in greater detail.

Respiratory syncytial virus

Human respiratory syncytial virus (RSV) was first isolated from a laboratory chimpanzee with upper respiratory tract infection (URTI) in 1956 [39]. RSV is today recognized as the leading viral agent in upper respiratory tract disease in infancy and childhood. The spectrum of RSV-caused diseases includes rhinitis, otitis media, pneumonia and bronchiolitis. The latter two diseases can be associated with a substantial morbidity and mortality. In addition, there is growing recognition for its importance as a causative agent for diseases in elderly and immunocompromised patients [40]. The World Health Organization estimates that RSV causes 64 million infections and 160000 deaths annually [41]. A bovine RSV (BRSV) has been described causing economically important respiratory diseases in cattle [42]. Another animal RSV is the pneumonia virus of mice (PVM) [43], suggesting that there was an interspecies spread in the evolution of these viruses. However, an animal reservoir for human RSV has not been described so far [44]. Despite the importance of RSV as a leading cause for respiratory diseases, the pathogenesis of RSV infection is not fully understood and efficacious vaccines are not available.

Taxonomy, structure and replication

RSV is a member of the order *Mononegavirales*, which includes several non-segmented negative-strand RNA viruses. RSV is a member of the family of *Paramyxoviridae*, subfamily *Pneumovirinae* and represents the type species for the genus Pneumovirus [43].

RSV virions consist of an envelope and a nucleocapsid. The viral gene expression and nucleic acid replication occur in the cytoplasm. The envelope is acquired by cell budding. Virions are spherical to pleomorphic; filamentous and other forms are common. They measure 150–300 nm in diameter and up to 1000–10 000 nm in length [45]. The surface of the virion is covered by projections (spikes) formed by fusion (F) glycoproteins. The spikes are 11–20 nm long and are spaced 6–10 nm apart; they mediate attachment and penetration. The helical nucleocapsid is filamentous with a length of 600–800(1000) nm and a width of 12–15 nm [40]. The nucleocapsid does not enter the cells by surface fusion typical for paramyxoviruses but rather by membrane fusion which may involve clathrin-mediated endocytosis [46].

The unsegmented genome contains a single molecule of linear negative-sense, single-stranded RNA. Virions occasionally contain a positive-sense single-stranded copy of the genome (partial self-annealing of extracted RNA may occur). The complete genome is approximately 15 300 nucleotides long and fully sequenced. The genome has the accession number(s) [D00386] – [D00397] [43]. The RNA genome has a 3'-extragenic leader region, followed by the ten viral genes and a 5' trailer region. Each gene is transcribed into a separate mRNA encoding for a single viral protein with the exception of the M2 mRNA. This contains two overlapping ORF, expressed by a ribosomal stop-restart mechanism into two proteins, M2-1 and M2-2 [47]. Although gene expression is consistent with that of other members of the order of *Mononegavirales* M2-1 and M2-2 have some regulatory features unique to RSV [44].

The five nucleocapsid-associated proteins are the N (nucleocapsid) protein, the phosphoprotein P (co-factor for RNA synthesis), the L protein (large, a 2165-amino acid subunit of viral polymerase), the M2-1 (transcription processivity factor) and the M2-2 protein (which possesses regulatory functions) [44, 48]. The N protein binds the genomic and the antigenomic (positive-sense intermediate) RNA and protects is against degradation. In addition, it reduces the detection and responses by the host's immune system (for instance Toll-like receptors, TLRs) and intracellular RNA recognition helicases, which initiate innate immune responses [44, 49, 50].

The viral envelope is formed by four RSV proteins that associate with the lipid bilayer: a matrix (M) protein that is located at the inner surface and is important for the assembly of the virion [51], a glycosylated (G) protein, a fusion (F) protein and a small hydrophobic (SH) protein. Two other RSV proteins, the NS1 and NS2 proteins are a minor part of the virion [44]. NS1 and NS2 are thought to modulate the host response to RSV infection. The G glycoprotein (~90 kDa) has a peptide backbone with 24–25 side chains and is important for viral attachment to the host cell [52]. A second secretory form of the G protein exists that arises from a second initiation codon in the G ORF. Proteolytic trimming removes additional amino acids, and the final protein lacks the 65 N-terminal residues, including the membrane anchor [44, 52]. The ectodomain of the G protein has a mucin-like structure that differs from attachment proteins of other paramyxovirus. Its function is not clear but it is thought to contribute to virus spread or to prevent trapping by mucus [44].

The F protein has two distinct functions: penetration into the host cell by membrane fusion and a syncytia-forming property. The F protein matures by activation through a furin-like intracellular protease that cleaves the precursor, F_0 into three fragments, F_1, F_2 and p27. F_1 and F_2 are linked by a disulfide bond and represent the active form of F [53]. The hydrophobic N terminus of F_1 is conserved within the RSV and it is thought that this domain inserts into the host cell membrane when fusion occurs [44].

NS1 and NS2 are thought to modulate the host's immune response to RSV [44]. Lack of M2-1 results in reduced expression of NS1 and NS2, and it is thought that this down-regulation of the host-defense antagonists may help to facilitate persistent RSV infection [44].

Pathogenesis, immunology and clinical symptoms

Infection occurs through direct contact, through large respiratory droplets and, to a lesser extent, through small droplets. The site of the first replication is the nasopharynx. After an incubation period of 4–5 days the virus spreads to the lower respiratory tract [54, 55]. The clinical signs include cough, rhinitis, fever and signs of bronchiolitis like air trapping, wheezing and increased airway resistance. The most prominent clinical symptoms are cough and rhinorrhea, which occur in approximately 90% of primary RSV infections in infants and to some lesser extent in reinfected adults [56]. Fever occurs in 30–40% of both infected infants and adults and otitis media is reported in approximately 20% of infected infants. Ear and sinus pain is reported in 20–30% of infected adults. Symptoms of LRTI, including bronchiolitis, pneumonia, croup, wheeze and tracheobronchitis, are observed in 30–40% of infected infants and to some lesser extent in adults, with wheeze and tracheobronchitis being the most prominent disease symptoms. Hospitalization is necessary in approximately 3% of infected children and below 0.1% of infected adults. RSV is the single most important agent in children younger than 3 years of age. Importantly, children with a mild RSV disease have also been reported to have recurrent wheezing for up to 10 years after the primary acute disease [57].

Extrapulmonary dissemination may occur in immunocompromised patients [58]. The virus may spread to kidneys, liver, the central nervous system and the heart. Virus can be isolated from the nasopharynx of children for up to 14 days. In immunocompromised patients, virus recovery is possible for up to 1 month or even longer. In immunocompetent individuals the viral infection is usually restricted to the superficial cells of the epithelia and viral spread outside the respiratory tract is uncommon [54, 59]. An exception, however, is the middle ear: the virus frequently causes otitis media [60].

The typical pathological findings in RSV-infected tissue include epithelial necrosis and infiltrates of monocytes, T cells and neutrophils [61]. Airways appear obstructed due to sloughed cells, mucus secretion, proliferation of bronchoalveolar epithelium or cellular infiltration. Formation of syncytia in the bronchoalveolar epithelium is sometimes observed [61]. However, giant cell pneumonia or syncytia formation are related to severe T cell-deficient patients [44].

Specific host factors that may influence the clinical signs and outcome of RSV infection including the general health status, the nutritional status [56, 62, 63], gender, ethnic group, levels of maternal antibodies [64], age of first RSV infection [65] and underlying cardiac or pulmonary diseases [66]. In addition, there are several environmental factors (e.g., tobacco use in household, stress, day care) that may influence the course of the disease or severity of symptoms. The role of inflammation and a bias of the host's immune response towards a humoral Th2 response (the typical cytokines are IL-4, IL-5, IL-10 and IL-13) are discussed controversially in the literature. A strong inflammatory response does not seem to be determinative for the severity of clinical symptoms [67], a finding supported by the fact that in many clinical studies patients receiving anti-inflammatory therapy did not significantly benefit from that treatment [68]. However, strong inflammatory responses also have been suggested to enhance the severity of clinical symptoms in RSV disease. The role of inflammatory chemokines in RSV pathogenesis has been supported by many preclinical and clinical studies (reviewed in [44]). For example, genetic polymorphisms that increase IL-8, a major chemoattractant for neutrophils, and CCR5 expression have been associated with increased RSV disease [69]. A link between an increased ratio of Th2/Th1 immune response (a bias toward the humoral vs the classical cytotoxic response) has been suggested by several authors. This discussion is based on evidence for elevated Th2/Th1 response ratios in clinical studies, the role of key Th2 cytokines in the pathogenesis of asthma and the experience with a formalin-inactivated RSV vaccine in the 1960s [70–72]. This vaccine was poorly protective and vaccinated children and infants developed dramatically enhanced disease compared to naive patients upon natural RSV reinfection [48]. Subsequent preclinical studies confirmed a bias toward a Th2-specific $CD4^+$ T cell response in animals treated with formalin-inactivated RSV vaccine vs naturally infected animals [73]. IL-4 and IL-13 support isotype switching to IgE, which is bound to mast cells and eosinophils and, upon antigen contact, induces release of inflammatory mediators like histamine or leukotrienes by these cells. These mediators contribute to the development of the typical clinical symptoms associated with RSV disease.

Several viral proteins play an important role in the pathogenesis of RSV disease (reviewed in [44]). The soluble G protein has been suggested to modulate the innate immune response by down-regulating inflammatory mediators such as IL-6 or IL-8 in epithelial cells as a response to RSV infection [74]. G protein also modulates inflammatory responses of monocytes by acting as a general antagonist for TLR activity [75]. The G-mediated suppression of TLR-4 signaling appears to be counteracted by the F protein, which has been described to induce signaling through this TLR [76], although the significance of this activity is unclear.

Importantly, RSV infection can block the maturation of dendritic cells (DC), which serve as major antigen-presenting cells (reviewed in [44]). This alteration of DC biology may support the shift of the Th2/Th1 balance towards Th2, reduce antiviral interferon activity and limit the mobility of mature antigen-presenting cells, thus qualitatively altering the immune response to RSV infection (reviewed in [44]).

In summary, there are several host factors or viral factors that play roles in the pathogenesis of RSV infection. The picture, however, is highly complex and relative contributions of the various factors to RSV pathogenesis are not entirely understood.

Epidemiology, diagnosis and treatment

As mentioned above RSV is a leading cause of respiratory diseases in children and has increasing importance as a causative agent for respiratory diseases in elderly. In a prospective study of infants and children in the Unites States, RSV was detected in 43% of pediatric hospitalizations for bronchiolitis, 25% for pneumonia, 11% for bronchitis and 10% for croup [54]. Approximately 90% of infants have been infected at least once by 2 years of age [44, 77]. Although RSV is represented by one serotype, a protective immunity against RSV is generally weak and reinfection occurs. Virus-neutralizing antibodies, including secretory IgA found in the respiratory tract, contribute to viral clearance and may play a role in protection against reinfection [54]. However, the IgA response is short [44, 54]. In the lower respiratory tract, the IgG response has been described as more efficient. The role of antibodies as a down-modulator of clinical symptoms has been confirmed by the clinical experience with palivizumab.

In temperate regions, RSV circulates quickly during winter/early spring, but timing varies more elsewhere. Effective vaccines are not available and effective therapies are not available. However, an RSV-neutralizing humanized monoclonal antibody, palivizumab, reduces RSV-associated hospitalization if used as a passive immunoprophylaxis [78].

RSV infection is assumed to be frequently misdiagnosed, particularly in adults [56], because the symptoms are similar to those caused by other respiratory viruses like influenza. Laboratory diagnostic tests are usually performed on secretion samples obtained from the nasopharynx. Novel rapid ELISA-based or RT-PCR-based tests are useful particularly in a hospital setting to identify outbreaks, prevent further transmission, initiate therapies or reduce inappropriate use of antibiotics [56].

Experimental models

Animal models are comprehensively reviewed by Moore and Stokes Peebles [79]. RSV is species specific; however, some animal species exhibit semi-permissive infection with RSV. Chimpanzees were productively infected with RSV and exhibited upper respiratory tract illness, whereas adult squirrel monkeys, newborn rhesus monkeys, and infant cebus monkeys did not show symptoms but shed low levels of virus [80]. Bonnet monkeys, which are more widely available than chimpanzees, can be infected with RSV [81]. Non-human primate models of RSV infection, especially chimpanzee, have advantages but certainly limitations associated with the high cost and genetic variability, which limits the reproducibility of results.

The cotton rat which is susceptible to both URTI and LRTI with RSV is seen as one of the best animal models of RSV infection and disease [79, 82]. In these animals, RSV infection led to histologically confirmed proliferative rhinitis, bronchiolitis, and the pulmonary infiltration of lymphocytes and neutrophils [82–84]. The cotton rat model was used to study the mechanism of antibody-mediated clearance of RSV [84].

The advantages of mouse models are obvious: they are inexpensive, inbred strains are available and a wealth of reagents (e.g., antibodies), arrays, probes or information (e.g., the genome sequence) is available. Although there is variability between the strains regarding susceptibility and viral load, viral load does not vary much within the strains [79]. BALB/c is the most widely used inbred mouse strain to study RSV infection [79]. RSV-infected BALB/c mice show signs of clinical illness including weight loss, ruffled fur and ataxia peaking at day 8 after infection [85]. Interestingly, the susceptibility to RSV replication in nose and lung increased with age. The predominant histological findings in RSV-infected 3-week-old BALB/c mice were peribronchiolar and perivascular accumulations of mononuclear cells [86].

The role of Th1 and Th2 cell response to RSV infection has been the dominant focus of the BALB/c mouse studies in this context [79]. RSV infection induces a Th1 response dominated by high IFN-γ levels in the lungs of infected mice, abundant IFN-γ-producing cells in the bronchoalveolar lavage fluid (BALF) and RSV-specific cytotoxic T cell (CTL) response [87, 88].

STAT1$^{(-/-)}$ mice with a BALB/c background have been described as having an excellent RSV disease phenotype (reviewed in [79]). Although this model has the limitation that it probably does not exactly mirror the complexity of a natural infection in humans, it is regarded as an attractive tool to study RSV pathogenesis and evaluating novel therapies.

In addition to other mouse models and the infection in chinchillas [89], infection of natural hosts has been studied in detail. Bovine respiratory syncytial virus is a major cause of respiratory illness in calves and has been studied in this context. The clinical signs after experimental infection include cough, lung sound, dyspnea, fever, increased respiratory rate and pulmonary resistance. Prominent histological findings include proliferative bronchiolitis, alveolitis, syncytia, and, to some extent, emphysema [90]. RSV infection of calves might be useful for evaluating vaccination strategies; however, it is not an animal model for the evaluation of novel therapies.

The list of experimental models also includes pneumonia virus infection of mice (PVM) [91]. Although the PVM model of respiratory disease is interesting because it shows the phenotype of a natural infection, PVM differs from RSV including the G and the NS1 proteins that fulfill important functions during RSV infection.

Human parainfluenza virus

Human parainfluenza viruses (HPIV) are important causes of respiratory diseases in infants and children. They usually cause URTI of which 30–50% may be accompanied by otitis media. HPIV may also cause LRTI, about 0.3% of which require hospitalization. HPIV1–3 infections are second to RSV infections as the viral cause of serious acute respiratory infections in young children that occur primarily in the first 6 months of life [92, 93]. HPIV3 may cause severe diseases. Approximately 80% of infants and children infected with HPIV3 developed febrile illness and one third of these infected individuals developed LRTI, resulting in bronchitis or pneumonia [93–95]. Most children have been infected with HPIV3 by the age of 2 years.

Croup is the main clinical manifestation of infection with parainfluenza viruses, especially HPIV1 and 2, and these infections may extend to the lower respiratory tract and result in pneumonia [94]. HPIV4 mainly causes mild URTI in children and adults [93]. Along with RSV, HPIV are also a leading causative agent of serious acute respiratory infections and community-acquired respiratory disease requiring hospitalization in adults.

The proportions of hospitalizations associated with HPIV infection vary widely in hospital-based studies. According to the WHO, HPIV1 is estimated to account for 5800–28 900 annual hospitalizations in the USA,

HPIV2 for 1800–15 600 hospitalizations, and HPIV3 for 8700–52000 hospitalizations [92].

Taxonomy, structure and replication

Parainfluenza viruses belong to the order of *Mononegavirales*, family *Paramyxoviridae*, subfamily *Paramyxovirinae*. HPIV1 and 3 belong to the genus Respirovirus, and HPIV2 and 4 to the genus Rubulavirus [96]. The virions are spherical enveloped particles of approximately 150–250 nm in diameter with an internal helical nucleocapsid. Virions are enveloped by a lipid bilayer membrane that bears spike-like projections composed of hemagglutinin-neuraminidase (HN) and fusion (F) protein [97].

As for other paramyxoviruses, all HPIVs contain a negative strand, ~15500-nucleotide-long non-segmented RNA genome [93] encoding two envelope glycoproteins, the HN, and the F protein, a matrix protein (M), a nucleocapsid protein (NP) and several nonstructural proteins including a polymerase-associated protein (P/V) and the viral replicase (L) (reviewed in [93]). The replication of PIV is similar to that of other paramyxoviruses with the RNA genome serving as a template for the transcription of the mRNAs.

Binding of the HN glycoprotein to its cell receptor initiates the infection [98]. In addition to having this function, HN is thought to enhance the fusion activity of F, which, following virus attachment to the host cell, mediates the fusion of virus and subsequent penetration. F also mediates fusion of infected and uninfected cells, allowing virus to spread. F is synthesized as an inactive precursor (F_0) that is post-translationally cleaved by a host cell protease to yield two subunits, F_1 and F_2 that remain linked by a disulfide bond [93].

Pathogenesis, immunology and clinical symptoms

The mucous membranes of the upper respiratory tract are the common sites of infection. Prominent clinical symptoms of HPIV infection can be characterized by rhinitis, pharyngitis and bronchitis. The incubation period is about 4 days [95]. Coughing, hoarseness and fever that last for approximately 2–3 days are frequent. Involvement of the trachea results in croup and extension to the lower respiratory tract may lead to pneumonia. Severe disease characterized as bronchopneumonia or bronchiolitis has been observed with HPIV3 infections [93–95].

Specific virus and host properties that determine the severity of HPIV-related disease are not yet understood. Infection with PIV induces an immune response to HN and F. Neutralizing antibodies to PIV correlate with partial resistance to infection or clinical symptoms but usually do not prevent re-infection [99]. Secretory IgA neutralizing antibodies are more important in adults than in children [100].

Epidemiology, diagnosis and treatment

As mentioned above, the HPIVs are important causes of respiratory tract diseases in infants and children. Epidemics of HPIV3 usually occur in the early spring [101]. Viruses do not persist for a long time in the environment [93]. The seasonal peak of HPIV1 and 2 infections is reflected in the seasonality of croup, which is the highest in autumn in the USA [102]. Croup during the winter months is more likely to be caused by other viruses, such as influenza virus or RSV [93].

The diagnosis of PIV infection is mainly clinical, and molecular diagnostic procedures are usually not performed. There is no specific antiviral treatment against PIV available, and therapeutic intervention is mainly targeted against symptoms of croup. Early treatment will reduce the severity of the symptoms, the rates at which patients return to a health care practitioner for additional medical attention, visits to the emergency department, and admission to the hospital [103].

Effective vaccines are currently not available. Attenuated strains have been studied and a virosomal formulation of an HPIV3 vaccine is currently under development [92]. The National Institute of Allergy and Infectious Diseases (NIAID) is studying the safety and immunogenicity of a recombinant live-attenuated chimeric bovine/human parainfluenza type 3 virus, rB/hPIV3, vaccine in a Phase I study. The test vaccine is delivered as nose drops to adults 18–49 years of age, HPIV3-seropositive children 15–59 months of age, and HPIV3-seronegative infants and children 6–36 months of age [104]. HPIV vaccines are also developed by some companies [105].

Adenovirus

Adenoviruses cause infections of the respiratory and gastrointestinal tract, kidney, eye and other organs, the latter mostly as a consequence of immunosuppression [106]. They are known to frequently cause respiratory infections among people in institutional environments – outbreaks among children are reported at boarding schools and summer camps [107]. Outbreaks have also been reported in military camps [108]. Most infections with adenovirus result in infections of the upper respiratory tract. In addition, adenovirus infections may result in conjunctivitis, tonsillitis, ear infection or croup [106–109]. Adenoviruses are responsible for approximately 5% of acute respiratory infections in children under the age of 5 [107, 109]. The Centers for Disease Control (CDC) reported in the November 16, 2007, issue of the Morbidity and Mortality Weekly Report [MMWR 56(45):1181–1184] an unusual number of cases of severe pneumonia and deaths caused by adenovirus serotype 14 (Ad14) infection among civilian and military communities.

Taxonomy, structure and replication

Adenoviruses belong to the family *Adenoviridae*, genus Mastadenovirus. There are 6 species including human adenovirus A–F with 51 immunologically distinct human adenovirus serotypes [110]. The most common human adenoviral pathogens belong to the C adenoviruses and those mainly infect the upper respiratory tract [107].

The virions are not enveloped. They consist of a capsid and a core with proteins associated to it. The icosahedral capsid has a diameter of 70–100 nm [111, 112]. All capsids consist of 252 capsomers. The surface structure reveals a regular pattern with distinctive features. Surface projections are often lost during preparation. Distinct filaments protrude from the 12 vertices/pentons [112–114].

The genome is not segmented and contains a single molecule of linear double-stranded DNA with terminally redundant sequences, which have inverted terminal repetitions (ITR). The complete genome of mastadenoviruses is approximately 31–36 kpb long and has a guanine + cytosine content of 48–61%. The genome has a terminal protein, which is covalently linked to the 5'-end of each DNA strand [114, 115].

The viral genome encodes structural proteins and non-structural proteins. Virions consist of 11 proteins located in the capsid, fibers, and core. The capsid is comprised of seven polypeptides, polypeptide II which is the basis for the hexon (three tightly associated proteins). Polypeptides VI, VIII, IX are associated with the hexon, polypeptides VI and VIII serve as bridge between the capsid and the core. Five polypeptide III copies are the basis for the penton. Polypeptide IV forms the trimeric fiber [116], which has a knob domain that serves as a viral receptor for the target host cell. The cell receptor is the receptor for coxsackie B virus and adenovirus (CAR) for adenoviruses A, C, D, E and F and CD46 for adenoviruses B with the exception of serotypes 3 and 7 [117]. The core consists of four proteins (V, VII, mu and the terminal protein, which is covalently linked to the 5´ end of the DNA) and the DNA (reviewed in [112]).

The replication cycle of adenoviruses is divided into two phases. The early phase includes adsorption of the virus to the host cell, penetration, transcription and translation of early genes. The early gene products mediate gene expression and DNA replication, block apoptosis and promote the cell cycle progression. In addition, they possess potent immunomodulatory functions (reviewed in [112]).

The viral E1A gene product should briefly be mentioned: In the nucleus, E1A activates the expression of a number of genes by interacting with cellular transcription factors and other cellular regulatory proteins [112]. E1A has been postulated to play role in the pathogenesis of chronic obstructive pulmonary disease (COPD) [118–120].

Pathogenesis and clinical symptoms

Human adenovirus A–F can cause human infections ranging from respiratory disease, and conjunctivitis (B and D), to gastroenteritis (F serotypes 40 and 41) [106, 112]. The most common clinical picture after adenovirus infection of the respiratory tract is mild self-limiting upper respiratory disease with nasal congestion, coryza and cough [106, 113]. Some patients develop exsudative tonsillitis that is clinically indistinguishable from streptococcus tonsillitis [120]. These infections are commonly caused by serotype 1, 2, 5 and 6 C adenoviruses and serotype 3 B adenovirus [107, 109]. Respiratory symptoms may be accompanied by systemic manifestations including generalized malaise, chills, fever and headache [106]. However, adenoviruses may infect alveolar and bronchiolar epithelial cells [121] and cause pneumonia, bronchiolitis or bronchiolitis obliterans [122–124]. Adenoviruses account for approximately 10% of pneumonias in children [106].

In contrast to many other respiratory viruses, both persistent and latent infections have been described, particularly in lymphocytes [106]. Adenoviral DNA may persist in the nuclei of infected cells or even integrate into the host DNA. Adenoviral E1A protein has been postulated to play a role in the pathogenesis of COPD [121]. Adenoviral DNA was found in the lungs of COPD patients and expression of E1A correlated with disease severity [125–127]. In response to inflammatory stimuli, E1A increases ICAM-1 and IL-8 expression along with nuclear factor-κB (NF-κB) activation in lung epithelial cells ([128], reviewed in [113]). While these factors support emphysema, E1A up-regulates transforming growth factor-β1 (TGF-β1) in bronchiolar epithelial cells [129], supporting a role for E1A in airway remodeling [130].

In summary, adenoviruses are pathogens that frequently cause mild or severe acute infections of the respiratory tract. The importance of adenovirus infections, however, goes beyond acute airway disease.

Epidemiology, diagnosis and treatment

Adenoviruses are non-enveloped pathogens and thus very stable to chemical or physical agents and adverse pH conditions. It is believed that respiratory adenoviruses are mainly spread *via* aerosols; however, other routes (fecal, waterborne) also frequently lead to infection. Antibodies to one or more adenoviruses are found in approximately 50% of infants and nearly 100% of adults and since there are many different types of adenovirus, repeated adenoviral infections can occur [109, 131, 132].

Although adenovirus infections can occur at any time of the year, respiratory tract disease caused by adenovirus is more common in late winter, spring, and early summer [106].

Virological diagnosis can be performed using a variety of molecular or immunological approaches. This is, however, only important in the context of severe or epidemic diseases. Development efforts for vaccines were discontinued [133]. Antiviral therapy is only important in infected immunocompromised patients. In these patients, cidofovir has shown some promise [122].

Human metapneumovirus

Human metapneumovirus (HMPV) was identified in 2001 [134], and is today considered as a major cause of acute respiratory infections worldwide, especially in children. Virtually all children have experienced an infection with HMPV by the age of 5–10 years (reviewed in [135]).

Taxonomy, structure and replication

HMPV is a member of the order *Mononegavirales*, family *Paramyxoviridae*, subfamily *Pneumovirinae* (as is RSV), genus Metapneumovirus [136]. There are two major groups and at least four subgroups of HMPV [137–140]. HMPV particles are enveloped, pleomorphic, filamenteous and spherical and have a mean diameter of approximately 210 nm [137]. The genome consists of a single-stranded negative RNA of approximately 13.3 kb and contains eight genes in the order 3'N-P-M-F-M2-SH-G-L-5' coding for a nucleoprotein (N), a phosphoprotein (P), matrix protein (M), fusion protein (F), a transcription elongation factor (M2-1), a protein regulating RNA synthesis (M2-2), a small hydrophobic protein (SH), attachment protein (G), a polymerase subunit (L) and probably additional proteins [141, 142]. The F protein is the major immunogenic viral protein [143]. Replication is generally comparable to that of other members of *Mononegavirales*.

Pathogenesis, immunology and clinical symptoms

This virus infection occurs primarily during winter months or early spring and can manifest as both upper and lower respiratory tract disease [144]. After a severe HMPV infection, virus was detected in alveolar and airway epithelial cells [145]. It was also reported in this study that the virus caused acute organizing lung injury, tissue damage and, which is not observed in other paramyxovirus infections, induction of smudge cell formation.

The clinical symptoms associated with HMPV infection are indistinguishable from those of RSV infection [146] and range from common cold to pneumonia. Otitis media is observed in up to 50% of the infected individuals (reviewed in [135]). As for other respiratory viruses, HMPV may cause exacerbation of underlying chronic diseases like asthma, congestive heart disease or chronic obstructive pulmonary disease. The importance of coinfections with RSV or influenza viruses is not clear (reviewed in [135]). As for many other respiratory viruses, serious disease caused by HMPV is observed among immunosuppressed patients. Results from a recent retrospective study suggested that HMPV infection may be an important cause of idiopathic pneumonia syndrome after stem cell transplantation [147].

Epidemiology, diagnosis and treatment

HMPV is thought to be the second or third cause of severe acute respiratory tract infection in children, just ranking behind RSV and influenza virus [146, 148]. Infections occur very early in life and up to 100% of children have experienced an HMPV infection by the age of 10 years. Reinfections occur frequently. Incidences in hospitalized children with acute respiratory tract infection range from 5% to 10%. Incidence is up to 20% in patients consulting at an outpatient clinic (reviewed in [135]).

The routes of transmission are believed to be similar to those of RSV (respiratory droplets, hand-to mouth or hand-to eye contact) [149, 150].

The diagnosis of HMPV infection is mainly clinical. Molecular diagnostic procedures are usually not performed routinely but are possible using standard technologies like RT-PCR or immunological techniques.

There is no specific antiviral treatment available. However, ribavirin has shown some promise [151] and monoclonal antibodies are under development that could potentially be used to prevent HMPV infections [152]. Several vaccines are being developed but are still in an early stage.

Human bocavirus

Human bocavirus (HBoV), a parvovirus, was detected in children with LRTI in 2005 using random amplification methods [153]. HBoV infection is predominantly associated with respiratory and/or gastrointestinal symptoms in children at around 2 years of age [154]. Seroprevalence reaches 95% in adults [155]. However, the role of HBoV in the pathogenesis of human respiratory disorders is not yet fully understood – HBoV infections are frequently accompanied by coinfections with other viral and bacterial pathogens [154].

Taxonomy, structure and replication

HBoV is classified into the *Parvoviridae* family, subfamily *Parvovirinae*, genus Bocavirus. As other parvoviruses, HBoV virions are icosahedral non-enveloped particles with a diameter of 21–25 nm [154]. The HBoV genome (a linear single-stranded DNA that encompasses approximately 5.2 kb) is organized like that of other parvoviruses: conserved genes encoding for the two non-structural proteins are located in the 5' region and genes for two structural proteins are located in the 3' region of the genome [156]. The structural proteins VP1 and VP2 are identical in sequence but differ in an N-terminal extension that is only present in VP1 (VP1 unique region, VP1u) and possesses a phospholipase A2-like activity (PLA2) [157]. The functions of the two nonstructural proteins NS1 and NP1 of HBoV are not known; however, regulatory functions of NS1 of other parvoviruses have been described [154].

Pathogenesis, immunology and clinical symptoms

HBoV has been detected in children with respiratory disease. The range of clinical manifestations is broad. Diseases of the upper (rhinitis or coughing) and the lower respiratory tract (including pneumonia, bronchiolitis and wheezing) or even the gastrointestinal disease have been described (reviewed in [154]). Other symptoms include fever or rashes [158]. However, HBoV infections are linked frequently with coinfections with viral and bacterial pathogens in up to approximately 69% of HBoV DNA-positive individuals [159] which makes it rather difficult to distinguish between symptoms that have been caused by HBoV or by other pathogens. The role of vertical transmission, seen with other parvoviruses, is not known.

Antibodies against the viral structural protein VP1 have been detected in approximately 95% of children older than 2 years and adults [155]. In addition, IgG1 subclass antibodies against HBOV VP2-virus-like particles (VLP) were detected in approximately 98% of samples that were obtained from healthy adult blood donors [154]. The same authors found IgM antibodies in 41.7% of sera from HBoV DNA-positive children but not in samples from DNA-negative children. Cellular immunity also plays a role in HBoV infections and frequent $CD4^+$ T helper cell reactions have been observed against HBoV VLP [160].

Epidemiology, diagnosis and treatment

Many epidemiological aspects have been discussed above. However, it is noteworthy that the majority of the analyses have been performed in symptomatic individuals and more data from asymptomatic healthy children and adults would add to the understanding of the HBoV epidemiology.

Diagnosis of HBoV infection is mainly done by PCR amplification of viral DNA or the detection of anti-HBoV antibodies by ELISA [154, 161].

At present, no specific treatment of HBoV infections is available.

Human Coronavirus

Coronaviruses are known to cause a variety of diseases in animals [161]. Human coronaviruses are mainly associated with respiratory disorders; some may cause enteric infections [162]. The human coronaviruses HCoV-229E and HCoV-OC43 were identified in the 1960s [163–165]. A coronavirus causing a severe acute human respiratory syndrome (SARS), the SARS-CoV, was first described in 2003 [166, 167] and two additional human coronaviruses, HCoV-NL61 and HCoV-HKU1 that were both linked to respiratory disorders have been identified recently [168, 169].

Because of the economic importance of coronaviruses in veterinary medicine (for instance in swine), development of vaccines is more advanced in veterinary medicine than in human medicine. However, with the appearance of the SARS coronavirus, human coronaviruses gained a greater share of interest.

Taxonomy, structure and replication

Coronaviruses belong to the order *Nidovirales*, family *Coronaviridae*, genus: Coronavirus. In addition to the five human coronaviruses (HCoV-229E, HCoV-HKU1, HCoV-NL 63, HCoV-OC43 and SARS-CoV), a specific human enteric coronavirus has been reported [170].

Coronaviruses have been assigned to three groups based on antigenic relationships between species of different groups (reviewed in [171]). HCoV-229E and HCoV-NL63 are included in group 1, HCoV-HKU1 and HCoV-OC43 in group 2 and SARS-CoV represents an early split from group 2 [172].

Coronaviruses are enveloped viruses, approximately 120 nm in diameter with large (20 nm) club-shaped surface projections (spike protein, S). The structure and function of the S protein have been reviewed elsewhere [173]. Apart from S, coronaviruses have a smaller membrane protein, M (reviewed in [174]). In addition, coronaviruses have a third envelope protein, the very small, non-glycosylated E protein [175]. E and M have been found to be essential for virus particle formation (reviewed in [176]). Group 2 coronaviruses also have an HE (hemagglutinin esterase) protein that forms a layer of approximately 7 nm [175]. HE is a neuraminic acetylesterase that hydrolyses the 9-O-acetylated sialic acid on erythrocytes, thus potentially destroying receptors [177]. Another coronavirus protein, N, is closely linked to the RNA genome (and forms a ribonucleoprotein, RNP). N, which may have a functional role in replication and transcription, is phosphorylated (reviewed in [178]).

Coronaviruses have positive-sense single-stranded RNA genomes of about 30 kb. The genome is generally organized in the following manner: 5'-UTR-polymerase gene-structural protein genes-UTR3' where the UTR are untranslated regions each up to 500 nucleotides. The structural proteins are encoded in the following order: HE (only group 2 coronaviruses) – S – E – M - N [171].

The infection is initiated by binding of the S protein to the cell receptor [179]. CD13 (human aminopeptidase N, APN), a metalloproteinase located on the surface of epithelial cells, has been identified as the cell receptor for HCoV-229E [180]. A metallopeptidase, angiotensin converting enzyme 2 (ACE 2) may be the cell receptor for SARS-CoV [181]. Binding of the S protein to the cell receptor induces conformational changes in S that triggers fusogenic activity [182]. The coronavirus genome can only be released into the cytoplasm after fusion of the envelope with the cell membrane which is mediated through the S2 region of the S protein [173, 183]. Replication occurs within the cytoplasm. Early during infection the genomic RNA is released and acts as an mRNA for the translation of the first gene, the polymerase. mRNAs for the other genes are generated subsequently. In general, coronaviruses have several 3' co-terminal subgenomic mRNAs, so-called 'nested set'. The unique part of each mRNA (which is not within the next smaller mRNA) is translated during the replication cycle. At the 5' end of each gene there is a sequence that is common to all genes, the so-called 'transcription-associated sequence', which, as the name implies, is associated with the discontinuous transcription process (reviewed in [171]). The various mechanisms that have been proposed for the production of subgenomic mRNAs have been reviewed elsewhere [184].

Pathogenesis, immunology and clinical symptoms

Human coronaviruses are generally thought of as common cold agents. This role was confirmed when healthy volunteers were infected with HCoV-OC43 and HCoV-229E and developed classical common cold symptoms [185]. Whereas most infections result in mild disease or are even asymptomatic, additional factors like immunosuppression or coinfections might cause severe disease, even pneumonia [186, 187]. It is not clear whether HCoV-229E and HCoV-OC43 infect the lower respiratory tract in otherwise healthy people, because only URTI was observed in this population. It has been suggested that the lower respiratory tract is more susceptible to HCoV infection in children [187]. Most studies were performed in healthy adults and there is less information about the most susceptible and vulnerable population, children and elderly. However, HCoV-229E and HCoV-OC43 nucleic acid were frequently detected in children with respiratory tract disease (11%) using RT-PCR, whereas in an otherwise healthy control group (asymptomatic bone marrow recipients) only one sample tested positive (0.37%, $p < 0.01$) [188]. This finding suggests that these coronaviruses cause upper and lower respiratory tract diseases in children that are more severe than in adults. It has been suggested that up to 30% of wheezing episodes in asthmatic children may be due to coronavirus infections [189].

HCoV-NL63 was detected in young hospitalized children with severe LRTI [190]. This virus has also been detected in elderly patients with fatal respiratory disease [191]. The risk of developing croup was about 6.6 times higher in children shown to be positive for HCoV-NL63 than in those who tested negative [192, 193]. HCoV-HKU1 was first detected in elderly and children with underlying disease [194]. Symptoms of HCoV-HKU1 include rhinorrhea, fever, coughing, and wheezing as well as bronchiolitis and pneumonia [195]. HCoV-HKU1 might also cause gastrointestinal disease [196].

HCoV infection results in antibody titers in serum. Secretory antibodies can be detected in the respiratory and enteric tracts (and in milk or colostrum) [197].

Epidemiology, diagnosis and treatment

Infections with HCoV peak during winter season [198]. It is estimated that approximately 25% of common cold cases are caused by coronaviruses [162]. Outbreaks of different human coronaviruses have found to alternate every 2–3 years [197]. Although early studies demonstrated that antibodies against coronaviruses are frequently present in adults [199], new studies suggest that there are differences with respect to the HCoV species. Hofmann et al. [200] demonstrated that infections with HCoV-229E occur less frequently than with HCoV-NL63 by measuring specific antibodies neutralizing either HCoV-NL63 or HCoV-229E. In addition, co-detection of coronaviruses with other viruses is common [187]. As with most coronaviruses, human coronaviruses are species specific. However, the SARS coronavirus probably originated from an animal reservoir, presumably bats [201, 202] but was transmitted to humans by civet cats.

The transmission of human coronaviruses from human to human occurs *via* secretions like aerosols and respiratory droplets (or, in case of enteric infection, feces) [197]. Adults with acute symptomatic or inapparent infection transmit the virus to infants who develop clinical disease [162].

Diagnosis of HCoV infection is more clinical; an etiological diagnosis, however, can be performed using molecular or immunological techniques.

Vaccines against coronavirus diseases have been developed for domestic animals because of the economic importance [197], but not for humans. Recent antiviral strategies against coronavirus infection have been reviewed elsewhere [203]. These strategies explore small interfering RNA, blocking of viral entry (e.g., using carbohydrate-binding agents) or neutralizing antibodies. In addition, viral enzymes like protease or helicase are studied as potential targets for novel antivirals (reviewed in [203]).

Influenza virus

According to estimates from the WHO, the burden of influenza in the USA is currently estimated to be 25–50 million cases per year, leading to 150000 hospitalizations and 30000–40000 deaths per year. If these numbers are extrapolated to the rest of the world, influenza virus would infect 5–15% of the world population, causing 3–5 million cases of severe disease and approximately 0.5 million deaths per year. Although this number is high, it would only characterize inter-pandemic influenza [204]. Epidemics and outbreaks of influenza follow a seasonal pattern, which differs according to the region in the world: in temperate climate zones, seasonal epidemics typically begin in the late fall with a peak in late winter. The seasonal pattern is less pronounced in tropical zones (reviewed in [205]).

The focus of this book is on 'common cold'. For details on influenza and influenza viruses, further reading of standard literature is recommended.

Taxonomy, structure and replication

Influenza viruses are members of the *Orthomyxoviridae*, genus Influenzavirus and include influenza virus types A, B and C. The viruses are enveloped pleomorphic particles with a size ranging from 100 to >300 nm, their genome is organized on eight (influenza virus A and B) or seven (influenza virus C) negative-sense single-stranded RNA segments [206]. Spikes consist of hemagglutinin (HA) and neuraminidase (NA). The nomenclature for human influenza virus includes type, geographic location of the first isolation, isolate number and year of isolation. In addition, subtypes of influenza A are described by their HA and NA designations. To date, 16 HA and 9 NA types have been described. The viral envelope is also associated with a matrix protein (M) that, after infection, forms a tetrameric ion channel. Several polymerase proteins (PB1, PB2, PA) form, together with the nucleoprotein (NP) and the RNA, a ribonucleoprotein (RNP) complex (reviewed in [206]). Influenza viruses are transmitted *via* the respiratory route and bind to a cell receptor that consists of oligosaccharides and that is present on the surface of respiratory epithelial cells. The sialic acid-α2,6-galactose linkage (SAα2,6Gal) that is associated with binding to human influenza virus HA is present in the human respiratory tract (reviewed in [207]). After binding, the virus enters the host cell by endocytosis [208]. Further steps include fusion of the virus to the endosome [206] and the release of the RNP into the nucleus through an ion channel that is formed by M2 [209]. The viral RNA is a template for complementary RNA and the mRNA. The non-structural NEP/NS2 as well as M1 play a role in the nuclear export of novel RNA. Assembly occurs at the apical surface of the cell, budding occurs and the novel virus is released (reviewed in [206]).

Pathogenesis, immunology and clinical symptoms

Influenza viruses are transmitted *via* the respiratory route [206]. Host specificity is largely determined by the availability of host cell receptors on the surface of epithelial cells [210]. Usually, influenza in humans is an URTI that is characterized by cough, headache, malaise and fever [211]. However, complications are frequent, and encephalitis, Reye's syndrome, myelitis [212] as well as muscular manifestations of the infection including myocarditis [213], disseminated intravascular coagulation and toxic and septic shock [214] may occur.

Major airway congestion, inflammation and necrosis have been found in histopathological examinations [215].

Although much progress in the understanding of the pathogenesis of human influenza has been made during the past decade, the molecular mechanisms responsible for the virulence of particular strains of influenza virus are not yet understood.

Epidemiology, diagnosis and treatment

Influenza A virus can infect humans as well as waterfowl and chickens, swine, horses, and other species. Influenza B virus, on the other hand, has a restricted host range and circulates predominantly in humans. However, influenza B virus was recently isolated from seals [216]. Different types of HA mediate species-specific binding of the virus [217, 218]. It would be beyond the scope of this book on common cold to review all the recent literature that has been published regarding the epidemiology of influenza viruses. However, one important aspect should be mentioned here. Influenza virus is a changing virus and the repetitive occurrence of the yearly epidemic is supported by 'antigenic drift', an accumulation of point mutations in the viral receptors (HA and NA). The drift is attributed to a low fidelity of the viral RNA polymerase [219]. These new variants then infect a population without pre-existing immunity (reviewed in [206]). A second process that contributes to the emergence of new influenza variants is called 'antigenic shift'. An antigenic shift may occur during co-infection with other influenza viruses. Such a co-infection may lead to a viral reassortment (an exchange of genome segments between different virus strains) [206]. If this process leads to a new virus strain that is able to effectively spread from individual to individual, a worldwide outbreak, a pandemic, may occur [207]. There have been several pandemics in the past century including the so-called "Spanish flu" in 1918/1919, infecting about the half of the world population at that time and killing approximately 20–50 million people [204]. Current pandemic concerns are focused on the highly pathogenic variants of the strain A/H5N1 or H1N1. The epidemiology of influenza has been comprehensively reviewed [220, 221].

Influenza is typically diagnosed clinically, but laboratory diagnosis has been established and organized according to standardized procedures as part of national and global pandemic plans.

Several effective vaccines exist today (reviewed in [222]) and a pre-pandemic vaccine has been licensed recently.

References

1 Couch RB (1996) Rhinoviruses. In: BN Fields, DM Knipe, PM Howley et al. (eds): *Fields Virology*, 3rd edn. Lippincott-Raven, New York, 713 ff

2 Virus Taxonomy 2008. International Committee on Taxonomy of Viruses. http://www.ictvonline.org/virusTaxonomy.asp, retrieved June 11, 2008

3 Stanway G (1999) Rhinoviruses (Picornaviridae). In: A Granoff, RG Webster (eds): *Encycloedial of Virology*, 2nd edn. Academic Press, London

4 Rossmann MG, Arnold E, Erickson JW, Frankenberger EA, Griffith JP, Hecht HJ, Johnson JE, Kamer G, Luo M, Mosser AG et al. (1985) Structure of a human common cold virus and functional relationship to other picornaviruses. *Nature* 317: 145–153

5 Olson NH, Kolatkar PR, Oliveira MA, Cheng RH, Greve JM, McClelland A, Baker TS, Rossmann MG (1993) Structure of a human rhinovirus complexed with its receptor molecule. *Proc Natl Acad Sci USA* 90: 507–511

6 Abraham G, Colonno RJ (1984) Many rhinovirus serotypes share the same cellular receptor. *J Virol* 51: 340–345

7 Staunton DE, Merluzzi VJ, Rothlein R, Barton R, Marlin SD, Springe, TA (1989) A cell adhesion molecule, ICAM-1 is the major surface receptor for rhinoviruses. *Cell* 56: 849–853

8 Rossmann MG, Bella J, Kolatkar PR, He Y, Wimmer E, Kuhn RJ, Baker TS (2000) Cell recognition and entry by rhino- and enteroviruses. *Virology* 269: 239–247

9 Matthews DA, Smith WW, Ferre RA, Condon B, Budahazi G, Sisson W, Villafranca JE, Janson CA, McElroy HE, Gribskov CL et al. (1994) Structure of human rhinovirus 3C protease reveals a trypsin-like polypeptide fold, RNA-binding site, and means for cleaving precursor polyprotein. *Cell* 77: 761–771

10 Hendley JO, Wenzel RP, Gwaltney JM Jr (1973) Transmission of rhinovirus colds by self-inoculation. *N Engl J Med* 288: 1361–1364

11 Reed SE (1975) An investigation of possible transmission of rhinovirus colds through indirect contact. *J Hyg* 75: 249–258

12 Gwaltney JM Jr, Moskalski PB, Hendley JO (1978) Hand-to-hand transmission of rhinovirus colds. *Ann Intern Med* 88: 463–367

13 Couch RB, Cate TR, Douglas RC Jr, Gerone JP, Knight V (1966) Effect of route of inoculation on experimental respiratory viral disease in volunteers and evidence for airborne transmission. *Bacteriol Rev* 30: 517–529

14 Douglas RG Jr, Cate TR, Gerone JP, Couch RB (1966) Quantitative rhinovirus shedding patterns in volunteers. *Am Rev Respir Dis* 94: 159–167

15 Arruda E, Mifflin TE, Gwaltney JM, Winther B, Hayden FG (1991) Localization of rhinovirus replication *In vitro* with *in situ* hybridization. *J Med Virol* 34: 38–44

16 Winther B, Gwaltney JM Jr, Hendley JO (1990) Respiratory virus infection of monolayer cultures of human nasal epithelial cells. *Am Rev Respir Dis* 141: 839–845

17 Winther B, Farr B, Turner RB, Hendley JO, Gwaltney JM Jr, Mygind N (1984) Histopathologic examination and enumeration of polymorphonuclear leukocytes in the nasal mucosa during experimental rhinovirus colds. *Acta Otolaryngol (Stockh)* (Suppl) 413: 19–24

18 Arruda E, Boyle TR, Winther B, Pevear DC, Gwaltney JM Jr, Hayden FG (1995) Localization of human rhinovirus replication in the upper respiratory tract by *in situ* hybridization. *J Infect Dis* 171: 1329–1333

19 Turner RB, Hendley JO, Gwaltney JM Jr (1982) Shedding of infected ciliated epithelial cells in rhinovirus colds. *J Infect Dis* 145 849–853

20 Turner RB, Weingand KW, Yeh C-H, Leedy D (1998) Association between nasal secretion interleukin–8 concentration and symptom severity in experimental rhinovirus colds. *Clin Infect Dis* 26: 840–846

21 Proud D, Gwaltney JM Jr, Hendley JO, Dinarello CA, Gillis S, Schleimer RP (1994) Increased levels of interleukin-1 are detected in nasal secretions of volunteers during experimental rhinovirus colds. *J Infect Dis* 169: 1007–1013

22 Zhu Z, Tang W, Ray A, Wu Y, Einarsson O, Landry ML, Gwaltney J Jr, Elias JA (1996) Rhinovirus stimulation of interleukin-6 *in vivo* and *In vitro*: Evidence for nuclear factor kB-dependent transcriptional activation. *J Clin Invest* 97: 421–430

23 Papadopoulos NG, Bate PJ, Bardin PG, Papi A, Leir SH, Fraenkel DJ, Meyer J, Lackie PM, Sanderson G, Holgate, TS et al. (2000) Rhinoviruses infect the lower airways. *J Infect Dis* 181: 1875–1884

24 Mertsola J, Ziegler T, Ruuskanen O, Vanto T, Koivikko A, Halonen P (1991) Recurrent wheezy bronchitis and viral respiratory infections. *Arch Dis Child*hood 66: 124–129

25 Minor TE, Dick EC, Baker JW, Quellette JJ, Cohen M, Reed CE (1976) Rhinovirus and influenza type A infections as precipitants of asthma. *Am Rev Respir Dis* 113: 149–153

26 Corne JM, Marshall C, Smith S, Schreiber J, Sanderson G, Holgate ST, Johnston SL (2002) Frequency, severity, and duration of rhinovirus infections in asthmatic and non-asthmatic individuals: A longitudinal cohort study. *Lancet* 359: 831–834

27 Wark PA, Johnston SL, Moric I, Simpson JL, Hensley MJ, Gibson PG (2002) Neutrophil degranulation and cell lysis is associated with clinical severity in virus-induced asthma. *Eur Respir J* 19: 68–75

28 Nicolson KG, Kent J, Ireland DC (1993) Respiratory viruses and exacerbations of asthma in adults. *BMJ* 307: 982–986

29 Wark PA, Johnston SL, Bucchieri F, Powell R, Puddicombe S, Laza-Stanca V, Holgate ST, Davies DE (2005) Asthmatic bronchial epithelial cells have a deficient innate immune response to infection with rhinovirus. *N Engl J Med* 201: 937–957

30 Fox JP, Cooney MK, Hall CE, Foy HM (1985) Rhinoviruses in Seattle families, 1975–1979. *Am J Epidemiol* 101: 122–143

31 Turner RB, Hayden FG (2003) Rhinovirus. In: H Ruebsamen-Waigmann, K Deres, G Hewlett, R Welker (eds): *Viral infections and treatment.* Marcel Dekker, New York, 139–164

32 Hamparian VV, Ketler A, Hilleman MR (1961) Recovery of new viruses (coryzavirus) from cases of common cold in human adults. *Proc Soc Exp Biol Med* 108: 444–453

33 Jackson GG, Muldoon RL (1973) Viruses causing common respiratory infections in man. *J Infect Dis* 127: 328–355

34 Kisch AL, Webb PA, Johnson KM (1964) Further properties of five new organized picornaviruses (rhinoviruses) Am *J Hyg* 79: 125–135

35 Yin FH, Lomax NB (1986) Establishment of a mouse model for human rhinovirus infection. *J Gen Virol* 67: 2335–2340

36 Dick EC (1968) Experimental infections of chimpanzees with human rhinovirus types 14 and 43. *Proc Soc Exp Biol Med* 127: 1079–1081

37 Pinto CA, Haff RF (1969) Experimental infection of gibbons with rhinovirus. *Nature* 224: 1310–1311

38 Bartlett NW, Walton RP, Edwards MR, Aniscenko J, Caramori G, Zhu J, Glanville N, Choy KJ, Jourdan P, Burnet J et al. (2008) Mouse models of rhinovirus-induced disease and exacerbation of allergic airway inflammation. *Nat Med* 14: 199–204

39 Morris JA Jr, Blount RE, Savage RE (1956) Recovery of cytopathogenic agent from chimpanzees with coryza. *Proc Soc Exp Biol Med* 92: 544–550

40 Collins PL, McIntosh K, Chanock RM (1996) Respiratory syncytial virus. In: BN Fields, DM Knipe, PM Howley et al. (eds): *Fields Virology,* 3rd edn. Lippincott-Raven, New York, 1313 ff

41 Initiative for Vaccine Research: Respiratory syncytial virus, World Health Organization. http: //www.who.int/vaccine_research/diseases/ari/en/index3.html, retrieved on August 15, 2008

42 Stott EJ, Taylor G (1985) Respiratory syncytial virus. Brief review. *Arch Virol* 84: 1–52

43 Virus Taxonomy 2008. International Committee on Taxonomy of Viruses. http: //www.ictvonline.org/virusTaxonomy.asp, retrieved August 15, 2008

44 Collins PL, Graham BS (2008) Viral and host factors in human respiratory syncytial virus pathogenesis. *J Virol* 82: 2040–2055

45 Bachi T, Howe C (1973) Morphogenesis and ultrastructure of respiratory syncytial virus. *J Virol* 12: 1173–1180

46 Kolokoltsov AA, Deniger D, Fleming EH, Roberts NJ Jr, Karpilow JM, Davey RA (2007) siRNA profiling reveals key role of clathrin-mediated endocytosis

and early endosome formation for infection by respiratory syncytial virus. *J Virol* 81: 7786–7800
47 Gould PS, Easton AJ (2007) Coupled translation of the second ORF of the M2 mRNA is sequence dependent and differs significantly in the subfamily Pneumovirinae. *J Virol* 81: 8488–8496
48 Collins PL, Crowe JEJ (2007) Respiratory syncytial virus and metapneumovirus, In: DM Knipe, PM Howley, DE Griffin, RA Lamb, MA Martin, B Roizman, SE Straus (eds): *Fields virology*, 5th edn. Lippincott Williams & Wilkins, Philadelphia, 1601 ff
49 Akira S, Uematsu S, Takeuchi O (2006) Pathogen recognition and innate immunity. *Cell* 124: 783–801
50 Liu P, Jamaluddin M, Li K, Garofalo RP, Casola A, Brasier AR (2007) Retinoic acid-inducible gene I mediates early *Antiviral Res*ponse and Toll-like receptor 3 expression in respiratory syncytial virus-infected airway epithelial cells. *J Virol* 81: 1401–1411
51 Teng MN, Collins PL (1998) Identification of the respiratory syncytial virus proteins required for formation and passage of helper-dependent infectious particles. *J Virol* 72: 5707–5716
52 Teng MN, Collins PL (2002) The central conserved cystine noose of the attachment G protein of human respiratory syncytial virus is not required for efficient viral infection *In vitro* or *in vivo*. *J Virol* 76: 6164–6171
53 Gonzalez-Reyes L, Ruiz-Arguello MB, Garcia-Barreno B, Calder L, Lopez JA, Albar JP, Skehel JJ, Wiley DC, Melero JA (2001) Cleavage of the human respiratory syncytial virus fusion protein at two distinct sites is required for activation of membrane fusion. *Proc Natl Acad Sci USA* 98: 9859–9864
54 Collins PL, Crowe JEJ (2007) Respiratory syncytial virus and metapneumovirus. In: DM Knipe, PM Howley, DE Griffin, RA Lamb, MA Martin, B Roizman, SE Straus (eds): *Fields Virology*, 5th edn. Lippincott Williams & Wilkins, Philadelphia, 1601 ff
55 McNamara PS, Smyth RL (2002) The pathogenesis of respiratory syncytial virus disease in childhood. *Br Med Bull* 61: 13–28
56 Wyde PR, Piedra PA (2003) Respiratory syncytial virus. In: H Ruebsamen-Waigmann, K Deres, G Hewlett, R Welker (eds): *Viral infections and treatment.* Marcel Dekker, New York, 91–137
57 Stein RT, Sherill, D Morgan WJ, Holberg CJ, Halonen M, Taussig LM, Wright AL, Martinez FD (1999) Respiratory syncytial virus in early life and risk of wheeze and allergy by age of 13. *Lancet* 354: 541–545
58 Whimbey E, Gosh S (2000) Respiratory syncytial virus infections in immunocompromised adults. *Curr Clin Topics Infect Dis* 20: 232–255
59 Gardner PS, Mc Quillan J, Court SD (1970) Speculation on pathogenesis in death from respiratory syncytial virus infection. *Br Med J* 1: 327–330
60 Heikkinen T, Thint M, Chonmaitree T (1999) Prevalence of various respiratory viruses in the middle ear during acute otitis media. *N Engl J Med* 340: 260–264
61 Aherne W, Bird T, Court SDM, Gardner PS, McQuillin J (1970) Pathological changes in virus infections of the lower respiratory tract in children. *J Clin Pathol* 23: 7–18

62 Hall CB, McCarthy CA (2000) Respiratory syncytial virus. In: GL Mandell, JE Bennett, K Dolin (eds): *Mandell, Douglas and Bennetts principles and practice in infectious diseases.* Churchill Livingston, Philadelphia, 1782–1801
63 Krilov LR (2001) Respiratory syncytial virus: Update on infection, treatment and prevention. *Curr Infect Dis Rep* 3: 242–246
64 Selwyn BJ (1990) The epidemiology of acute respiratory tract infection in young children. *Res Infect Dis* 12: 5870–5888
65 Glezen WP, Paredes A, Allison JE, Tabe, LH (1981) Risk of respiratory syncytial virus infection for infants from low-income families in relationship to age, sex, ethnic group and maternal antibody level. *Pediatrics* 98: 708–715
66 Hall CB (1998) Respiratory syncytial virus. In: RD Feigin, JD Cherry (eds): *Textbook of pediatric infectious diseases.* WB Saunders, Philadelphia. 2084–2111
67 Laham FR, Israele V, Casellas JM, Garcia AM, Lac Prugent CM, Hoffman SJ, Hauer D, Thumar B, Name MI, Pascual A et al. (2004) Differential production of inflammatory cytokines in primary infection with human metapneumovirus and with other common respiratory viruses of infancy. *J Infect Dis* 189: 2047–2056
68 Broughton S, Greenough A (2003) Effectiveness of drug therapies to treat or prevent respiratory syncytial virus infection-related morbidity. *Expert Opin Pharmacother* 4: 1801–1808
69 Hull J (2007) Genetic susceptibility to RSV disease, In PA Cane (ed): *Respiratory syncytial virus*, vol. 14. Elsevier, Amsterdam, 115–140
70 Kim C K, Kim SW, Park CS, Kim BI, Kang H, Koh YY (2003) Bronchoalveolar lavage cytokine profiles in acute asthma and acute bronchiolitis. *J Allergy Clin Immunol* 112: 64–71
71 Lee FE, Walsh EE, Falsey AR, Lumb ME, Okam NV, Liu N, Divekar AA, Hall CB, Mosmann TR (2007) Human infant respiratory syncytial virus (RSV)-specific type 1 and 2 cytokine responses *ex vivo* during primary RSV infection. *J Infect Dis* 195: 1779–1788
72 Legg JP, Hussain IR, Warner JA, Johnston SL, Warner JO (2003) Type 1 and type 2 cytokine imbalance in acute respiratory syncytial virus bronchiolitis. *Am J Respir Crit Care Med* 168: 633–639
73 Graham BS, Henderson GS, Tang YW, Lu X, Neuzil KM, Colley DG (1993) Priming immunization determines T helper cytokine mRNA expression patterns in lungs of mice challenged with respiratory syncytial virus. *J Immunol* 151: 2032–2040
74 Arnold R, Konig B, Werchau H, Konig W (2004) Respiratory syncytial virus deficient in soluble G protein induced an increased proinflammatory response in human lung epithelial cells. *Virology* 330: 384–397
75 Polack FP, Irusta PM, Hoffman SJ, Schiatti MP, Melendi GA, Delgado MF, Laham FR, Thumar B, Hendry RM, Melero JA et al. (2005) The cysteine-rich region of respiratory syncytial virus attachment protein inhibits innate immunity elicited by the virus and endotoxin. *Proc Natl Acad Sci USA* 102: 8996–9001
76 Kurt-Jones EA, Popova L, Kwinn L, Haynes LM, Jones LP, Tripp RA, Walsh EE, Freeman MW, Golenbock DT, Anderson LJ, Finberg RW (2000) Pattern

recognition receptors TLR4 and CD14 mediate response to respiratory syncytial virus. *Nat Immunol* 1: 398–401
77 Karron RA, Singleton RJ, Bulkow L, Parkinson A, Kruse D, DeSmet I, Indorf C, Petersen KM, Leombruno D, Hurlburt D et al. (1999) Severe respiratory syncytial virus disease in Alaska native children. *J Infect Dis* 180: 41–49
78 Cardenas SA, Auais A, Piedimonte G (2005) Palivizumab in the prophylaxis of respiratory syncytial virus infection. *Expert Rev Anti Infect Ther* 3: 719–726
79 Moore ML, Stokes Peebles R Jr (2006) Respiratory syncytial virus disease mechanisms implicated by human, animal model, and *In vitro* data facilitate vaccine strategies and new therapeutics. *Pharmacol Ther* 112: 405–424
80 Belshe RB, Richardson LS, London WT, Sly DL, Lorfeld JH, Camargo E, Prevar DA, Chanock RM (1977) Experimental respiratory syncytial virus infection of four species of primates. *J Med Virol* 1: 157–162
81 Simoes EA, Hayward AR, Ponnuraj EM, Straumanis JP, Stenmark KR, Wilson HL, Babu PG (1999) Respiratory syncytial virus infects the bonnet monkey, *Macaca radiata*. *Pediatr Dev Pathol* 2: 316–326
82 Prince GA, Jenson AB, Horswood RL, Camargo E, Chanock RM (1978) The pathogenesis of respiratory syncytial virus infection in cotton rats. *Am J Pathol* 93: 771–791
83 Prince GA, Jenson AB, Hemming VG, Murphy BR, Walsh EE, Horswood RL, Chanock RM (1986) Enhancement of respiratory syncytial virus pulmonary pathology in cotton rats by prior intramuscular inoculation of formalin-inactivated virus. *J Virol* 57: 721–728
84 Prince, GA, Hemming, VG, Horswood, RL, Baron, PA, Murphy, BR, Chanock, RM (1990) Mechanism of antibody-mediated viral clearance in immunotherapy of respiratory syncytial virus infection of cotton rats. *J Virol* 64: 3091–3092
85 Graham BS, Perkins MD, Wright PF, Karzon DT (1988) Primary respiratory syncytial virus infection in mice. *J Med Virol* 26: 153–162
86 Taylor G, Stott EJ, Hughes M, Collins AP (1984) Respiratory syncytial virus infection in mice. *Infect Immun* 43: 649–655
87 Hussell T, Openshaw PJ (1998) Intracellular IFN-gamma expression in natural killer cells precedes lung $CD8^+$ T cell recruitment during respiratory syncytial virus infection. *J Gen Virol* 79: 2593–2601
88 Graham BS, Johnson TR, Peebles RS (2000) Immune-mediated disease pathogenesis in respiratory syncytial virus infection. *Immunopharmacology* 48: 237–247
89 Gitiban N, Jurcisek JA, Harris RH, Mertz SE, Durbin RK, Bakaletz LO, Durbin JE (2005) Chinchilla and murine models of upper respiratory tract infections with respiratory syncytial virus. *J Virol* 79: 6035–6042
90 Woolums AR, Anderson ML, Gunther RA, Schelegle ES, LaRochelle DR, Singer RS, Boyle GA, Friebertshauser KE, Gershwin LJ (1999) Evaluation of severe disease induced by aerosol inoculation of calves with bovine respiratory syncytial virus. *Am J Vet Res* 60: 473–480
91 Krempl CD, Lamirande EW, Collins PL (2005) Complete sequence of the RNA genome of pneumonia virus of mice (PVM). *Virus Genes* 30: 237–249
92 Initiative for Vaccine Research: Parainfluenza viruses. World Health

Organization. http: //www.who.int/vaccine_research/diseases/ari/en/index2.html, retrieved on August 26, 2008
93 Collins PL, Chanock RM, McIntosh K (1996) Parainfluenza viruses. In: BN Fields, DM Knipe, PM Howley et al. (eds): *Fields Virology*, 3rd edn. Lippincott-Raven, New York, 1205 ff
94 Parrott RH, Vargosko AJ, Kim HW, Bell JA, Channock RM (1962) Myxoviruses. III Parainfluenza. *Am J Public Health* 52: 907–917
95 Channock RM, Parrott RH, Johnson KM, Kapikian AZ, Bell JA (1963) Myxoviruses: Parainfluenza. *Am Rev Respir Dis* 88: 152–166
96 Virus Taxonomy 2008. International Committee on Taxonomy of Viruses. http: //www.ictvonline.org/virusTaxonomy.aspref, retrieved on September 03, 2008
97 Choppin PW, Scheid A (1980) The role of viral glycoproteins in adsorption, penetration, and pathogenicity of viruses. *Rev Infect Dis* 1: 40–61
98 Markwell MAK (1991) New frontiers opened by the exploration of host cell receptors. In: DW Kingsbury (ed): *The paramyxoviruses*. Plenum Press, New York, 407–426
99 Kasel JA, Frank AL, Keitel WA, Taber LH, Glezen WP (1984) Acquisition of serum antibodies to specific glycoproteins of parainfluenza virus 3 in children. *J Virol* 52: 828–832
100 Yanagihara R, McIntosh K (1980) secretory immunological response in infants and children to parainfluenza virus types 1 and 2. *Infect Immun* 30: 23–28
101 de Silva LM, Cloonan MJ (1991) Brief report: Parainfluenza virus type 3 infections: Finding in Sydney and some observations on variations in seasonality world-wide. *J Med Virol* 35: 19–21
102 Denny FW, Murphy TF, Clyde WA Jr, Collier AM, Henderson FW (1983) Croup: An 11 year study in pediatric practice. *Pediatrics* 71: 871–876
103 Leung AK, Kellner JD, Johnson DW (2004) Viral croup: A current perspective. *J Pediatr* Health Care 18: 297–301
104 http: //clinicaltrials.gov/ct2/show/NCT00366782?term=vaccine+NIAID&recr=Open&rank=16, retrieved on September , 03, 2008
105 http: //www.clinicaltrials.gov/ct2/show/NCT00508651?term=parainfluenza+virus&rank=6, retrieved on September , 03, 2008
106 Horwitz MS (2001) Adenoviruses. In: DM Knipe, PM Howley (eds): *Fields Virology*, 4th edn. Lippincott, Williams & Wilkins, New York, 2310–2326
107 Schmitz H, Wiegand R, Heinrich W (1983) Worldwide epidemiology of human adenovirus infections. *Am J Epidemiol* 117: 455–466
108 Hilleman MR, Werner JH (1954) Recovery of new agents from patients with acute respiratory illness. *Proc Soc Exp Biol Med* 85: 183–188
109 Brandt CD, Kim HW, Vargosdo AJ, Jeffries BC, Arrobio JO, Rindge B, Parrott RH, Chanock RM (1969) Infections in 18,000 infants and children in a controlled study of respiratory tract disease. I. Adenovirus pathogenicity in relation to serologic type and illness syndrome. *Am J Epidemiol* 90: 484–500
110 Virus Taxonomy 2008. International Committee on Taxonomy of Viruses. http: //www.ictvonline.org/virusTaxonomy.asp, retrieved on September 03, 2008
111 Horne RW, Bonner S, Waterson AP, Wildy P (1959) The icosahedral form of an adenovirus. *J Mol Biol* 1: 84–86
112 Shenk T (2001) Adenoviruses. The viruses and their replication. In: DM Knipe,

PM Howley (eds): *Fields Virology*, 4th edn. Lippincott, Williams & Wilkins, New York, 2265–2300
113 Goncalves MA, de Vries AA (2006) Adenovirus: From foe to friend. *Rev Med Virol* 16: 167–186
114 Ginsberg HS, Pereira HG, Valentine RC, Wilcox WC (1966) A proposed terminology for the adenovirus antigens and virion morphological subunits. *Virology*, 28: 782–783
115 ICTVdB Management (2006) 00.001.0.01.001. Human adenovirus C. In: C Büchen-Osmond (ed): *ICTVdB – The Universal Virus Database, version 4.* Columbia University, New York
116 ICTVdB – The Universal Virus Database, version 4. http: //www.ncbi.nlm.nih.gov/ICTVdb/ICTVdB/ retrieved on September, 03, 2008
117 van Oostrum J, Burnett RM (1985) The molecular composition of the adenovirus type 2 virion. *J Virol* 56: 439–448
118 Martilla M, Persson D, Gustafsson D, Liszewski MK, Atkinson JP, Wadell G, Arnberg N (2005) CD46 is a cellular receptor for all species B adenoviruses except types 3 and 7. *J Virol* 79: 14429–14436
119 Shenk T, Flint SJ (1991) Transcriptional and transforming activities of the adenovirus E1A proteins. *Adv Cancer Res* 57: 47–85
120 Hayashi S (2002) Latent adenovirus infection in COPD. Chest 121: 183S–187S
121 Ginsberg HS, Gold E, Jordan WS Jr, Katz S, Badger GF, Dingle JH (1955) Relations of the new respiratory agents to acute respiratory diseases. *Am J Public Health* 45: 915–922
122 Hayashi S, Hogg JC (2007) Adenovirus infections and lung disease. *Curr Opin Pharmacol* 7: 237–243
123 Hogg JC, Irving WL, Porter H, Evans M, Dunnill MS, Fleming K (1989) In situ hybridization studies of adenoviral infections of the lung and their relationship to follicular bronchiectasis. *Am Rev Respir Dis* 139: 1531–1535
124 Bencroft DM (1967) Histopathology of adenovirus infection of the respiratory tract in young children. *J Clin Pathol* 20: 561–569
125 Pichler MN, Reichenbach J, Schmidt H, Hermann G, Zielen S (2000) Severe adenovirus bronchiolitis in children. *Acta Paediatr* 89: 1387–1389
126 Matsuse T, Hayashi S, Kuwano K, Keunecke H, Jefferies WA, Hogg HC (1992) Latent adenoviral infection in the pathogenesis of chronic airways obstruction. *Am Rev Respir Dis* 146: 177–184
127 Elliott WM, Hayashi S, Hogg JC (1995) Immunodetection of adenoviral E1A proteins in human lung tissue. *Am J Respir Cell Mol Biol* 12: 642–648
128 Retamales I, Elliott WM, Meshi B, Coxson HO, Pare PD, Sciurba FC, Rogers RM, Hayashi S, Hogg JC (2001) Amplification of inflammation in emphysema and its association with latent adenoviral infection. *Am J Respir Crit Care Med* 164: 469–473
129 Ogawa E, Elliott WM, Hughes F, Eichholtz TJ, Hogg JC, Hayashi S (2004) Latent adenoviral infection induces production of growth factors relevant to airway remodeling in COPD. *Am J Physiol Lung Cell Mol Physiol* 286: L189-L197
130 Hogg JC, Chu F, Utokaparch S, Woods R, Elliott WM, Buzatu L, Cherniack RM, Rogers RM, Sciurba FC, Coxson HO et al. (2004) The nature of small

airway obstruction in chronic obstructive pulmonary disease. *N Engl J Med* 350: 2645–2653

131 Huebner RJ, Rowe WP, Ward TG, Parrott RH, Bell JA (1954) Adenoidal-pharyngeal-conjunctival agents: A newly recognized group of common viruses of the respiratory system. *N Engl J Med* 251: 1077–1086

132 Badger GF, Curtiss C, Dingle JH, Ginsberg HS, Gold E, Jordan WS Jr (1956) A study of illness in a group of Cleveland families. X. The occurrence of adenovirus infections. *Am J Hyg* 64: 336–348

133 Top FH Jr, Buescher EL, Bancroft WH, Russell PK (1971) Immunization with live types 7 and 4 adenovirus vaccines. II. Antibody response and protective effect against acute respiratory disease due to adenovirus type 7. *J Infect Dis* 124: 155–160

134 van den Hoogen BG, de Jong JC, Groen J, Kuiken T, de Groot R, Fouchier, RA, Osterhaus AD (2001) A newly discovered human pneumovirus isolated from young children with respiratory tract disease. *Nat Med* 7: 719–724

135 Deffrasnes CD, Hamelin ME, Boivin G (2007) Human metapneumovirus. *Semin Respir Crit Care Med* 28: 213–221

136 Virus Taxonomy 2008. International Committee on Taxonomy of Viruses. http: //www.ictvonline.org/virusTaxonomy.asp, retrieved September 10, 2008

137 Peret TC, Boivin G, Li Y, Couillard M, Humphrey C, Osterhaus AD, Erdman DD, Anderson LJ (2002) Characterization of human metapneumoviruses isolated from patients in North America. *J Infect Dis* 185: 1660–1663

138 Boivin G, Mackay I, Sloots TP, Madhi S, Freymuth F, Wolf D, Shemer-Avni Y, Ludewick H, Gray GC, LeBlanc E (2004) Global genetic diversity of human metapneumovirus fusion gene. *Emerg Infect Dis* 10: 1154–1157

139 Mackay IM, Bialasiewicz S, Waliuzzaman Z, Chidlow GR, Fegredo DC, Laingam S, Adamson P, Harnett GB, Rawlinson W, Nissen MD, Sloots TP (2004) Use of the P gene to genotype human metapneumovirus identifies 4 viral subtypes. *J Infect Dis* 190: 1913–1918

140 Huck B, Scharf G, Neumann-Haefelin D, Puppe W, Weigl J, Falcone V (2006) Novel human metapneumovirus sublineage. *Emerg Infect Dis* 12: 147–150

141 van den Hoogen GB, Bestebroer TM, Osterhaus AD, Fouchier RA (2002) Analysis of the genomic sequence of a human metapneumovirus. *Virology* 295: 119–132

142 Hall CB (2001) Respiratory syncytial virus and parainfluenzavirus. *N Engl J Med* 344: 1917–1928

143 Skiadopoulos MH, Biacchesi S, Buchholz, UJ, Amaro-Carambot E, Surman SR, Collins PL, Murphy BR (2006) Individual contributions of the human metapneumovirus F, G, and SH surface glycoproteins to the induction of neutralizing antibodies and protective immunity. *Virology* 345: 492–501

144 Williams JV, Harris PA, Tollefson SJ, Halburnt-Rush LL, Pingsterhaus JM, Edwards KM, Wright PF, Crowe JE Jr (2004) Human metapneumovirus and lower respiratory tract disease in otherwise healthy infants and children. *N Engl J Med* 350: 443–450

145 Sumino KC, Agapov E, Pierce RA, Trulock EP, Pfeifer JD, Ritter JH, Gaudreault-Keener M, Storch GA, Holtzman MJ (2005) Detection of severe

human metapneumovirus infection by real-time polymerase chain reaction and histopathological assessment. *J Infect Dis* 192: 1052–1060
146 Boivin G, De Serres G, Côté S, Gilca R, Abed Y, Rochette L, Bergeron MG, Déry P (2003) Human metapneumovirus infections in hospitalized children. *Emerg Infect Dis* 9: 634–640
147 Englund JA, Boeckh M, Kuypers J, Nichols WG, Hackman RC, Morrow RA, Fredricks DN, Corey L (2006) Brief communication: Fatal human metapneumovirus infection in stem-cell transplant recipients. *Ann Intern Med* 144: 374–375
148 Sloots TP, Mackay IM, Bialasiewicz S, Jacob KC, McQueen E, Harnett GB, Siebert DJ, Masters BI, Young PR, Nissen MD (2006) Human metapneumovirus, Australia, 2001–2004. *Emerg Infect Dis* 12: 1263–1266
149 Mahalingam S, Schwarze J, Zaid A, Nissen M, Sloots T, Tauro S, Storer J, Alvarez R, Tripp RA (2006) Perspective on the host response to human metapneumovirus infection: What can we learn from respiratory syncytial virus infections? *Microbes Infect* 8: 285–293
150 Kahn JS (2006) Epidemiology of human metapneumovirus. Clin *Microbiol Rev* 19: 546–557
151 Wyde PR, Chetty SN, Jewell AM, Boivin G, Piedra PA (2003) Comparison of the inhibition of human metapneumovirus and human respiratory syncytial virus by ribavirin and immune serum globulin *In vitro*. *Antiviral Res* 60: 51–59
152 Ulbrandt ND, Ji H, Patel NK, Riggs JM, Brewah YA, Ready S, Donacki NE, Folliot K, Barnes AS, Senthil K et al. (2006) Isolation and characterization of monoclonal antibodies which neutralize human metapneumovirus *In vitro* and *in vivo*. *J Virol* 80: 7799–7806
153 Allander T, Tammi MT, Eriksoson M, Bjerkner A, Tiveljung-Lindell A, Andersson B (2005) Cloning of a human parvovirus by molecular screening of respiratory tract samples. *Proc Natl Acad Sci USA* 102: 12891–12896
154 Lindner J, Modrow S (2008) Human Bocavirus – A novel parvovirus to infect humans. *Intervirology* 51: 116–122
155 Endo R, Ishiguro N, Kikuta H, Teramoto S, Shirkoohi R, Ma X, Ebihara T, Ishiko H, Ariga T (2007) Seroepidemiology of human bocavirus in Hokkaido prefecture, Japan. *J Clin Microbiol* 45: 3218–3223
156 Chieochasnin T, Chutinimitkul S, Payungporn S, Hiranras T, Samransamruajkit R, Theamboolers A, Poovorawan Y (2007) Complete coding sequences and phylogenetic analysis of human bocavirus (HBoV). Virus Res 129: 54–57
157 Qu XW, Duan ZJ, Qi ZY, Xie ZP, Gao HC, Liu WP, Huang CP, Peng FW, Zheng LS, Hou YD (2007) Human bocavirus infection, People's Republic of China. *Emerg Infect Dis* 13: 165–168
158 Arnold JC, Singh KK, Spector SA, Sawyer MH (2006) Human bocavirus: Prevalence and clinical spectrum at a children's hospital. *Clin Infect Dis* 6: 109
159 Hindiyeh M, Keller N, Mandelboim M, Ram D, Rubinov J, Regev L, Levy V, Orzitzer S, Shaharabani H, Aza, R et al. (1008) High rate of human bocavirus and adenovirus co-infection in hospitalized Israeli children. *J Clin Microbiol* 46: 334–337
160 Lindner J, Zehentmaier S, Franssila R, Schroeder J, Barabas S, Deml L, Modrow

S (2008) CD4+ T helper cell responses against human bocavirus VP2 virus-like particles in healthy adults. *J Infect Dis* 198: 1677–1684

161 Choi JH, Chung YS, Kim KS, Lee WJ, Chung IY, Oh HB, Kang C (2008) Development of real time PCR assays for detection and quantification of human bocavirus. *J Clin Virol* 42: 249–253

162 McIntosh K (1996) Coronaviruses. In: BN Fields, DM Knipe, PM Howley et al. (eds): *Fields Virology*, 3rd edn. Lippincott-Raven, New York, 1095–1103

163 Tyrrell DA, Bynoe ML (1965) Cultivation of a novel type of common-cold virus in organ cultures. *Br Med J* 1: 1467–1470

164 Hamre D, Procknow JJ (1966) A new virus isolated from the human respiratory tract. *Proc Soc Exp Biol Med* 121: 190–193

165 McIntosh K, Dees JH, Becker WB, Kapikian AZ, Chanock RM (1967) Recovery in tracheal organ cultures of novel viruses from patients with respiratory disease. *Proc Natl Acad Sci USA* 57: 933–940

166 Drosten C, Günther S, Preiser W, van der Werf S, Brodt HR, Becker S, Rabenau H, Panning M, Kolesnikova L, Fouchier RA et al. (2003) Identification of a novel coronavirus in patients with acute respiratory syndrome. *N Engl J Med* 348: 1967–1976

167 Ksiazek TG, Erdman D, Goldsmith CS, Zaki SR, Peret T, Emery S, Tong S, Urbani C, Comer JA, Lim W et al. (2003) A novel coronavirus associated with severe acute respiratory syndrome. *N Engl J Med* 348: 1953–1966

168 van der Hoek L, Pyrc K, Jebbink MF, Vermeulen-Oost W, Berkhout RJ, Wolthers KC, Wertheim-van Dillen PM, Kaandorp J, Spaargaren J, Berkhout B (2004) Identification of a new human coronavirus. *Nat Med* 10: 368–373

169 Woo PC, Lau SK, Chu CM, Chan KH, Tsoi HW, Huang Y, Wong BH, Poon RW, Cai JJ, Luk WK et al. (2005) Characterization and complete genome sequence of a novel coronavirus, coronavirus HKU1, from patients with pneumonia. *J Virol* 79: 884–895

170 Virus Taxonomy 2008. International Committee on Taxonomy of Viruses. http://www.ictvonline.org/virusTaxonomy.aspref, retrieved on September 30, 2008

171 Cavanagh D (2005) *Coronaviridae: A review of coronaviruses and torovirus*. Birkhäuser, Basel, 1–54

172 Eickmann M, Becker S, Klenk HD, Doerr HW, Stadler K, Censini S, Guidotti S, Masignani V, Scarselli M, Mora M et al. (2003) Phylogeny of the SARS coronavirus. *Science* 302: 1504–1505

173 Cavanagh D (1995) The coronavirus surface glycoprotein. In: SG Siddell (ed): *The Coronaviridae*. Plenum Press, New York, 73–113

174 Rottier PJM (1995) The coronavirus membrane glycoprotein. In: SG Siddell (ed): *The Coronaviridae*. Plenum Press, New York, 115–139

175 Siddell SG (1995) The small membrane protein. In: SG Siddell (ed): *The Coronaviridae*. Plenum Press, New York, 181–189

176 Brian DA, Hogue BG, Kienzle TE (1995) The coronavirus hemagglutinin esterase glycoprotein. In: SG Siddell (ed): *The Coronaviridae*. Plenum Press, New York, 141–163

177 Vlasak R, Luytjes W, Spaan W, Palese P (1988) Human and bovine coronaviruses recognize sialic acid-containing receptors similar to those of influenza C viruses. *Proc Natl Acad Sci USA* 85: 4526–4529

178 Laude H, Masters, PS (1995) The coronavirus nucleocapsid protein. In: SG Siddell (ed): *The Coronaviridae*. Plenum Press, New York, 141–163
179 Schultze B, Wahn K, Klenk HD, Herrler G (1991) Isolated HE protein from hemagglutinating encephalomyelitis virus and bovine coronavirus has receptor-destroying and receptor-binding activity. *Virology* 180: 221–228
180 Tresnan DB, Levis R, Holmes KV (1996) Feline aminopeptidase N serves as a receptor for feline, canine, porcine and human coronaviruses in serogroup 1. *J Virol* 70: 8669–8674
181 Li W, Moore MJ, Vasilieva N, Soi J, Wong SK, Berne MA, Somasunduran M, Sullivan JL, Luzuriaga K, Greenough TC et al. (2003) Angiotensin-converting enzyme 2 is a functional receptor for the SARS coronavirus. *Nature* 426: 450–454
182 Zelus BD, Schickli JH, Blau DM, Weiss SR, Holmes KV (2003) Conformational changes in the spike glycoprotein of murine coronavirus are induced at 37 degrees C either by soluble murine CEACAM1 receptors or by pH 8. *J Virol* 77: 830–840
183 Gallagher TM, Buchmeier MJ (2001) Coronavirus spike proteins in viral entry and pathogenesis. *Virology* 279: 371–374
184 Lai MMC, Cavanagh D (1997) The molecular biology of coronaviruses. *Adv Virus Res* 48: 1–100
185 Bradburne AF, Bynoe ML, Tyrrell DA (1967) Effects of a "new" human respiratory virus in volunteers. *Br Med J* 3: 767–769
186 Pene F, Merlat A, Vabret A, Rozenberg F, Buzyn A, Dreyfus F, Cariou A, Freymuth F, Lebon P (2003) Coronavirus 229E-related pneumonia in immunocompromised patients. *Clin Infect Dis* 37: 920–932
187 van der Hoek L, Pyrc K, Berkhout B (2006) Human coronavirus NL 63, a new respiratory virus. *FEMS Microbiol Rev* 30: 760–737
188 van Elden LJ, van Loon AM, van Alphen F, Hendriksen KA, Hoepelman AI, van Kraaij MG, Oosterheert JJ, Schipper P, Schuurman R, Nijhuis M (2004) Frequent detection of human coronaviruses in clinical specimens from patients with respiratory tract infection by use of a novel real-time reverse-transcriptase polymerase chain reaction. *J Infect Dis* 189: 652–657
189 McKean MC, Leech M, Lambert PC, Hewitt C, Myint S, Silverman M (2001) A model of viral wheeze in nonasthmatic adults: Symptoms and physiology. *Eur Respir J* 18–23–32
190 Fouchier RA, Hartwig NG, Bestebroer TM, Niemeyer B, de Jong JC, Simon JH, Osterhaus AD (2004) A previously undescribed coronavirus associated with respiratory disease in humans. *Proc Natl Acad Sci USA* 101: 6212–6216
191 Bastien N, Anderson K, Hart L, Van Caeseele P, Brandt K, Milley D, Hatchette T, Weiss EC, Li Y (2005) Human coronavirus NL63 infection in Canada. *J Infect Dis* 191: 503–506
192 Forster J, Ihorst G, Rieger CH, Stephan V, Frank HD, Gurth H, Berner R, Rohwedder A, Werchau H, Schumacher M et al. (2004) Prospective population-based study of viral lower respiratory tract infections in children under 3 years of age (the PRI.DE study). *Eur J Pediatr* 163: 709–716
193 Konig B, Konig W, Arnold R, Werchau H, Ihorst G, Forster J (2004) Prospective

study of human metapneumovirus infection in children less than 3 years of age. *J Clin Microbiol* 42: 4632–4635
194 Woo PC, Lau SK, Tsoi HW, Huang Y, Poon RW, Chu CM, Lee RA, Luk WK, Wong GK, Wong BH et al. (2005) Clinical and molecular epidemiological features of coronavirus HKU1-associated community-acquired pneumonia. *J Infect Dis* 192: 1898–18907
195 Sloots TP, Mc Erlean P, Speicher DJ, Arden KE, Nissen MD, Mackay IM (2006) Evidence of human coronavirus HKU1 and human bocavirus in Australian children. *J Clin Virol* 35: 99–102
196 Vabret A, Dina J, Gouarin S, Petitjean J, Corbet S, Freymuth F (2006) Detection of the new human coronavirus HKU1: A report of 6 cases. *Clin Infect Dis* 42: 634–639
197 Holmes KV (1999) Coronaviruses. In: A Granoff, RG Webster (1999) *Encyclopedia of Virology,* 2nd edn. Academic Press, San Diego, 291–298
198 Cavanagh D (2004) Coronaviruses and toroviruses. In: AJ Zuckerman, JE Banatvala PD Griffiths JR Pattison BD Schoub (eds): *Principles and Practice of Clinical Virology,* 5th edn. John Wiley & Sons, Chichester, 379–397
199 Bradburne AF, Somerset BA (1972) Coronative antibody titers in sera of healthy adults and experimentally infected volunteers. *J Hyg (Lond)* 70: 235–244
200 Hoffmann H, Pyrc K, van der Hoek L, Geier M, Berkhout B, Pohlmann S (2005) Human coronavirus NL63 employs the severe acute respiratory syndrome coronavirus receptor for cellular entry. *Proc Natl Acad Sci USA* 102: 7988–7993
201 Li W, Shi Z, Yu M, Ren W, Smith C, Epstein JH, Wang H, Crameri G, Hu Z, Zhang H et al. (2005) Bats are natural reservoirs of SARS-like coronaviruses. *Science* 310: 676–679
202 Lau SK, Woo PC, Li KS, Huang Y, Tsoi HW, Wong BH, Wong SS, Leung SY, Chan KH, Yuen KY (2005) Severe acute respiratory syncytial virus in Chinese horseshoe bats. *Proc Natl Acad Sci USA* 102: 14040–14045
203 Golda A, Pyrc K (2008) Recent antiviral strategies against coronavirus-related respiratory illnesses. *Curr Opin Pulm Med* 14: 248–253
204 Initiative for Vaccine Research: Influenza virus, World Health Organization, http: //www.who.int/vaccine_research/diseases/ari/en/index.html#disease%20burden, retrieved on October 20, 2008
205 Lofgren E, Fefferman N, Naumov YN, Gorski J, Naumova EN (2007) Influenza seasonality: Underlying causes and modeling theories. *J Virol* 81: 5429–5436
206 Shaw ML, Palese P (2007) Orthomyxoviridae: The viruses and their replication. In: DM Knipe, PM Howley (eds): *Fields Virology*, 5th edn. Lippincott Williams & Wilkins, Philadelphia, 1647–1689
207 Mubareka S, Palese P (2008) Influenza virus: The biology of a changing virus. In: R Rappuoli, G Del Giudice (eds): *Influenza vaccines for the future.* Birkhäuser, Basel, 9–30
208 Nunes-Correia I, Eulalio A, Nir S, Pedroso de Lima MC (2004) Caveolae as an additional route for influenza virus endocytosis in MDCK cells. *Cell Mol Biol Lett* 9: 47–60
209 Takeda M, Pekosz A, Shuck K, Pinto LH, Lamb RA (2002) Influenza A

virusM2 ion channel activity is essential for efficient replication in tissue culture. *J Virol* 76: 1391–1399
210 Suzuki Y, Ito T, Suzuki T, Holland RE Jr, Chambers TM, Kiso M, Ishida H. Kawaoka Y (2000) Sialic acid species as a determinant of the host range of influenza A viruses. *J Virol* 74: 11825–11831
211 Call SA, Vollenweider MA, Hornung CA, Simel DL, McKinney WP (2005) Does this patient have influenza? JAMA 293: 987–997
212 Studahl M (2003) Influenza virus and CNS manifestations. *J Clin Virol* 28: 225–232
213 Bhat N, Wright JG, Broder KR, Murray EL, Greenberg ME, Glover MJ, Likos AM, Posey DL, Klimov A, Lindstrom SE et al. (2005) Influenza-associated deaths among children in the United States, 2003–2004. *N Engl J Med* 353: 2559–2567
214 Jaimovich DG, Kumar A, Shabino CL, Formoli R (1992) Influenza B virus infection associated with non-bacterial septic shock-like illness. *J Infect* 25: 311–315
215 Guarner J, Paddock CD, Shieh WJ, Packard MM, Patel M, Montague JL, Uyeki TM, Bhat N, Balish A, Lindstrom S et al. (2006) Histopathologic and immunohistochemical features of fatal influenza virus infection in children during the 2003–2004 season. *Clin Infect Dis* 43: 132–140
216 Osterhaus AD, Rimmelzwaan GF, Martina BE, Bestebroer TM, Fouchier RA (2000) Influenza B virus in seals. *Science* 288: 1051–1053
217 Rogers GN, Pritchett TJ, Lane JL, Paulson JC (1983) Differential sensitivity of human, avian, and equine influenza A viruses to a glycoprotein inhibitor of infection: Selection of receptor specific variants. *Virology* 131: 394–408
218 Rogers GN, Paulson JC (1983) Receptor determinants of human and animal influenza virus isolates: Differences in receptor specificity of the H3 hemagglutinin based on species of origin. *Virology* 127: 361–373
219 Fitch WM, Leiter JM, Li XQ, Palese P (1991) Positive Darwinian evolution in human influenza A viruses. *Proc Natl Acad Sci USA* 88: 4270–4274
220 Simonsen L, Viboud C, Taylor RJ, Miller MA (2008) The epidemiology of influenza and its control. In: R Rappuoli, G Del Giudice (eds): *Influenza vaccines for the future*. Birkhäuser, Basel, 65–93
221 Edwards KM (2008) Influenza and influenza vaccination In: R Rappuoli, G Del Giudice (eds): *Influenza vaccines for the future*. Birkhäuser, Basel, 95–111
222 Rappuoli R, Del Giudice G (2008) Waiting for a pandemic. In: R Rappuoli, G Del Giudice (eds): *Influenza vaccines for the future*. Birkhäuser, Basel, Boston, Berlin, 261–279

Common Cold
ed. by R. Eccles and O. Weber

Etiology of the common cold: Modulating factors

William J. Doyle[1] and Sheldon Cohen[2]

[1]*Department of Otolaryngology, University of Pittsburgh, 3000 Mt Royal Blvd, Glenshaw PA 15116, USA*
[2]*Department of Psychology, Carnegie Mellon University, Pittsburgh, PA 15213, USA*

Abstract

The development of a "cold-like illness" (CLI) usually requires infection with an upper respiratory virus such as rhinovirus, influenza virus, respiratory syncytial virus, parainfluenza virus, coronavirus or adenovirus, among others, and the development of sufficient signs, symptoms and pathophysiologies to qualify as being ill based on personal and cultural definitions. A viral upper respiratory tract infection (vURTI) in the absence of overt illness (subclinical vURTI) will not be made manifest to the individual or to observers and, therefore, will not be diagnosed as a CLI. The degree of illness occurring during a vURTI is directly related to the extent of provoked inflammation, which in turn depends on the engagement of antiviral defense systems. Thus, risk factors for CLI can modulate either the vURTI risk by affecting virus exposure and/or susceptibility to infection, or the CLI risk given a vURTI by affecting immunocompetence, the provoked inflammation and/or the interpretation of illness as a CLI. In this chapter, we review published studies for evidence of CLI risk-modulating factors and report that climate, crowding and perhaps female gender can affect the probability of exposure to vURTI viruses, that extant immunological factors and age can affect the probability of virus infection given exposure, that stress levels (moderated by social environment), health practices (exercise, tobacco and alcohol consumption, sleep efficiency) and genetics contribute to CLI risk most probably by modulating the immune-inflammatory response to infection, and that other factors such as pollution, home environment and certain personality traits affect CLI risk by biasing illness interpretation for a given set of symptoms and signs.

Introduction

This chapter reviews those factors that are suspected or proven to influence an individual's susceptibility to the 'common cold'. Because the common cold is an illness attributable to a viral upper respiratory infection (vURTI), we need to consider factors that moderate an individual's risk for infection with a common cold virus as well as those that moderate illness expression in infected individuals. Before reviewing the results of specific studies that address these issues, it is necessary to present a general background for purposes of establishing definitions and introducing certain concepts that lay the foundation for that discussion.

Definition of the 'common cold'

The first reported use of 'a cold' as an illness descriptor was in 1537 and reflected the noted similarities between the symptoms and signs of the 'disease condition' and the physiological responses to cold temperature exposure [1]. Indeed, a belief that cold air exposure caused the common cold was widespread during the time of Benjamin Franklin (1706–1790), who countered that developing the illness depended on contact with ill persons [2]. Much later it was shown that most illnesses recognized as a common cold were caused by viruses that infect the upper respiratory tract [3]. Recent definitions for the common cold note its infectious etiology, but still focus on a listing of the signs and symptoms characteristic of the illness. For example, the Merriam-Webster Medical dictionary defines the common cold as: "an acute contagious disease of the upper respiratory tract that is marked by inflammation of the mucous membranes of the nose, throat, eyes and Eustachian tubes with a watery then purulent discharge and is caused by any of several viruses" [4]. Thus, in discussing the common cold, we are referring to a culturally accepted constellation of upper respiratory symptoms (if perceptible only by the affected person) and signs (if perceptible by both affected persons and observers) [5] that signals the presence of a vURTI caused by rhinovirus (RV), respiratory syncytial virus (RSV), adenovirus, influenza virus, parainfluenza virus, coronavirus and metapneumovirus, among others [6–10]. While usually self-limiting and of short duration, vURTIs can be associated with a variety of complications [8, 11, 12] that include otitis media [10, 13, 14], sinusitis [15], bronchiolitis [11], asthma exacerbations [16, 17] and pneumonia [18]. Because the use of 'common cold' as an illness descriptor often carries the implicit connotation of RV infection, here we use the more inclusive term, cold-like illness (CLI) in referring to upper respiratory illness during a vURTI.

Definition of the viral symptom/sign complex

The viral symptom/sign complex (vSSC) is a summary measure of illness during a suspected vURTI and can be defined by the magnitudes and durations for a set of commonly expressed symptom and/or sign elements [19]. Most simply, the vSSC is measured as the area under the curve (AUC) relating the sum of vSSC element magnitudes to time for a specified period. In research, a commonly used vSSC element set is that originally defined by Jackson to include sneezing, runny nose, nasal congestion, sore-throat, cough, malaise, chills and headache [20, 21]. In other vSSC constructions, these elements are supplemented with additional symptoms/signs of an uncomplicated vURTI (e.g., confusion, insomnia, anorexia, fever, muscle ache and joint pain, among others) and/or the symptoms/signs associated with vURTI complications such as earache (otitis media), sinus pain/fullness (sinusitis), wheezing (bronchiolitis, asthma exacerbation) and chest congestion/difficulty breathing (pneumonia) [22]. While the viruses that cause vURTIs are diverse, the vSSC for all viruses is similar with few consistently expressed elements that would allow for assignment of an illness episode to a particular virus or group of viruses in the absence of additional information such as seasonality [5, 23–25].

CLI, vSSC and vURTI relationships

The vSSC is not equivalent to a CLI, but rather the vSSC is used by an assessor to define the presence of a CLI based on past experiences and cultural context. The symptom vSSC is used by affected individuals in making judgments as to whether or not they have a CLI, while the sign vSSC is used by others to mark an individual as 'ill' for possible contact avoidance [26]. Thus, persons assign themselves (and others) as to whether or not they 'have' a CLI based on selected aspects of vSSC and not on the presence/absence of vURTI. Importantly, a vSSC and the derived CLI assignment are not prerequisite expressions of a vURTI [27–31]. For example, experimental exposure of susceptible adults to usual vURTI viruses (influenza A virus, RV, RSV) causes a CLI in only about 60% of those with documented infection [32–34] and nasal/nasopharyngeal detection of vURTI viruses in children is associated with a parent-identified CLI for the child in only about 60–85% of the detections [35]. Moreover, the frequencies of vURTI complications are only partially conditioned by the vSSC or presence of a CLI [10, 14, 36]. These relationships are illustrated in the Venn diagram presented as Figure 1 where the CLI set is a subset of the vSSC set, which, in turn, is a subset of the vURTI set, but the intersection of the complication set with that for either the vSSC or CLI is not unity.

CLI assignments

Figure 2a shows an idealized vSSC (sum of element magnitudes *versus* time) for a vURTI. There, the onset of increased vSSC magnitude occurs at a variable time after virus infection and the vSSC magnitude shows a curvilinear increase to a plateau and then a decrease to baseline [19]. This type of curve embeds a number of signals that can be abstracted by an individual for purposes of assigning the presence of a CLI. These include, the AUC, the rate of change in vSSC magnitude between days or over a period of days after illness onset (slope of the vSSC rise), the maximum vSSC magnitude and the time

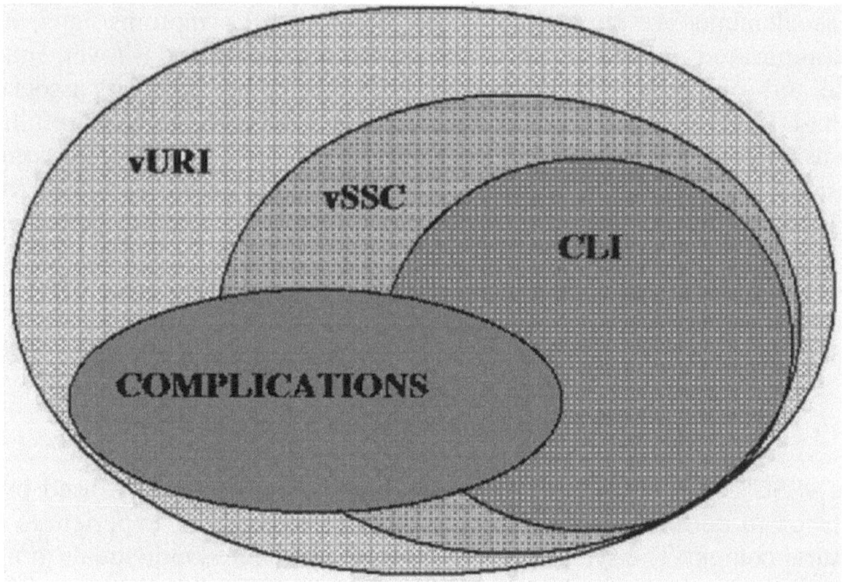

Figure 1. Modified Venn diagram depicting the nested relationships among a vURTI, the vSSC, a CLI and complications.

during which the vSSC magnitude exceeds a certain value (width of the time-window bounding the vSSC at a specified vSSC magnitude). Studies of CLI assignments made by adult subjects with experimental vURTIs and by parents for their children with natural vURTIs show that different persons may use different signals to make their CLI assignments [19, 22] and document a relative weighting of the vSSC elements (e.g., greater weight for rhinorrhea and nasal congestion when compared to other elements) used in vSSC construction that is not uniform across the population. For these reasons, there is not a 1:1 correspondence between an objectively measured vSSC and an individual's subjectively constructed vSSC or between either type of vSSC and an individual's CLI assignment. This is made explicit in the Jackson definition of a clinical 'cold', which requires either an individual's assignment of a CLI and the concurrent presence of specific symptom vSSC elements or a symptom vSSC that conforms to certain criteria [20, 21]. Recognizing that perceived symptoms need not scale linearly with objectively measured signs [37–39], some investigators differentiate subjective and objective CLIs (clinical colds). For example, Cohen and colleagues defined a subjective CLI using the Jackson criteria as modified by Gwaltney and colleagues [40] and an objective CLI using measurable vSSC sign elements [41].

Figure 2b shows a more realistic vSSC that includes a discrepancy between the subjective (dashed curve) and objective vSSCs (solid curve), a pre-exposure, basal SSC (bSSC) and two (T1 and T2) subjective vSSC magnitude thresholds for assigning a CLI. From this vSSC representation, it

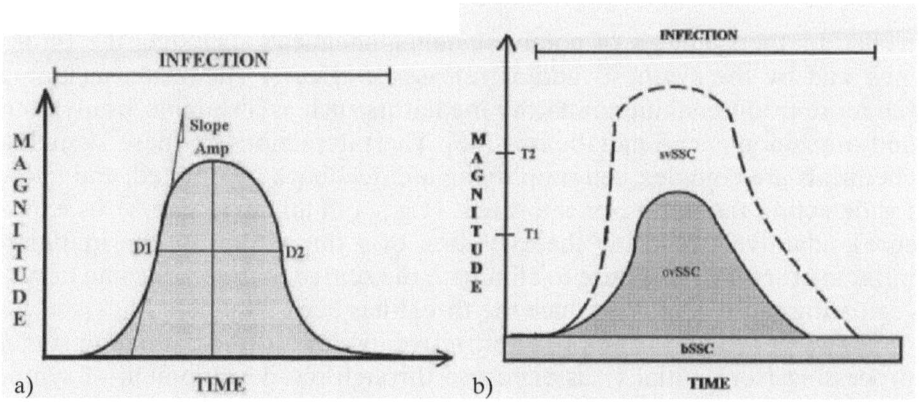

Figure 2. (a) Simple depiction of a vSSC represented by the function relating the sum of symptom or sign element magnitudes to time. Signals for extracting the presence or absence of a CLI include the slope of the vSSC rise (Slope), the maximum vSSC magnitude (Amp), the width of the time-window bounding the vSSC at a specified vSSC magnitude (D2-D1) and the AUC (shaded area). (b) A more realistic vSSC that includes a discrepancy between the subjective (svSSC, dashed curve) and objective vSSCs (ovSSC, solid curve), a pre-exposure, basal SSC (bSSC) and two (T1 and T2) subjective vSSC magnitude thresholds for assigning a CLI.

is clear that CLI assignment can be affected by the chosen threshold criterion (either T1 or T2), by the subjective vSSC bias (difference between the subjective and objective vSSC) and by the magnitude of the bSSC. Also, the objective vSSC can be modified by changes in the inflammatory reactivity of the upper respiratory tract as measured by the magnitude of provoked inflammation for a given stimulus intensity. For example, reactivity can be dramatically increased by pre-exposure to certain inflammatory stimuli (e.g., allergy, pollutants, cold air), a phenomenon termed 'priming' [42]. Priming by a non-vURTI stimulus would be manifest as an increased objective vSSC and a higher probability of CLI assignment during a vURTI. Alternatively, a vURTI can 'prime' the upper respiratory tract to other inflammatory stimuli such as cold air [43], which would increase the objective vSSC and possibly transform a subclinical vURTI into a CLI. These effects may partly explain modulation of CLI risk by certain personality traits (e.g., positive subjective vSSC bias attributable to neuroticism [38]), adverse environments (e.g., increased bSSC attributable to air pollution [44]), allergy (e.g., priming of the vSSC by household mold [45]), cold weather (e.g., priming of the inflammatory response to cold air by a vURTI [43]) and by other factors described in the Results section.

Interpretive model

Numerous studies document that the immune-inflammatory responses of the upper respiratory tract to a noxious stimulus are orchestrated and controlled by the synthesis of potent signaling chemicals, including the cytokines, and by the synthesis and/or release of effector chemicals, including the more traditional inflammatory mediators such as histamine, bradykinin and arachidonic acid metabolites [46]. The interactions of these signaling chemicals are complex, self-amplifying and feedback modulated, and allow for detecting the nature of the threat (e.g., pollutant, allergen, virus exposure), adaptively tailoring the evolution of a threat-appropriate immune-inflammatory host response to eliminate the source of the threat, and down-regulating those responses once the threat has been eliminated.

Figure 3 presents a simple interpretive model for understanding signal processing from initial virus exposure through the development of symptoms, signs and complications during the course of a vURTI and for defining the various nodes at which modulating factors can act. Briefly, virus exposure is processed by a set of biological filters that may or may not prevent infection and/or limit viral replication and viral spread to adjacent cells. These filters are tuned by environmental factors (e.g., air pollution, cigarette smoke exposure), genetic factors (e.g., HLA haplotypes), the functionality of existing physical barriers to infection (e.g., mucociliary clearance system) and the immune status of the host (e.g., extant presence of non-specific antiviral chemicals, homotypic sIgA antiviral antibody titers). If infection is established, viral sensors detect the event and trigger the activation and/or up-regulation of the innate immune system and of both the humoral and cellular components of the adaptive immune systems. In turn, these systems up-regulate the activities of the biological filters with the teleological goals of progressively decreasing viral load, limiting viral spread to adjacent anatomical compartments, eliminating infected cells, preventing secondary bacterial infections, establishing immune memory to prevent re-infection with the same virus and healing the damaged mucosa [26]. Failure to achieve threat-appropriate responses or to adequately coordinate the up- and down-regulation of these responses can lead to the development of an exaggerated inflammatory response as well as to vURTI complications.

Activation of these signaling pathways generates an inflammatory response that is expressed as the symptom and sign elements of the vSSC [5]. Because that inflammatory response provides feedback modulation to the biological filters, many of the vSSC elements can be considered to be protective. For example, nasal congestion can prevent further inhalation of aerosolized virus, rhinorrhea can provide a vehicle for the delivery of specific and nonspecific antiviral chemicals and effector cells to the infected mucosa, sneezing and cough can forcibly expel virus laden secretions from the upper and lower respiratory tracts, respectively, fever can create an inhospitable environment for viral replication and anorexia may modulate T-helper (Th1/Th2) balance [26, 47–49]. However, pharmacological interventions that moderate selected aspects of the inflammatory response are not associated with either delayed viral clearance or delayed CLI resolution

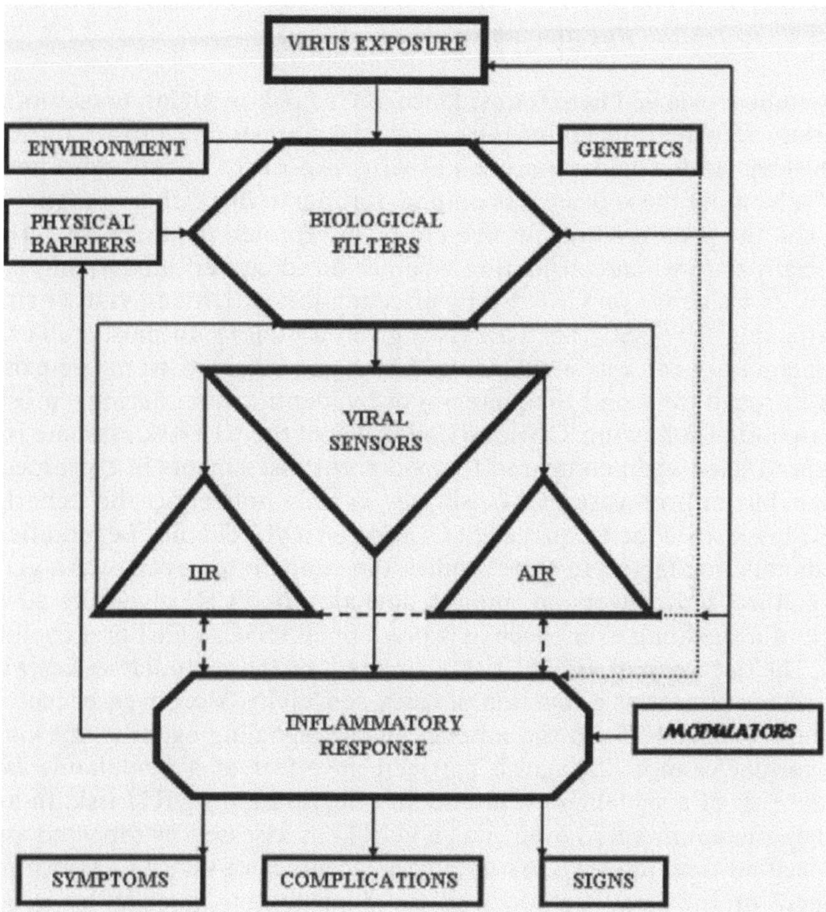

Figure 3. A simple interpretive model illustrating the pathways for signal processing from initial virus exposure through the development of symptoms, signs and complications during the course of a vURTI and for defining the various nodes at which modulating factors act (AIR, adaptive immune response; IIR, innate immune response).

[50–52] and vURTI resolution is not delayed in persons who fail to develop a vSSC or a CLI [32, 53]. Thus, much of the inflammatory response represented as the vSSC may be peripheral to host defense and modifiable by CLI risk factors independent of an effect on immunocompetence.

Modulators that affect CLI risk can act on a variety of nodes in these pathways, e.g., by reducing/enhancing the risk of virus exposure, modifying the initial state of the biological filters, modifying the innate and/or adaptive immune responses and controlling the inflammatory response as reflected in the objective vSSC. Also, as discussed above, these modulators could affect the interpretation of the objective vSSC as a subjective vSSC and as a CLI.

Caveats to results interpretation

The studies reviewed here for evidence of CLI risk-modulating factors used a variety of formats including retrospective cohort studies, prospective natural history studies and experimental virus exposures in otherwise healthy adults. None of these designs is optimal for identifying risk-modulating factors and the presented results need to be interpreted in perspective. This is especially true when considering whether an identified modulating factor exerts its influence on CLI risk by affecting the underlying vURTI risk or by affecting the vSSC (i.e., CLI risk) given a vURTI. In most studies, the enumerated event was a subjective CLI as ascertained from pre-existing data by recall for a past time interval or by identification during a prospective period of follow-up. Obviously, accuracy of the CLI risk estimate is less for recall data when compared to concurrent assessments in a prospective design, but in both cases, CLI risk may or may not reflect the underlying vURTI risk since the frequency of CLIs given a vURTI may be modified by the modulating factor. In some studies, the enumerated event was a vURTI (by culture, seroconversion, antigen detection or PCR) given the co-existence of a signaling event such as a predefined vSSC, a CLI or a complication. The accuracy of vURTI risk estimates for these studies varies within and across viruses as a function of assay sensitivity. Moreover, because the frequency of vURTIs in the absence of the signaling event is not known, this format cannot distinguish between an effect of a modulating factor on the risk of a signaling event and an effect on the vURTI risk. In a few studies, the enumerated event was a vURTI as assessed by repeated assays at specified time intervals. As noted, the accuracy of vURTI risk estimates depends on the assay method used and documenting an event by seroconversion alone is troublesome since modulating factors may affect the rate of seroconversion given a vURTI. Nonetheless, this study format provides reasonable estimates of vURTI risk for evaluating the effects of potential modulating factors. A number of the reviewed studies used experimental virus challenge (exposure) in adult humans to evaluate the effect of modulating factors on CLI and vURTI risk. That format provides good control over subject susceptibility to the challenge virus, virus exposure dose and potential confounding factors, accurate pre-exposure assessments of the risk factor(s) under study, and the capability for accurate assessments of the provoked subjective and objective vSSC, CLIs and vURTIs. However, in many of the reviewed studies, a relatively high frequency of virus infection in the challenged population was documented. Thus, for this format, it is often difficult to evaluate the effect of modulating factors on vURTI risk and most, but not all, studies report the effect of those factors on CLI risk given a vURTI. In the presented review, an attempt is made to distinguish between the effects of a modulating factor on CLI and vURTI risks by using CLI risk to indicate the relative incidence of CLIs without attempted confirmation of viral infection, CLIv risk to indicate the relative incidence of CLIs with confirmed viral infection, and vURTI risk to indicate the relative incidence of confirmed viral infections with/without CLIs and/or complications.

Results

In this section, evidence supporting the effects of different modulators on the vSSC and on the CLI and vURTI risks in humans is reviewed. The section is organized under general headings of Environmental and Host factors and, within each, nested listings of factors with evidence supporting CLI risk modulation. This organization follows a simple logical outline but is somewhat arbitrary in that the position of a given modulator could be reasonably reassigned to a different category. Also, the presented list of modulators should be considered to be representative and not necessarily exhaustive.

Environmental modulators

Climate

Early research documented a pronounced CLI seasonality for temperate climates with the incidence of illness in a community being relatively low in the warmer, summer months and high in the colder months [54]. After the introduction of assays for specific viruses, this effect was shown to mirror seasonal patterns in vURTIs caused by RV, influenza virus, RSV and parainfluenza virus, among other viruses [27, 55–59]. For example, while rvURTIs were detected year round, but with a major peak in the fall and a minor peak in the spring, vURTIs caused by each of the other viruses showed a more discrete fall-winter, winter, or winter-spring peak and more restricted temporal activity [60, 61]. Slight shifts in the months of peak rvURTI incidence were noted for different geographical areas and the seasonality of all vURTI viruses worldwide was shown to be different for temperate, cold or rainy climates [61–64].

Recent developments including PCR for virus detection and determination of phylogenetic relationships among virus strains [65], advanced computer modeling of viral spread [66, 67] and the establishment of multisite consortiums covering a wide range of climates [68] have led to a better, although still incomplete, understanding of the role played by climate in determining vURTI and CLI risks. Current models of climate effects on CLI and vURTI incidence involve a complex, virus-specific interplay among meteorological variables [68–71], physiochemical properties of the virus [72–74], virus reservoir [75–77], mechanism of virus transmission [67], spatial density of the population [78], distribution of 'susceptibility' to infection in the population [66, 67] and human behavior [65]. Nonetheless, for a given virus such as RSV [68] or influenza [69], meteorological variables including temperature, relative humidity, barometric pressure and ultraviolet radiation can explain as much as 40% of the variance in vURTI risk and this appears to be closely related to the physical conditions favoring virus survival [72–74].

Crowding

Crowding, a measure of population density at the community (e.g., persons per square mile), housing (e.g., people per room) and congregational (e.g., preschool, school) levels, can increase CLI incidence by increasing virus-exposure rates. Cross-sectional studies of populations living in crowded communities support this effect. For example, Bang and colleagues [79] compared CLI incidence among three low income communities in West Bengal and reported the highest incidence for a 'crowded' urban community, an intermediate incidence for a suburban village and the least incidence in an isolated village. While other CLI risk factors were reported to be similar for the three settings, in general, these types of studies are characterized by problems with CLI documentation and with control over confounding factors [e.g., socioeconomic status (SES), air pollution, malnutrition]. However, crowding was also demonstrated to increase vURTI risk in family studies where vURTI incidence within the family was directly proportional to the number of children sharing a bedroom [80] and CLI spread from child to mother was common [81]. Day care or preschool, school, shared work areas, community homes and hospitals can be considered to be environments characterized by crowding. Day care is consistently identified as a CLI risk factor [11, 82–85], opening of the school year is coincident with the peak in rvURTI incidence [61], sharing an office with one or more colleagues was reported to significantly increase CLI risk [86] and nosocomial vURTIs are common in the hospital and nursing home environments [87–89].

Pollution

Air pollution is associated with generalized upper and lower respiratory symptoms and signs [44, 90, 91], and has been identified as a possible CLI risk factor in a number of studies. For example, a study conducted in northern Finland compared the CLI incidence rates measured in children over a 1-year period among three cities and within two regions of one city with different levels of air pollution. CLI incidence was higher in the more polluted city when compared to the less polluted cities and in the more polluted region of a city when compared to the less polluted region [92]. A cross-sectional survey of upper respiratory illness in children from Swiss communities that had a documented decrease in particulate air pollution over a 9-year period reported a corresponding decrease in CLI incidence over that period, and this difference was retained after controlling for SES and other potential CLI risk factors [93]. Similar results were reported for a second cross-sectional community study where CLI incidence decreased as air quality improved [94].

An effect of indoor air pollution on CLI incidence was reported in a prospective study done in an industrial area of Delhi, India. There, mean indoor particulates was greater than outdoor particulates and was significantly higher in homes of children with a positive history of frequent respiratory illness (including CLIs) when compared to homes of children with a negative history [95]. Other studies reported a direct relationship between CLI incidence and the presence of moisture and mold in the home environment [45, 96].

Stress

Stress is a generalized set of diverse host responses to external or internal stimuli (stressors) that are or are perceived to be harmful [97]. Stress causes changes in immune function [98, 99] and higher levels of stress were reported to be associated with an increased risk for infectious and non-infectious diseases [100]. Stress (both physical and psychological) may be the integrating factor for such diverse influences on CLI risk as low SES [101, 102], crowding [79], intense exercise [103, 104] and job-related factors [105–108], among others.

A large body of work has focused on the CLI risk of psychological stress [109] defined as occurring when life events and demands exceed coping ability [110]. A number of studies documented a positive correlation between psychological stress levels and the vSSC. For example, in a prospective family study of life events and CLIs in 58 children, Boyce and colleagues [111] reported a significant association between negative life events and the vSSC. In an early study of experimental RV exposure in 52 adults, Totman and colleagues [112] reported a significant positive correlation between a measure of stress, the Totman Change Index, and the magnitude of virus shedding, and between a second measure of stress, the Totman Loss Index, and the provoked vSSC. A later study of 55 subjects experimentally infected with influenza A virus reported that the level of perceived stress was directly related to the provoked objective and subjective vSSC and to the post-exposure nasal IL-6 concentration [113].

Other prospective cohort studies documented a direct relationship between CLI risk and negative life events and/or perceived stress [114–121]. Using experimental virus challenge as a vURTI model, Cohen and colleagues [53] exposed 394 adult subjects to 1 of 5 upper respiratory viruses (RV types 2, 9 and 14, RSV and coronavirus) and then assessed infection and illness. Prior to exposure, they assessed the frequency of major negative life events in the past year, perceived stress and negative affect, which were combined to form a stress index for each subject. After adjusting for control variables, the rates of both provoked vURTIs and CLIvs increased with increasing values of the stress index. In a subsequent analysis of those data, they reported that that negative life events were the only significant predictor of CLIv risk, whereas perceived stress and negative affect were significant predictors of vURTI risk [122]. This pattern was reproduced in a smaller study of 17 subjects experimentally infected with RV that reported a significant positive correlation between major negative life events, but not perceived stress or negative affect, and CLIv risk [123]. In a later study, the frequency and severity of acute and chronic negative life events in the previous year was measured in 276 adult subjects who were subsequently exposed to RV and followed for the development of a CLIv [33]. The results documented that severe chronic negative life events (primarily underemployment or unemployment and enduring interpersonal difficulties with family and/or friends), but not severe acute negative life events, were associated with an increased CLIv risk.

Cohen and colleagues [41] reported that one marker of stress, urinary epinephrine, but not two others (urinary norepinephrine and cortisol), measured before RV challenge predicted CLIv risk. However, controlling for epinephrine level did not decrease the effect of the chronic negative life events on CLIv risk, suggesting independent contributions. In a prospective study of 115 adult subjects, negative life events were measured, and the physiological responses to an acute stressor assessed. The subjects were then monitored over a 12-week period for the development of a natural CLI [124]. The results documented an interaction between the cortisol response to acute stress and negative life events in predicting CLI risk, such that those who produced high levels of cortisol to the acute stressor (reactors) and had high levels of negative life events were at greater risk for a CLI than were high reactors with low levels of negative life events and low reactors irrespective of their life events. Also reported was the observation that baseline immunological measures of reactivity [$CD8^+$ number, natural killer (NK) cell number, and NK cell cytotoxicity] interacted with weekly perceived stress levels in predicting concurrent self-reported CLI episodes. For these outcomes, it was low immune reactors who were more likely to experience a CLI during high stress than low stress weeks, while high immune reactors did not exhibit differences in weekly CLIs as a function of weekly stress level. Three earlier studies in children reported that measures of the physiological response (increase in heart rate, increase in CD19 white blood cells and decreased serum antibody response to vaccination) to acute stress modulated the CLI risk associated with background stress levels [125, 126]. However, while suggestive that certain measures of the physiological response to acute stressors can discriminate between groups at high and low risk for CLIs under stressful conditions, the results of these studies were not consistent regarding the measure of the acute stress response that interacts with background stress levels to predict CLI susceptibility, and further work in this area is needed.

Social environment

There has been considerable interest in the role played by social network structure, quality and quantity of social interactions and social support in maintaining health. Past literature reviews document abundant evidence that higher levels of social support and more positive social relationships improve immunoregulation and are associated with less chronic illnesses and less all-cause mortality [127–129]. One hypothesized mechanism to explain this relationship is that quality social interactions and social supports dissipate stress, thereby attenuating the harmful effects of stress on immunity and other physiological functions [127], but this mechanism does not explain all of the beneficial health effects of social support, suggesting the existence of other linkage pathways [130]. For example, one recent study reported that adults with smaller social networks had a poorer immunological response to influenza vaccination [131].

Evidence that social support moderates CLI risk during stress was provided by the results of two longitudinal cohort studies. Evans and colleagues [118] enrolled 100 subjects in a daily diary study of desirable and undesirable events and CLIs. Desirable events were significantly decreased in frequency in the 4 days before CLI onset and individual item analyses showed that perceived intimacy, social support and self-esteem moderated the effect. Smith and colleagues [116] followed 92 asthmatic adults over 1 year for asthmatic exacerbations during a CLI. Eighty percent of the population developed at least one event, and, of those, persons reporting more negative life events and lesser levels of social support had a greater frequency of episodes. However, two studies of stress, social support and CLI risk in adults and children reported that, while higher life event stress was associated with increased CLI risk, social support buffered that risk only in those with low background stress [120, 121].

Cohen and colleagues [41] used an experimental model of virus infection to explore the role of social ties in moderating CLIv susceptibility. Two hundred and seventy-six otherwise healthy adults provided information on their participation in 12 types of social ties and were assessed for typical health practices, negative mood states and urinary cortisol and catecholamine concentrations. Then, all subjects were experimentally exposed to RV and followed for the development of CLIvs. Results showed that those participating in a greater number of social ties had significantly less virus shedding, lesser vSSCs and fewer CLIvs. The magnitude of the effect on CLIv risk was not modified after controlling for pre-challenge viral specific antibody, standard demographic variables, magnitude of viral shedding, serum levels of cortisol and catecholamines or absolute number of contacts.

Host modulators

Demographic factors

Sex, age and race

Analyses of the data from a large community study conducted between 1965 and 1981 reported that CLIvs were more frequent in males prior to the age of 3 years and in females after that age [81, 132]. Also, CLIvs were less frequent in women who worked outside of the home when compared to those who did not, an effect most likely mediated by the more frequent contact with ill children in the latter group [81]. However, sex was not identified as a predictor of CLIv risk in experimental studies of virus exposure in men and women aged 18–54 years [41, 53, 133, 134].

In the community study and in an earlier family study of CLI transmission, the CLIv incidence decreased with advancing age from a high of two to ten episodes/year in the youngest children to a low of two to four episodes per year in the oldest adults [54, 132]. More recently, Ball and colleagues [84] reported a significant interaction between day care attendance and age on CLI incidence in children. There, compared to young children raised "at home" with their mothers, children in day care experienced more CLIs/year at younger ages (<6 years) but fewer CLIs/year at older ages (>6 years). An age-dependent pattern for CLI incidence was found in a 1996 survey of illness in the United States that reported CLI (including influenza) incidences of 1.73, 0.92, 0.65, 0.64 and 0.37 CLIs/year/person for individuals aged <5 years, 5–17 years, 18–24 years, 25–44 years and >45 years, respectively [135]. However, an analysis of the data for studies of experimental viral exposure in adults aged 18–54 years did not find associations between age and CLIs [41, 53, 133, 134].

There are few comparative data for natural vURTIs and/or CLIs to determine if race influences CLIv or vURTI risk. However, analyses of the data from several large cohorts experimentally exposed to upper respiratory viruses did not evidence an association between self-assigned race (primarily White vs Black) and CLIv risk [41, 53, 133, 134].

Socioeconomic status

SES is a composite measure of economic, social and occupational status as reflected by income, education and occupation [136]. When assessed over its full scale from poverty to affluence, SES is an inverse predictor of mortality and of the risks for both acute and chronic diseases [136–138]. The effect of SES on health is believed to be mediated in part by the relationships between SES and nutrition, population demographics, health practices, daily environment, stress levels, social interactions and personality structure [136]. For example, one recent study of 196 adults reported that lower SES was associated with higher levels of two markers of ongoing stress, salivary cortisol and urinary epinephrine, with less diverse social networks and with poorer health behaviors such as higher rates of smoking, associations that were independent of race [101].

Few studies have evaluated the effect of SES on CLI risk. In an early community study, Monto and Ulman reported a higher annual CLIv incidence in persons with low family incomes when compared to those with middle or high family incomes [132]. In contrast, Alper and colleagues [139] prospectively followed 60 children from two communities aged 1–4 years by daily parental diary for CLIs over the 8 months of the typical CLI season (October through April) and recorded a total of 267 CLIs. Multivariate analysis documented a significant effect on CLI risk of age (younger > older), gender (male > female) and the CLI burden in the child's sibling (higher > lower) but no effect of SES as measured by parental education and occupation, despite significant variability in those measures for the population.

Cohen and colleagues conducted two studies of the effect of SES on the response of adult subjects to experimental virus exposure [102, 134], but neither documented an effect of concurrent SES as measured by income, education or home ownership on vURTI or CLIv risk. However, in the second study that enrolled 193 adults aged 21–55 who were exposed to influenza or RV, perceived SES as measured by where a subject believes that they rank in terms of income, education and occupation with respect to the United States population was a significant inverse predictor of CLIv risk.

There is a growing literature indicating that early childhood SES influences susceptibility to disease in adults [140]. In a study that experimentally exposed 334 adults to RV, a significant negative correlation between childhood SES as measured by years of parental home ownership and adult vURTI and CLIv risks was observed. The effect of childhood SES on CLIv susceptibility was fixed by the time of adolescence since subjects whose parents did not own their home early in life but did during adolescence were at the same increased CLIv risk as those whose parents never owned their home.

Health behaviors

Diet

A study of 1600 children in India reported a direct association between malnutrition and the incidence of CLIs with and without complications [141]. Analyses of the data from two studies of poverty in the United States (the Community Childhood Hunger Identification Project and the third National Health and Nutrition Examination Survey) documented an increased risk for CLIs in poor, food-insufficient (hungry) children when compared to poor, food-sufficient children [142].

Relatively few studies have evaluated diet as a risk factor for vURTIs and CLIs in food-sufficient persons. Cohen and colleagues [41] collected dietary data by standard questionnaire on 276 healthy volunteers who were subsequently exposed to RV. Of the dietary items (e.g., zinc, selenium, vitamins), only intake of ≤85 mg vitamin C was an independent predictor of CLIv risk. However, in a cohort study of 4273 faculty and staff at Spanish universities, daily dietary intake of vitamin C and zinc assessed by questionnaire did not predict CLI risk during the 1-year period of follow-up [143]. Also, analyses of the data for a cohort of 21 796 male smokers drawn from the Alpha-Tocopherol Beta-Carotene Cancer Prevention Study did not document an effect of dietary vitamin C and E and beta-carotene on CLI risk [144].

There is a wide variety of conventional and alternative dietary supplements that are promoted as being effective in reducing CLI risk [145, 146]. Nonetheless, there is little convincing evidence that dietary supplementation with vitamin C [144, 147], beta-carotene [144], vitamin E [144], zinc [143, 148] or *Echinacea* [149] affects CLI or vURTI risk in the general population of otherwise healthy adults. However, there is limited evidence for reduced CLI risk attributable to some of these supplements in certain subpopulations such as the elderly (vitamin E) [144, 150] and those engaged in strenuous activities (vitamin C) [151, 152]. Other studies reported prophylactic efficacy with respect to CLIs of such diverse dietary supplements as probiotic bacteria plus vitamins and minerals [153], *Camellia sinensis* (green tea) capsules [154], micronutrient-fortified beverages [155] and hydrolyzed rice bran [156], but these studies need to be replicated before the findings can be accepted.

Alcohol and tobacco use

Tobacco smoke is a major health risk and both tobacco smoke and nicotine have immunosuppressive effects [157, 158]. While debated, alcohol is considered to be immunoenhancing in low doses and immunosuppressive in high doses [159, 160] and low doses of alcohol may have anti-inflammatory effects [161]. These observations suggest that exposure to tobacco smoke will be associated with a greater risk for both vURTIs and CLIs, while moderate alcohol consumption will be associated with a lesser vSSC magnitude and a lesser frequency of CLIs when compared to populations of teetotalers or alcohol abusers.

Population-based studies focused on both passive and active tobacco smoke exposure as risk factors for CLIs and vURTIs have reported mixed results. For example, an analysis of Australian health survey data did not establish a relationship between mother, father and combined tobacco smoking and CLI risk in their children [162], but an analysis of the Women's Health Study data reported a slightly increased CLI risk in women passively exposed to cigarette smoke [163]. Interestingly, the latter study did not document an increased risk for CLIs among heavy smokers when compared to non-smokers. In contrast, a cohort study focusing on job demands and CLI risk identified cigarette smoking as a significant, independent predictor of CLI risk [105]. The results of epidemiological studies on tobacco smoking and vURTI risk are inconsistent with influenza vURTIs linked to tobacco smoking, but not vURTIs caused by other viruses [55, 164–166].

Three cohort studies reported that compared to teetotalers, persons who consumed alcoholic beverages were at decreased risk for CLIs. The first followed 92 asthmatic adults for CLIs complicated by asthma exacerbations and reported that the subgroup with no qualifying events consumed more alcohol when compared to the subgroup with qualifying events [116]. The second followed 4272 faculty and staff at five Spanish universities for CLIs after assessing each individual's 'usual' alcohol consumption by means of a questionnaire. The results showed that consumption of wine (but not total alcohol, beer or spirits intake) was associated with a lower risk for CLIs [167]. The third followed 107 adults over a 15-week period for investigator verified CLIs and reported that subjects who consumed alcohol were at significantly less risk of developing a verified CLI when compared to non-drinkers and that, for those who consumed alcohol, CLI risk was indirectly related to the amount of alcohol consumed [120].

In a study of experimental virus exposure in adults, Cohen and colleagues [168] collected data for 'typical' smoking and alcohol consumption on 322 subjects who were subsequently exposed to one of five viruses and followed for the development of a vURTI and a CLIv. Effects analyses controlled for demographics, virus type, personality, stress, antibody titer, allergy and other study variables and showed that smoking was associated with greater vURTI and CLIv risks, that alcohol consumption decreased the CLIv risk in a dose-response manner, but that 'smokers' were not protected from CLIvs by drinking alcohol. These effects of 'typical' alcohol consumption and tobacco smoking on CLIv risk were reproduced in a second study of 276 healthy adults experimentally exposed to RV [41].

Exercise

Exercise (and physical activity) affects immune function with moderate intensity, regular exercise being immunoenhancing and long-duration strenuous exercise being immunosuppressive [169–171]. These immunological effects were hypothesized to translate into an effect of exercise on vURTI and CLI risks characterized by a 'J' curve [104, 172]. There, CLI risk would be greatest in the strenuous exercisers, intermediate in sedentary persons and least in moderate exercisers. While some studies reported an increased risk for CLIs with strenuous exercise, most of these were limited to assessments of the difference between CLI incidence during training and after competition in 'elite athletes' [104]. However, inherent biases in the natural pre-selection of persons for membership in that group make generalization of any relationships to other populations tenuous [173]. Hemila and colleagues [151] reviewed those studies and noted that many were underpowered and that the results were inconsistent. Using cohort data collected on 14 401 male smokers enrolled in the Alpha-Tocopherol, Beta-Carotene Cancer Prevention Trial, they analyzed CLI risk for effects of exercise during leisure times and of physical activity at work but found no significant associations. In contrast, evidence supporting the J risk curve was provided by a recent study that prospectively assessed CLI and vURTI incidence over a 5-month period in 32 elite and 31 recreationally competitive triathletes and cyclists, and in 20 sedentary controls. As predicted by the J model, respective CLI incidences were 4.5, 0.7 and 1.9 CLIs per person for the three groups, but an infectious etiology could be documented in less than 30% of the CLIs despite the use of both culture and PCR methodologies [174].

With respect to the hypothesized effect of regular, moderate intensity exercise in lowering CLI and vURTI risks, Osterback and colleagues [175] followed school children who did and did not participate in organized sports for CLIs as assessed by maternal interview every 2 months and physical examinations every 3 months but found no between-group differences in the CLI incidence. Weidner and colleagues [176] randomly assigned 34 healthy adults to an exercise group and 16 healthy adults to a non-exercise control group and challenged all subjects with RV. Those assigned to the exercise group completed 40 minutes of supervised exercise every other day for a 10-day period and the vSSC was assessed on all subjects at 12-hour intervals. There were no significant differences in the vSSC between groups or within the exercise group before and after exercise, suggesting that moderate exercise during a vURTI does not affect the vSSC.

In contrast, regular exercise as assessed by history reduced the CLIv risk in a study of 276 healthy adults experimentally exposed to RV [41]. A later study of 61 healthy active volunteers aged 66–84 years estimated daily energy expenditure and leisure time sports activity by questionnaire at baseline and then assessed the vSSC daily by diary for 1 year. The results showed that the CLI burden (days/year with illness) and incidence were negatively correlated with both estimates of energy expenditure [177]. More recently, Chubak and colleagues [178] randomly assigned 115 overweight and obese, sedentary, postmenopausal women to either 45 minutes of moderate-intensity exercise 5 days per week or 45-minute stretching sessions once per week for 12 months and assessed CLI incidence by quarterly questionnaires. A significantly decreased CLI incidence for the exercise group relative to the control group was reported.

Sleep efficiency

Sleep deprivation is associated with altered immune function reflected as reduced NK cell activity and IL-2 production [179], increased levels of circulating pro-inflammatory cytokines [180] and poorer antibody responses to hepatitis A [181] and influenza [182] vaccinations. A cohort study comparing CLI risk assessed by retrospective questionnaire for the previous 4 months between day and shift workers reported that shift workers had poorer sleep quality, a greater number of days with fatigue and more CLI episodes [106]. Two studies of experimental RV exposure in 276 and 334 adults reported that poor sleep efficiency measured before challenge predicted increased CLIv risk [41, 133]. In a later study of 153 healthy adults aged 21–55 years, sleep duration and efficiency were measured for 14 consecutive days and then the subjects were challenged with RV and monitored for the development of vURTIs and CLIvs. The analysis documented that average sleep duration and efficiency, but not the percent of days feeling rested, were inversely related to CLIv risk. Those results were unaffected after controlling for pre-challenge virus-specific antibody, age, sex, season of the year, body mass, education, income, perceived socioeconomic rank, race and physical activity [183].

Pre-exposure virus-specific immune status

During a vURTI caused by a novel virus, the adaptive immune system participates in eliminating free virus and destroying virus-infected cells as well as in establishing an immune memory that ideally reduces the probability of reinfection with the same virus. A salient feature of the humoral component of immune memory is the development of specific antiviral antibodies resident in secretions (sIgA) and serum (IgG). In humans, the best correlate of protection from a vURTI caused by a specific virus is the pre-existing anti-virus-specific IgG antibody titer [184–186]. In animal models, virus-specific sIgA antibody protects from infection [187] but this is difficult to demonstrate in humans where the local sIgA titers are highly correlated with the respective serum IgG antibody titers [188–190]. Also, for established vURTIs, pre-existing serum IgG antibodies titers were shown to correlate inversely with the magnitude of viral shedding, the vSSC and the CLIv risk [32, 185, 186, 191, 192]. The cellular component of immune memory functions to reduce the duration of a subsequent vURTI caused by the same or related virus. Expectedly, this should be accompanied by a lesser recruitment of accessory inflammatory responses and thus a decreased vSSC and CLI risk, although this has not been conclusively demonstrated in humans.

Constitutional factors

Prospective studies reported that individuals with a history of frequent CLIs were highly likely to continue to experience frequent CLIs at later times [27, 193–196]. For example, Ball and colleagues [195] prospectively followed 858 children from birth to age 13 years. Parental recall data for child CLIs in the previous year were collected at 2, 3, 6, 8, 11 and 13 years of age. Children with more than 3 CLIs/year at 2 or 3 years of age were more likely to have frequent CLIs at the later assessment times when compared to children with infrequent CLIs at 2 or 3 years of age. This relationship held after controlling for confounding variables such as gender, ethnicity, maternal education, breast-feeding, number of persons in the household, smoking exposure and presence of pets in the household. Factors that could contribute to this CLI constitution are listed below.

Immunology

Higher than expected frequencies of deficiencies in the humoral and cellular components of the adaptive immune system were reported for patients with a history of frequent CLIs. For example, Cedzynski and colleagues [197] reported that of 335 patients aged 1–16 years with a history of recurrent CLIs, 93 (28%) had defects in the humoral immune response, 66 (20%) had disturbances in cellular immunity and 19 (6%) had both humoral and cellular abnormalities. These data suggest that children with functional immune deficiencies are at greater risk for re-infection with the same viral strain and for an exaggerated vSSC interpretable as a CLI during established vURTIs.

In persons exposed to a novel virus, a first line of defense against infection is the innate immune system. While local levels of nonspecific antiviral chemicals and other components of the innate immune system are expected to participate in protection from all vURTIs [198, 199], there are few data supporting this expectation for humans. However, a number of published studies suggest a role for the constitutional production of certain components of innate immunity as modulators of CLI risk. The majority of these studies focused on the interferons, a family of host-produced antiviral proteins that up-regulate epithelial cell resistance to virus infection [200], and reported that lower stimulated leukocyte production of interferon was associated with a higher frequency of CLIs in children [195, 201–203]. In contrast, Becker and colleagues [204] focused on ICAM-1, the epithelial cell receptor for the major RV subgroup (and other viruses), and reported an inverse relationship between CLI risk and ICAM-1 serum levels [205]. Because circulating ICAM-1 can serve as a decoy for RV attachment, they argued that protection was afforded by lowering the probability of RV attachment to epithelial cells.

Allergy and asthma are chronic diseases characterized by an altered Th1/Th2 balance of adaptive immunity [206]. Adequate Th1 function is required to eradicate viral infections and this suggests that allergic/asthmatic individuals may express a greater vSSC and thus be at greater risk for CLIs when compared to 'normal' individuals. Indeed, subtle differences between allergic and non-allergic subjects in the immune response to experimental RV, but not influenza virus, infection have been reported [207, 208]. However, the results of an experimental RV challenge study of 10 allergic and 10 non-allergic adult volunteers did not evidence between-group differences in the vSSC or in the CLIv frequency. This lack of effect was replicated in a second study that compared the upper and lower respiratory tract responses to RV infection between 11 allergic-asthmatic subjects and 10 non-allergic, non-asthmatic control subjects. No between-group differences were noted for the vSSC, cellular response, cytokine response or lower airway response to infection [209]. In a study that evaluated the possible effect of allergen priming on CLIv risk, allergic adult subjects were challenged with either allergen or placebo (10/group) three times in the week before experimental exposure to RV. No between-group differences in infection rate, vSSC magnitude, cellular response and local cytokine production were documented [210]. The results for these experimental studies are consistent with those reported for a study of natural RV infection in asthmatic and control subjects [211]. There, 76 cohabitating couples with one allergic-asthmatic and one healthy member were followed by daily diary for upper and lower respiratory symptoms, twice daily peak expiratory flow measurement and bimonthly collection of nasal secretions for RV detection. There were no between-group differences in rvURTI or CLI incidences or in the rvSSC.

Genetics

A possible genetic contribution to CLI risk is suggested by data collected during the Seattle Virus Watch where the spread of vURTIs in families was studied using nasopharyngeal virus cultures and data on CLIvs were collected from diaries [27]. Fox and colleagues reported that some families were characterized by a CLIv with every documented rvURTI, while others had no CLIvs despite frequent rvURTIs and concluded that a 'familial' factor, either environmental or genetic, controlled CLIv risk. While no studies have used twin methodologies to estimate the heritability of vURTIs or CLIs, there is evidence that genetic factors contribute to a 'CLI constitution' by affecting the vURTI risk, the CLIv risk and the risk of vURTI complications.

Human leukocyte antigens (HLAs) are encoded by genes of the major histocompatibility complex and play a prominent role in regulating the immune response to infection. Past studies reported that HLA genotype influences the humoral response to vaccination [212], while other studies attempted to associate HLA genotypes with resistance to different infectious diseases [213]. Coetzee and colleagues [214] genotyped 59 adult female members of the Bantu-speaking Tswana and collected retrospective data on the number of CLIs experienced in the previous year. HLA-B allele frequency was a significant predictor of CLI incidence but not of the number of total illnesses in the previous year. The more common HLA-B alleles in that population were associated with a lesser CLI incidence.

Mannose-binding protein (MBP) is a member of a host-produced family of collectins that plays a prominent role in innate immune defense. The gene coding for MBP is polymorphic in the population, with different genotypes being related to different levels of MBP production [215]. A number of studies investigated the role for these polymorphisms as a modifier of CLI susceptibility [216]. For example, Koch and colleagues [217] genotyped 252 children <2 years of age for MBP polymorphisms and followed the children for 2 years by weekly assessments of illness. MBP mutations associated with lesser levels of MBP production were significantly more frequent in children at high risk for CLIs, an effect that was more evident in children younger than 17 months of age.

As mentioned, the immune/inflammatory response during a vURTI is orchestrated by the synthesis of pro-inflammatory and anti-inflammatory cytokines [46]. Other studies showed that polymorphisms in the genes coding for many of these cytokines affect their synthesis [218]. Recent work focused on a possible role for these polymorphisms in determining CLI risk. Nieters and colleagues [214] genotyped 111 adults for polymorphisms in the

TNF-α (-308 G/A), IL-2 (-330 T/G), IL-10 (-1082 G/A, -819 T/C, -592 A/C), IL-6 (-174 G/C) and IFN-γ (+874 A/T) genes and assessed the frequency of CLIs by yearly interview over 2 consecutive years. They found significant associations between the IL-2 and IL-6 genotypes and CLI incidence. In a later study of 29 adults experimentally exposed to RSV and genotyped for the TNF-α, IL-10, IL-6 and IFN-γ polymorphisms, Gentile and colleagues [219] reported a significant association between the IL-6 genotype and the vSSC, and this was reproduced in a study of 31 adults experimentally exposed to RV (Doyle, unpublished). IL-6 is a cytokine whose local level during experimental vURTIs caused by RV, influenza virus and RSV correlates with the vSSC [46, 113, 220] and these results suggest that IL-6 gene polymorphisms affect CLIv risk by modifying the objective vSSC.

Other work focused on a possible role for these polymorphisms in determining the frequency of complications during a vURTI. Gentile and colleagues [221] genotyped 77 hospitalized infants <6 months of age with bronchiolitis secondary to confirmed RSV infection for TNF-α, IL-10, IL-6 and IFN-γ polymorphisms. They reported a significant association between the IL-6 genotype and length of hospital stay, between the IFN-γ genotype and presentation with otitis media and between the IL-10 genotype and presentation with pneumonia. Alper and colleagues [222] prospectively followed 230 children over the typical cold season for nasopharyngeal virus detected by PCR, CLIs by daily parental diary and otitis media by weekly otoscopy. All children were genotyped for the TNF-α, IL-10, IL-6 and IFN-γ polymorphisms. IL-10 and TNF-α genotypes were significant predictors of otitis media during rvURTIs and IL-10 genotype was a significant predictor of otitis media during rsvURTIs.

Personality

There is a growing body of evidence that an individual's personality influences basal immunity and illness risk [223], has a moderate heritability [224, 225] and is relatively stable over time [226]. Two early virus challenge studies reported that persons scoring high in introversion at entry developed a greater vSSC [112] and shed more virus [112, 227] after experimental RV exposure. Cohen and colleagues [41] measured each of the Goldberg Big 5 personality traits (extraversion, agreeableness, conscientiousness, neuroticism and openness to experience) in 276 adult subjects, exposed all subjects to RV and followed them for the development of a CLIv. Only extraversion was a predictor of CLIv risk with those scoring lower on that measure (higher on introversion) being at greater risk. In a second study, the same investigators explored whether extraversion, agreeableness and a variable combining these two traits (termed sociability) were associated with CLIv risk. There, they collected pre-exposure data for virus-specific antibody titers, demographics, health practices, social ties, salivary cortisol and urinary catecholamines in 334 healthy adults, measured the three traits and exposed all subjects to RV [133]. Increases in extraversion, agreeableness and their combination were all associated with decreasing CLIv risk. Although these traits were associated with more and higher-quality social interactions, participation in health-enhancing behaviors and better emotional regulation, controlling for those variables did not affect their relationship with CLIv risk.

Feldman and colleagues used pathway models to reanalyze the data collected in the Cohen and colleagues' study of the Big 5 Factors [41] with a focus on baseline symptoms and the subjective vSSC bias [38]. The analyses showed that neuroticism was positively correlated with unfounded symptoms both before and after virus exposure, that openness to experience was positively correlated with unfounded, post-exposure symptoms in those with a CLIv and that conscientiousness was positively correlated with unfounded, post-exposure symptoms in those without a documented CLIv. In a second study of 86 subjects experimentally exposed to either RV or influenza A virus, Cohen and colleagues [228] reported that a different measure of neuroticism, trait negative affect, was directly associated with an upwardly biased subjective vSSC.

As mentioned, negative emotional style or neuroticism was shown to be associated with greater unfounded symptoms before and after experimental virus exposure [38, 228]. In two more recent studies, Cohen and colleagues evaluated the effect on the provoked vSSC, vURTI risk and CLIv risk of a positive emotional style characterized by typically experiencing positive emotions such as "happy", "pleased" and "relaxed". The first study enrolled 334 adults, assessed positive and negative emotional styles, exposed all subjects to RV and followed the subjects for the development of a vURTI and a CLIv. The results showed that greater positive emotional style was associated with a lesser CLIv risk but not a lesser vURTI risk, that positive emotional style was associated with a downwardly biased subjective vSSC, that negative emotional style was associated with an upwardly biased subjective vSSC and that the effect of positive emotional style on CLIv risk was independent of negative emotional style [229]. In that study, data were also collected on nasal levels of three pro-inflammatory cytokines, IL-1β, IL-6, and IL-8. The temporal pattern for expression of all three cytokines tracked the vSSC, and lower positive emotional style was associated with greater levels of these cytokines and a greater vSSC. Controlling for IL-6 but not for IL-1β or IL-8 substantially decreased the relationship between positive emotional style and the vSSC, indicating the possibility that IL-6 mediated the association [220]. The relationships between positive emotional style and both the vSSC and CLIv risk were replicated in a second study that exposed 193 adult subjects to either influenza or RV. That study also showed that the relationship was independent of the personality traits of optimism, extraversion, mastery, self-esteem and purpose [39].

While emotional style is a measure of general disposition, mood reflects more transient emotional states. A number of studies have shown that negative moods can affect immunologic function [230] and that mood is adversely affected during a CLI [231–233]. In one study, Cohen and colleagues [228] assessed state negative affect (negative moods) on the day before virus challenge, exposed all subjects to influenza or RV and assessed the provoked subjective and objective vSSC. They reported that persons with higher negative mood scores had a greater, but unbiased, subjective vSSC when compared to those with lesser negative mood scores.

Conclusions

The development of a CLI requires four antecedent events: exposure to an upper respiratory virus at a potentially infectious dose, infection with the virus, the development of a vSSC and interpretation of the vSSC as a CLI. Factors that modulate CLI risk can moderate any of these sequential events. An ideal study of CLI risk factors would characterize the conditional probabilities of each of these sequential events for each potentially causal virus but this is clearly not feasible given that the 'denominators' (e.g.. CLIs/vSSCs/infections/exposures) for the rate calculation are difficult to estimate with accuracy. Nonetheless, it is possible to present hypothetical pathways for the action of some of the CLI risk factors suggested in the above review.

Virus exposure requires that a virus be circulating in a population, a precondition that is affected by climate, season, meteorological and other factors. Given the existence of a virus reservoir, the probability of exposure increases in proportion to the frequency of contacts with infected individuals (with or without a CLI). This is enhanced under community structures characterized by crowding (community, home, day care, school, work, hospital environments) and, perhaps, can be affected by certain personality characteristics. Given exposure to a virus, the probability of infection will depend on the functional status of the innate immune system, on the past experience of the individual with respect to the specific virus, and on the presence of immune memory as reflected in the specific antiviral antibodies. This will be affected by age given the increasing exposure to a greater repertoire of vURTI viruses with advancing age and by genetic polymorphisms and other factors that moderate the innate and adaptive immune response. Given a vURTI, whether or not an infected person expresses a vSSC depends on the extant immunocompetence of the host, which will determine the degree of inflammatory recruitment during the infection and on the propensity of the host to develop an inflammatory response. It is expected that a large number of the identified factors moderate immunocompetence including age, genetic background, past history of exposure to related viruses (cellular memory), social environment, diet, sleep efficiency, exercise frequency and intensity, tobacco use, mood states, some personality traits, childhood SES, perceived SES and both physical and psychological stress. Some of these factors such as poor sleep efficiency, strenuous exercise/work, childhood and perceived SES and crowding may operate in part by acting as stressors (be nested within the stress effect), while others such as certain personality traits, social support and physiological reactivity to acute stressors may operate by moderating the stress response (interact with the stress response). Moderate alcohol consumption, certain cytokine polymorphisms, exercise and other factors may act by affecting the propensity of the host to develop an inflammatory response, while others such as tobacco smoke exposure, mold (in allergic persons) and cold environments may act to prime the inflammatory response provoked by a vURTI. Finally, there are factors that most probably operate by modifying the interpretation of the vSSC as a CLI. For example, it is possible that air pollution, household mold and tobacco consumption increase the basal SSC with the effect of enhancing the vSSC and transforming subclinical vURTIs into CLIs. Personality factors can modify the vSSC threshold for CLI assignment and/or distort the basal SSC and the vSSC and affect the probability of assigning a CLI to a specific objective vSSC.

References

1 Ammer C (1997) The American Heritage® Dictionary of Idioms. Houghton Mifflin Company, Boston, MA

2 (2003) Encyclopædia Britannica Deluxe Edition. Encyclopædia Britannica, Inc., Chicago, IL

3 Eccles R (2002) An explanation for the seasonality of acute upper respiratory tract viral infections. *Acta Otolaryngol* 122: 183–191

4 (2002) *Merriam-Webster's Medical Dictionary*. Merriam-Webster, Inc

5 Eccles R (2005) Understanding the symptoms of the common cold and influenza. *Lancet Infect Dis* 5: 718–725

6 Makela MJ, Puhakka T, Ruuskanen O, Leinonen M, Saikku P, Kimpimaki M, Blomqvist S, Hyypia T, Arstila P (1998) Viruses and bacteria in the etiology of the common cold. *J Clin Microbiol* 36: 539–542

7 Nokso-Koivisto J, Pitkaranta A, Blomqvist S, Jokinen J, Kleemola M, Takala A, Kilpi T, Hovi T (2002) Viral etiology of frequently recurring respiratory tract infections in children. *Clin Infect Dis* 35: 540–546

8 Louie JK, Hacker JK, Gonzales R, Mark J, Maselli JH, Yagi S, Drew WL (2005) Characterization of viral agents causing acute respiratory infection in a San Francisco University Medical Center Clinic during the influenza season. *Clin Infect Dis* 41: 822–828

9 van Gageldonk-Lafeber AB, Heijnen ML, Bartelds AI, Peters MF, van der Plas SM, Wilbrink B (2005) A case-control study of acute respiratory tract infection in general practice patients in The Netherlands. *Clin Infect Dis* 41: 490–497

10 Winther B, Alper CM, Mandel EM, Doyle WJ, Hendley JO (2007) Temporal relationships between colds, upper respiratory viruses detected by polymerase chain reaction, and otitis media in young children followed through a typical cold season. *Pediatrics* 119: 1069–1075

11 Wald ER, Guerra N, Byers C (1991) Upper respiratory tract infections in young children: duration of and frequency of complications. *Pediatrics* 87: 129–133
12 Petersen I, Johnson AM, Islam A, Duckworth G, Livermore DM, Hayward AC (2007) Protective effect of antibiotics against serious complications of common respiratory tract infections: retrospective cohort study with the UK General Practice Research Database. *BMJ* 335: 982
13 Nokso-Koivisto J, Hovi T, Pitkaranta A (2006) Viral upper respiratory tract infections in young children with emphasis on acute otitis media. *Int J Pediatr Otorhinolaryngol* 70: 1333–1342
14 Winther B, Doyle WJ, Alper CM (2006) A high prevalence of new onset otitis media during parent diagnosed common colds. *Int J Pediatr Otorhinolaryngol* 70: 1725–1730
15 Alho OP (2005) Viral infections and susceptibility to recurrent sinusitis. *Curr Allergy Asthma Rep* 5: 477–481
16 Johnston SL, Pattemore PK, Sanderson G, Smith S, Lampe F, Josephs L, Symington P, O'Toole S, Myint SH, Tyrrell DA et al. (1995) Community study of role of viral infections in exacerbations of asthma in 9–11 year old children. *BMJ* 310: 1225–1229
17 Ahmed AH, Nicholson KG, Hammersley VS (1996) The contribution of respiratory viruses to severe exacerbations of asthma in adults. *Chest* 109: 588
18 Nicholson KG, Kent J, Hammersley V, Cancio E (1996) Risk factors for lower respiratory complications of rhinovirus infections in elderly people living in the community: prospective cohort study. *BMJ* 313: 1119–1123
19 Doyle WJ, Alper CM (2007) Use of diagnostic algorithms and new technologies to study the incidence and prevalence of viral upper respiratory tract infections and their complications in high risk populations. *Curr Opin Allergy Clin Immunol* 7: 11–16
20 Jackson GG, Dowling HF, Anderson TO, Riff L, Saporta J, Turck M (1960) Susceptibility and immunity to common upper respiratory viral infections – the common cold. *Ann Intern Med* 53: 719–738
21 Jackson GG, Dowling HF, Spiesman IG, Boand AV (1958) Transmission of the common cold to volunteers under controlled conditions. I. The common cold as a clinical entity. *AMA Arch Intern Med* 101: 267–278
22 Barrett B, Brown R, Mundt M, Safdar N, Dye L, Maberry R, Alt J (2005) The Wisconsin Upper Respiratory Symptom Survey is responsive, reliable, and valid. *J Clin Epidemiol* 58: 609–617
23 Nicholson KG, Kent J, Hammersley V, Cancio E (1997) Acute viral infections of upper respiratory tract in elderly people living in the community: comparative, prospective, population based study of disease burden. *BMJ* 315: 1060–1064
24 Boivin G, Hardy I, Tellier G, Maziade J (2000) Predicting influenza infections during epidemics with use of a clinical case definition. *Clin Infect Dis* 31: 1166–1169
25 Monto AS, Gravenstein S, Elliott M, Colopy M, Schweinle J (2000) Clinical signs and symptoms predicting influenza infection. *Arch Intern Med* 160: 3243–3247
26 Doyle WJ, Gentile DA, Skoner DP (2007) Viral and bacterial rhinitis. *Clin Allergy Immunol* 19: 177–195

27 Fox JP, Cooney MK, Hall CE (1975) The Seattle virus watch. V. Epidemiologic observations of rhinovirus infections, 1965–1969, in families with young children. *Am J Epidemiol* 101: 122–143
28 Foy HM, Cooney MK, Allan ID, Albrecht JK (1987) Influenza B in households: virus shedding without symptoms or antibody response. *Am J Epidemiol* 126: 506–515
29 Johnston SL, Sanderson G, Pattemore PK, Smith S, Bardin PG, Bruce CB, Lambden PR, Tyrrell DA, Holgate ST (1993) Use of polymerase chain reaction for diagnosis of picornavirus infection in subjects with and without respiratory symptoms. *J Clin Microbiol* 31: 111–117
30 Nokso-Koivisto J, Kinnari TJ, Lindahl P, Hovi T, Pitkaranta A (2002) Human picornavirus and coronavirus RNA in nasopharynx of children without concurrent respiratory symptoms. *J Med Virol* 66: 417–420
31 Graat JM, Schouten EG, Heijnen ML, Kok FJ, Pallast EG, de Greeff SC, Dorigo-Zetsma JW (2003) A prospective, community-based study on virologic assessment among elderly people with and without symptoms of acute respiratory infection. *J Clin Epidemiol* 56: 1218–1223
32 Doyle WJ, Skoner DP, Alper CM, Allen G, Moody SA, Seroky JT, Hayden FG (1998) Effect of rimantadine treatment on clinical manifestations and otologic complications in adults experimentally infected with influenza A (H1N1) virus. *J Infect Dis* 177: 1260–1265
33 Cohen S, Frank E, Doyle WJ, Skoner DP, Rabin BS, Gwaltney JM, Jr. (1998) Types of stressors that increase susceptibility to the common cold in healthy adults. *Health Psychol* 17: 214–223
34 Buchman CA, Doyle WJ, Pilcher O, Gentile DA, Skoner DP (2002) Nasal and otologic effects of experimental respiratory syncytial virus infection in adults. *Am J Otolaryngol* 23: 70–75
35 Alper CM, Doyle WJ, Winther B, Owen Hendley J (2008) Upper respiratory virus detection without parent-reported illness in children is virus-specific. *J Clin Virol* 43: 120–122
36 Doyle WJ, Alper CM, Buchman CA, Moody SA, Skoner DP, Cohen S (1999) Illness and otological changes during upper respiratory virus infection. *Laryngoscope* 109: 324–328
37 Clarke JD, Eccles R (2005) Paradoxical sensation of nasal airflow in patients with common cold. Are we measuring the correct modality? *Acta Otolaryngol* 125: 1307–1311
38 Feldman PJ, Cohen S, Doyle WJ, Skoner DP, Gwaltney JM, Jr. (1999) The impact of personality on the reporting of unfounded symptoms and illness. *J Pers Soc Psychol* 77: 370–378
39 Cohen S, Alper CM, Doyle WJ, Treanor JJ, Turner RB (2006) Positive emotional style predicts resistance to illness after experimental exposure to rhinovirus or influenza a virus. *Psychosom Med* 68: 809–815
40 Naclerio RM, Proud D, Kagey-Sobotka A, Lichtenstein LM, Hendley JO, Gwaltney JM Jr (1988) Is histamine responsible for the symptoms of rhinovirus colds? A look at the inflammatory mediators following infection. *Pediatr Infect Dis J* 7: 218–222
41 Cohen S, Doyle WJ, Skoner DP, Rabin BS, Gwaltney JM, Jr. (1997) Social ties and susceptibility to the common cold. *JAMA* 277: 1940–1944

42 Bousquet J, Vignola AM, Campbell AM, Michel FB (1996) Pathophysiology of allergic rhinitis. *Int Arch Allergy Immunol* 110: 207–218
43 Doyle WJ, Skoner DP, Seroky JT, Fireman P, Gwaltney JM (1994) Effect of experimental rhinovirus 39 infection on the nasal response to histamine and cold air challenges in allergic and nonallergic subjects. *J Allergy Clin Immunol* 93: 534–542
44 Ko FW, Lai CK, Woo J, Ho SC, Ho CW, Goggins W, Hui DS (2006) 12-year change in prevalence of respiratory symptoms in elderly Chinese living in Hong Kong. *Respir Med* 100: 1598–1607
45 Koskinen OM, Husman TM, Meklin TM, Nevalainen AI (1999) The relationship between moisture or mould observations in houses and the state of health of their occupants. *Eur Respir J* 14: 1363–1367
46 Doyle WJ, Skoner DP, Gentile D (2005) Nasal cytokines as mediators of illness during the common cold. *Curr Allergy Asthma Rep* 5: 173–181
47 Eccles R (1995) Rhinitis as a mechanism of respiratory defense. *Eur Arch Otorhinolaryngol* 252 (Suppl 1): S2–7
48 Eccles R (1996) A role for the nasal cycle in respiratory defence. *Eur Respir J* 9: 371–376
49 Bazar KA, Yun AJ, Lee PY (2005) "Starve a fever and feed a cold": feeding and anorexia may be adaptive behavioral modulators of autonomic and T helper balance. *Med Hypotheses* 64: 1080–1084
50 Mygind N (2001) Nasal inflammation and anti-inflammatory treatment. Semantics or clinical reality. *Rhinology* 39: 61–65
51 Gwaltney JM (2002) Viral respiratory infection therapy: historical perspectives and current trials. *Am J Med* 112 (Suppl) 6A: 33S–41S
52 Eccles R (2006) Efficacy and safety of over-the-counter analgesics in the treatment of common cold and flu. *J Clin Pharm Ther* 31: 309–319
53 Cohen S, Tyrrell DA, Smith AP (1991) Psychological stress and susceptibility to the common cold. *N Engl J Med* 325: 606–612
54 Badger GF, Dingle JH, Feller AE, Hodges RG, Jordan WS, Jr., Rammelkamp CH, Jr. (1953) A study of illness in a group of Cleveland families. II. Incidence of the common respiratory diseases. *Am J Hyg* 58: 31–40
55 Gwaltney JM, Jr., Hendley JO, Simon G, Jordan WS, Jr. (1966) Rhinovirus infections in an industrial population. I. The occurrence of illness. *N Engl J Med* 275: 1261–1268
56 Spigland I, Fox JP, Elveback LR, Wassermann FE, Ketler A, Brandt CD, Kogon A (1966) The Virus Watch program: a continuing surveillance of viral infections in metropolitan New York families. II. Laboratory methods and preliminary report on infections revealed by virus isolation. *Am J Epidemiol* 83: 413–435
57 Monto AS, Cavallaro JJ, Keller JB (1970) Seasonal patterns of acute infection in Tecumseh, Mich. *Arch Environ Health* 21: 408–417
58 Monto AS, Cavallaro JJ (1971) The Tecumseh study of respiratory illness. II. Patterns of occurrence of infection with respiratory pathogens, 1965–1969. *Am J Epidemiol* 94: 280–289
59 Monto AS, Koopman JS, Bryan ER (1986) The Tecumseh Study of Illness. XIV. Occurrence of respiratory viruses, 1976–1981. *Am J Epidemiol* 124: 359–367
60 Monto AS (2002) The seasonality of rhinovirus infections and its implications for clinical recognition. *Clin Ther* 24: 1987–1997

61 Monto AS (2002) Epidemiology of viral respiratory infections. *Am J Med* 112 (Suppl) 6A: 4S–12S
62 Chew FT, Doraisingham S, Ling AE, Kumarasinghe G, Lee BW (1998) Seasonal trends of viral respiratory tract infections in the tropics. *Epidemiol Infect* 121: 121–128
63 Shek LP, Lee BW (2003) Epidemiology and seasonality of respiratory tract virus infections in the tropics. *Paediatr Respir Rev* 4: 105–111
64 Moura FE, Nunes IF, Silva GB, Jr., Siqueira MM (2006) Respiratory syncytial virus infections in northeastern Brazil: seasonal trends and general aspects. *Am J Trop Med Hyg* 74: 165–167
65 Nelson MI, Simonsen L, Viboud C, Miller MA, Holmes EC (2007) Phylogenetic analysis reveals the global migration of seasonal influenza A viruses. *PLoS Pathog* 3: 1220–1228
66 Weber A, Weber M, Milligan P (2001) Modeling epidemics caused by respiratory syncytial virus (RSV). *Math Biosci* 172: 95–113
67 White LJ, Mandl JN, Gomes MG, Bodley-Tickell AT, Cane PA, Perez-Brena P, Aguilar JC, Siqueira MM, Portes SA, Straliotto SM et al. (2007) Understanding the transmission dynamics of respiratory syncytial virus using multiple time series and nested models. *Math Biosci* 209: 222–239
68 Welliver RC, Sr. (2007) Temperature, humidity, and ultraviolet B radiation predict community respiratory syncytial virus activity. *Pediatr Infect Dis J* 26: S29–35
69 Viboud C, Pakdaman K, Boelle PY, Wilson ML, Myers MF, Valleron AJ, Flahault A (2004) Association of influenza epidemics with global climate variability. *Eur J Epidemiol* 19: 1055–1059
70 Alonso WJ, Viboud C, Simonsen L, Hirano EW, Daufenbach LZ, Miller MA (2007) Seasonality of influenza in Brazil: a traveling wave from the Amazon to the subtropics. *Am J Epidemiol* 165: 1434–1442
71 Noyola DE, Mandeville PB (2008) Effect of climatological factors on respiratory syncytial virus epidemics. *Epidemiol Infect*: 1–6
72 Oliveira AC, Ishimaru D, Goncalves RB, Smith TJ, Mason P, Sa-Carvalho D, Silva JL (1999) Low temperature and pressure stability of picornaviruses: implications for virus uncoating. *Biophys J* 76: 1270–1279
73 Ausar SF, Rexroad J, Frolov VG, Look JL, Konar N, Middaugh CR (2005) Analysis of the thermal and pH stability of human respiratory syncytial virus. *Mol Pharm* 2: 491–499
74 Polozov IV, Bezrukov L, Gawrisch K, Zimmerberg J (2008) Progressive ordering with decreasing temperature of the phospholipids of influenza virus. *Nat Chem Biol* 4: 248–255
75 Light M (2007) Respiratory syncytial virus seasonality in southeast Florida: results from three area hospitals caring for children. *Pediatr Infect Dis J* 26: S55–59
76 Tang JW, Ngai KL, Lam WY, Chan PK (2008) Seasonality of influenza A(H3N2) virus: a Hong Kong perspective (1997–2006). *PLoS ONE* 3: e2768
77 Wong S, Pabbaraju K, Pang XL, Lee BE, Fox JD (2008) Detection of a broad range of human adenoviruses in respiratory tract samples using a sensitive multiplex real-time PCR assay. *J Med Virol* 80: 856–865

78 Greene SK, Ionides EL, Wilson ML (2006) Patterns of influenza-associated mortality among US elderly by geographic region and virus subtype, 1968–1998. *Am J Epidemiol* 163: 316–326
79 Bang FB, Bang MG, Bang BG (1975) Ecology of respiratory virus transmission: a comparison of three communities in West Bengal. *Am J Trop Med Hyg* 24: 326–346
80 Monto AS (1968) A community study of respiratory infections in the tropics. 3. Introduction and transmission of infections within families. *Am J Epidemiol* 88: 69–79
81 Monto AS, Sullivan KM (1993) Acute respiratory illness in the community. Frequency of illness and the agents involved. *Epidemiol Infect* 110: 145–160
82 Wald ER, Dashefsky B, Byers C, Guerra N, Taylor F (1988) Frequency and severity of infections in day care. *J Pediatr* 112: 540–546
83 Benediktsdottir B (1993) Upper airway infections in preschool children – frequency and risk factors. *Scand J Prim Health Care* 11: 197–201
84 Ball TM, Holberg CJ, Aldous MB, Martinez FD, Wright AL (2002) Influence of attendance at day care on the common cold from birth through 13 years of age. *Arch Pediatr Adolesc Med* 156: 121–126
85 Zutavern A, Rzehak P, Brockow I, Schaaf B, Bollrath C, von Berg A, Link E, Kraemer U, Borte M, Herbarth O et al. (2007) Day care in relation to respiratory-tract and gastrointestinal infections in a German birth cohort study. *Acta Paediatr* 96: 1494–1499
86 Jaakkola JJ, Heinonen OP (1995) Shared office space and the risk of the common cold. *Eur J Epidemiol* 11: 213–216
87 Wright SA, Bieluch VM (1993) Selected nosocomial viral infections. *Heart Lung* 22: 183–187
88 Mlinaric-Galinovic G, Varda-Brkic D (2000) Nosocomial respiratory syncytial virus infections in children's wards. *Diagn Microbiol Infect Dis* 37: 237–246
89 Aitken C, Jeffries DJ (2001) Nosocomial spread of viral disease. *Clin Microbiol Rev* 14: 528–546
90 Montnemery P, Popovic M, Andersson M, Greiff L, Nyberg P, Lofdahl CG, Svensson C, Persson CG (2003) Influence of heavy traffic, city dwelling and socio-economic status on nasal symptoms assessed in a postal population survey. *Respir Med* 97: 970–977
91 Thompson DJ, Lebowitz M, Cassell EJ, Wolter D, McCarroll J (1970) Health and the urban environment. 8. Air pollution, weather, and the common cold. *Am J Public Health Nations Health* 60: 731–739
92 Jaakkola JJ, Paunio M, Virtanen M, Heinonen OP (1991) Low-level air pollution and upper respiratory infections in children. *Am J Public Health* 81: 1060–1063
93 Bayer-Oglesby L, Grize L, Gassner M, Takken-Sahli K, Sennhauser FH, Neu U, Schindler C, Braun-Fahrlander C (2005) Decline of ambient air pollution levels and improved respiratory health in Swiss children. *Environ Health Perspect* 113: 1632–1637
94 Jaakkola JJ, Partti-Pellinen K, Marttila O, Miettinen P, Vilkka V, Haahtela T (1999) The South Karelia Air Pollution Study: changes in respiratory health in relation to emission reduction of malodorous sulfur compounds from pulp mills. *Arch Environ Health* 54: 254–263

95 Kumar R, Nagar JK, Kumar H, Kushwah AS, Meena M, Kumar P, Raj N, Singhal MK, Gaur SN (2007) Association of indoor and outdoor air pollutant level with respiratory problems among children in an industrial area of Delhi, India. *Arch Environ Occup Health* 62: 75–80
96 Pirhonen I, Nevalainen A, Husman T, Pekkanen J (1996) Home dampness, moulds and their influence on respiratory infections and symptoms in adults in Finland. *Eur Respir J* 9: 2618–2622
97 Selye H (1976) Forty years of stress research: principal remaining problems and misconceptions. *Can Med Assoc J* 115: 53–56
98 Cohen S, Miller GE, Rabin BS (2001) Psychological stress and antibody response to immunization: a critical review of the human literature. *Psychosom Med* 63: 7–18
99 Webster Marketon JI, Glaser R (2008) Stress hormones and immune function. *Cell Immunol* 252: 16–26
100 Cohen S, Williamson GM (1991) Stress and infectious disease in humans. *Psychol Bull* 109: 5–24
101 Cohen S, Doyle WJ, Baum A (2006) Socioeconomic status is associated with stress hormones. *Psychosom Med* 68: 414–420
102 Cohen S, Doyle WJ, Turner RB, Alper CM, Skoner DP (2004) Childhood socioeconomic status and host resistance to infectious illness in adulthood. *Psychosom Med* 66: 553–558
103 Angeli A, Minetto M, Dovio A, Paccotti P (2004) The overtraining syndrome in athletes: a stress-related disorder. *J Endocrinol Invest* 27: 603–612
104 Nieman DC (2003) Current perspective on exercise immunology. *Curr Sports Med Rep* 2: 239–242
105 Mohren DC, Swaen GM, Borm PJ, Bast A, Galama JM (2001) Psychological job demands as a risk factor for common cold in a Dutch working population. *J Psychosom Res* 50: 21–27
106 Mohren DC, Jansen NW, Kant IJ, Galama J, van den Brandt PA, Swaen GM (2002) Prevalence of common infections among employees in different work schedules. *J Occup Environ Med* 44: 1003–1011
107 Mohren DC, Swaen GM, Kant IJ, van Amelsvoort LG, Borm PJ, Galama JM (2003) Common infections and the role of burnout in a Dutch working population. *J Psychosom Res* 55: 201–208
108 Koh D, Yong Y, Ng V, Chia SE (2002) Stress, mucosal immunity, upper respiratory tract infections, and sickness absence. *J Occup Environ Med* 44: 987–988
109 Cohen S (2005) Keynote Presentation at the Eight International Congress of Behavioral Medicine: the Pittsburgh common cold studies: psychosocial predictors of susceptibility to respiratory infectious illness. *Int J Behav Med* 12: 123–131
110 Tache J, Selye H (1985) On stress and coping mechanisms. *Issues Ment Health Nurs* 7: 3–24
111 Boyce WT, Jensen EW, Cassel JC, Collier AM, Smith AH, Ramey CT (1977) Influence of life events and family routines on childhood respiratory tract illness. *Pediatrics* 60: 609–615
112 Totman R, Kiff J, Reed SE, Craig JW (1980) Predicting experimental colds in volunteers from different measures of recent life stress. *J Psychosom Res* 24: 155–163

113 Cohen S, Doyle WJ, Skoner DP (1999) Psychological stress, cytokine production, and severity of upper respiratory illness. *Psychosom Med* 61: 175–180
114 Spilken AZ, Jacobs MA (1971) Prediction of illness behavior from measures of life crisis, manifest distress and maladaptive coping. *Psychosom Med* 33: 251–264
115 Graham NM, Douglas RM, Ryan P (1986) Stress and acute respiratory infection. *Am J Epidemiol* 124: 389–401
116 Smith A, Nicholson K (2001) Psychosocial factors, respiratory viruses and exacerbation of asthma. *Psychoneuroendocrinology* 26: 411–420
117 Stone AA, Reed BR, Neale JM (1987) Changes in daily event frequency precede episodes of physical symptoms. *J Human Stress* 13: 70–74
118 Evans PD, Edgerton N (1991) Life-events and mood as predictors of the common cold. *Br J Med Psychol* 64 (Pt 1): 35–44
119 Takkouche B, Regueira C, Gestal-Otero JJ (2001) A cohort study of stress and the common cold. *Epidemiology* 12: 345–349
120 Cobb JM, Steptoe A (1996) Psychosocial stress and susceptibility to upper respiratory tract illness in an adult population sample. *Psychosom Med* 58: 404–412
121 Turner Cobb JM, Steptoe A (1998) Psychosocial influences on upper respiratory infectious illness in children. *J Psychosom Res* 45: 319–330
122 Cohen S, Tyrrell DA, Smith AP (1993) Negative life events, perceived stress, negative affect, and susceptibility to the common cold. *J Pers Soc Psychol* 64: 131–140
123 Stone AA, Bovbjerg DH, Neale JM, Napoli A, Valdimarsdottir H, Cox D, Hayden FG, Gwaltney JM Jr (1992) Development of common cold symptoms following experimental rhinovirus infection is related to prior stressful life events. *Behav Med* 18: 115–120
124 Cohen S, Hamrick N, Rodriguez MS, Feldman PJ, Rabin BS, Manuck SB (2002) Reactivity and vulnerability to stress-associated risk for upper respiratory illness. *Psychosom Med* 64: 302–310
125 Boyce WT, Chesterman EA, Martin N, Folkman S, Cohen F, Wara D (1993) Immunologic changes occurring at kindergarten entry predict respiratory illnesses after the Loma Prieta earthquake. *J Dev Behav Pediatr* 14: 296–303
126 Boyce WT, Chesney M, Alkon A, Tschann JM, Adams S, Chesterman B, Cohen F, Kaiser P, Folkman S, Wara D (1995) Psychobiologic reactivity to stress and childhood respiratory illnesses: results of two prospective studies. *Psychosom Med* 57: 411–422
127 Cobb S (1976) Presidential Address-1976. Social support as a moderator of life stress. *Psychosom Med* 38: 300–314
128 House JS, Landis KR, Umberson D (1988) Social relationships and health. *Science* 241: 540–545
129 Uchino BN, Cacioppo JT, Kiecolt-Glaser JK (1996) The relationship between social support and physiological processes: a review with emphasis on underlying mechanisms and implications for health. *Psychol Bull* 119: 488–531
130 Cohen S (2004) Social relationships and health. *Am Psychol* 59: 676–684
131 Pressman SD, Cohen S, Miller GE, Barkin A, Rabin BS, Treanor JJ (2005) Loneliness, social network size, and immune response to influenza vaccination in college freshmen. *Health Psychol* 24: 297–306

132 Monto AS, Ullman BM (1974) Acute respiratory illness in an American community. The Tecumseh study. *JAMA* 227: 164–169

133 Cohen S, Doyle WJ, Turner R, Alper CM, Skoner DP (2003) Sociability and susceptibility to the common cold. *Psychol Sci* 14: 389–395

134 Cohen S, Alper CM, Doyle WJ, Adler N, Treanor JJ, Turner RB (2008) Objective and subjective socioeconomic status and susceptibility to the common cold. *Health Psychol* 27: 268–274

135 Benson V, Marano MA (1998) Current estimates from the National Health Interview Survey, 1995. *Vital Health Stat* 10: 1–428

136 Adler NE, Boyce T, Chesney MA, Cohen S, Folkman S, Kahn RL, Syme SL (1994) Socioeconomic status and health. The challenge of the gradient. *Am Psychol* 49: 15–24

137 Anderson NB, Armstead CA (1995) Toward understanding the association of socioeconomic status and health: a new challenge for the biopsychosocial approach. *Psychosom Med* 57: 213–225

138 Naess O, Claussen B, Thelle DS, Smith GD (2005) Four indicators of socioeconomic position: relative ranking across causes of death. *Scand J Public Health* 33: 215–221

139 Alper CM, Winther B, Mandel EM, Doyle WJ (2007) Temporal relationships for cold-like illnesses and otitis media in sibling pairs. *Pediatr Infect Dis J* 26: 778–781

140 Galobardes B, Lynch JW, Smith GD (2008) Is the association between childhood socioeconomic circumstances and cause-specific mortality established? Update of a systematic review. *J Epidemiol Community Health* 62: 387–390

141 Kaushik PV, Singh JV, Bhatnagar M, Garg SK, Chopra H (1995) Nutritional correlates of acute respiratory infections. *Indian J Matern Child Health* 6: 71–72

142 Alaimo K, Olson CM, Frongillo EA, Jr., Briefel RR (2001) Food insufficiency, family income, and health in US preschool and school-aged children. *Am J Public Health* 91: 781–786

143 Takkouche B, Regueira-Mendez C, Garcia-Closas R, Figueiras A, Gestal-Otero JJ (2002) Intake of vitamin C and zinc and risk of common cold: a cohort study. *Epidemiology* 13: 38–44

144 Hemila H, Kaprio J, Albanes D, Heinonen OP, Virtamo J (2002) Vitamin C, vitamin E, and beta-carotene in relation to common cold incidence in male smokers. *Epidemiology* 13: 32–37

145 Roxas M, Jurenka J (2007) Colds and influenza: a review of diagnosis and conventional, botanical, and nutritional considerations. *Altern Med Rev* 12: 25–48

146 Ballabh B, Chaurasia OP (2007) Traditional medicinal plants of cold desert Ladakh – used in treatment of cold, cough and fever. *J Ethnopharmacol* 112: 341–349

147 Douglas RM, Hemila H, Chalker E, Treacy B (2007) Vitamin C for preventing and treating the common cold. *Cochrane Database Syst Rev*: CD000980

148 Fischer Walker C, Black RE (2004) Zinc and the risk for infectious disease. *Annu Rev Nutr* 24: 255–275

149 Turner RB, Bauer R, Woelkart K, Hulsey TC, Gangemi JD (2005) An evaluation of Echinacea angustifolia in experimental rhinovirus infections. *N Engl J Med* 353: 341–348

150 Meydani SN, Han SN, Hamer DH (2004) Vitamin E and respiratory infection in the elderly. *Ann NY Acad Sci* 1031: 214–222
151 Hemila H (1996) Vitamin C and common cold incidence: a review of studies with subjects under heavy physical stress. *Int J Sports Med* 17: 379–383
152 Hemila H, Douglas RM (1999) Vitamin C and acute respiratory infections. *Int J Tuberc Lung Dis* 3: 756–761
153 Winkler P, de Vrese M, Laue C, Schrezenmeir J (2005) Effect of a dietary supplement containing probiotic bacteria plus vitamins and minerals on common cold infections and cellular immune parameters. *Int J Clin Pharmacol Ther* 43: 318–326
154 Rowe CA, Nantz MP, Bukowski JF, Percival SS (2007) Specific formulation of Camellia sinensis prevents cold and flu symptoms and enhances gamma,delta T cell function: a randomized, double-blind, placebo-controlled study. *J Am Coll Nutr* 26: 445–452
155 Sarma KV, Udaykumar P, Balakrishna N, Vijayaraghavan K, Sivakumar B (2006) Effect of micronutrient supplementation on health and nutritional status of schoolchildren: growth and morbidity. *Nutrition* 22: S8–14
156 Maeda H, Ichihashi K, Fujii T, Omura K, Zhu X, Anazawa M, Tazawa K (2004) Oral administration of hydrolyzed rice bran prevents the common cold syndrome in the elderly based on its immunomodulatory action. *Biofactors* 21: 185–187
157 Sopori ML, Kozak W (1998) Immunomodulatory effects of cigarette smoke. *J Neuroimmunol* 83: 148–156
158 McAllister-Sistilli CG, Caggiula AR, Knopf S, Rose CA, Miller AL, Donny EC (1998) The effects of nicotine on the immune system. *Psychoneuroendocrinology* 23: 175–187
159 Diaz LE, Montero A, Gonzalez-Gross M, Vallejo AI, Romeo J, Marcos A (2002) Influence of alcohol consumption on immunological status: a review. *Eur J Clin Nutr* 56 (Suppl) 3: S50–53
160 Romeo J, Warnberg J, Nova E, Diaz LE, Gomez-Martinez S, Marcos A (2007) Moderate alcohol consumption and the immune system: a review. *Br J Nutr* 98 (Suppl 1): S111–115
161 Atkinson JP, Sullivan TJ, Kelly JP, Parker CW (1977) Stimulation by alcohols of cyclic AMP metabolism in human leukocytes. Possible role of cyclic AMP in the anti-inflammatory effects of ethanol. *J Clin Invest* 60: 284–294
162 Lister SM, Jorm LR (1998) Parental smoking and respiratory illnesses in Australian children aged 0–4 years: ABS 1989–90 National Health Survey results. *Aust NZ J Public Health* 22: 781–786
163 Bensenor IM, Cook NR, Lee IM, Chown MJ, Hennekens CH, Buring JE, Manson JE (2001) Active and passive smoking and risk of colds in women. *Ann Epidemiol* 11: 225–231
164 Finklea JF, Sandifer SH, Smith DD (1969) Cigarette smoking and epidemic influenza. *Am J Epidemiol* 90: 390–399
165 MacKenzie JS, MacKenzie IH, Holt PG (1976) The effect of cigarette smoking on susceptibility to epidemic influenza and on serological responses to live attenuated and killed subunit influenza vaccines. *J Hyg (Lond)* 77: 409–417
166 Monto AS, Ross H (1977) Acute respiratory illness in the community: effect

of family composition, smoking, and chronic symptoms. *Br J Prev Soc Med* 31: 101–108

167 Takkouche B, Regueira-Mendez C, Garcia-Closas R, Figueiras A, Gestal-Otero JJ, Hernan MA (2002) Intake of wine, beer, and spirits and the risk of clinical common cold. *Am J Epidemiol* 155: 853–858

168 Cohen S, Tyrrell DA, Russell MA, Jarvis MJ, Smith AP (1993) Smoking, alcohol consumption, and susceptibility to the common cold. *Am J Public Health* 83: 1277–1283

169 Moldoveanu AI, Shephard RJ, Shek PN (2001) The cytokine response to physical activity and training. *Sports Med* 31: 115–144

170 Gleeson M (2007) Immune function in sport and exercise. *J Appl Physiol* 103: 693–699

171 Brolinson PG, Elliott D (2007) Exercise and the immune system. *Clin Sports Med* 26: 311–319

172 Pedersen BK, Toft AD (2000) Effects of exercise on lymphocytes and cytokines. *Br J Sports Med* 34: 246–251

173 Malm C (2006) Susceptibility to infections in elite athletes: the S-curve. *Scand J Med Sci Sports* 16: 4–6

174 Spence L, Brown WJ, Pyne DB, Nissen MD, Sloots TP, McCormack JG, Locke AS, Fricker PA (2007) Incidence, etiology, and symptomatology of upper respiratory illness in elite athletes. *Med Sci Sports Exerc* 39: 577–586

175 Osterback L, Qvarnberg Y (1987) A prospective study of respiratory infections in 12-year-old children actively engaged in sports. *Acta Paediatr Scand* 76: 944–949

176 Weidner TG, Cranston T, Schurr T, Kaminsky LA (1998) The effect of exercise training on the severity and duration of a viral upper respiratory illness. *Med Sci Sports Exerc* 30: 1578–1583

177 Kostka T, Berthouze SE, Lacour J, Bonnefoy M (2000) The symptomatology of upper respiratory tract infections and exercise in elderly people. *Med Sci Sports Exerc* 32: 46–51

178 Chubak J, McTiernan A, Sorensen B, Wener MH, Yasui Y, Velasquez M, Wood B, Rajan KB, Wetmore CM, Potter JD et al. (2006) Moderate-intensity exercise reduces the incidence of colds among postmenopausal women. *Am J Med* 119: 937–942

179 Irwin M, McClintick J, Costlow C, Fortner M, White J, Gillin JC (1996) Partial night sleep deprivation reduces natural killer and cellular immune responses in humans. *Faseb J* 10: 643–653

180 Vgontzas AN, Zoumakis E, Bixler EO, Lin HM, Follett H, Kales A, Chrousos GP (2004) Adverse effects of modest sleep restriction on sleepiness, performance, and inflammatory cytokines. *J Clin Endocrinol Metab* 89: 2119–2126

181 Lange T, Perras B, Fehm HL, Born J (2003) Sleep enhances the human antibody response to hepatitis A vaccination. *Psychosom Med* 65: 831–835

182 Spiegel K, Sheridan JF, Van Cauter E (2002) Effect of sleep deprivation on response to immunization. *JAMA* 288: 1471–1472

183 Cohen S, Doyle WJ, Alper CM, Janicki-Deverts D, Turner RB (2009) Sleep habits and susceptibility to the common cold. *Arch Intern Med* 169: 62–67

184 Gwaltney JM Jr (1985) Virology and immunology of the common cold. *Rhinology* 23: 265–271
185 Reuman PD, Ayoub EM, Small PA (1987) Effect of passive maternal antibody on influenza illness in children: a prospective study of influenza A in mother-infant pairs. *Pediatr Infect Dis J* 6: 398–403
186 Falsey AR (2007) Respiratory syncytial virus infection in adults. *Semin Respir Crit Care Med* 28: 171–181
187 Renegar KB, Small PA Jr (1991) Passive transfer of local immunity to influenza virus infection by IgA antibody. *J Immunol* 146: 1972–1978
188 Murphy BR, Graham BS, Prince GA, Walsh EE, Chanock RM, Karzon DT, Wright PF (1986) Serum and nasal-wash immunoglobulin G and A antibody response of infants and children to respiratory syncytial virus F and G glycoproteins following primary infection. *J Clin Microbiol* 23: 1009–1014
189 Greenbaum E, Furst A, Kiderman A, Stewart B, Levy R, Schlesinger M, Morag A, Zakay-Rones Z (2001) Serum and mucosal immunologic responses in children following the administration of a new inactivated intranasal anti-influenza vaccine. *J Med Virol* 65: 178–184
190 Brandtzaeg P (2003) Role of mucosal immunity in influenza. *Dev Biol (Basel)* 115: 39–48
191 Alper CM, Doyle WJ, Skoner DP, Buchman CA, Cohen S, Gwaltney JM (1998) Prechallenge antibodies moderate disease expression in adults experimentally exposed to rhinovirus strain hanks. *Clin Infect Dis* 27: 119–128
192 Alper CM, Doyle WJ, Skoner DP, Buchman CA, Seroky JT, Gwaltney JM, Cohen SA (1996) Prechallenge antibodies: moderators of infection rate, signs, and symptoms in adults experimentally challenged with rhinovirus type 39. *Laryngoscope* 106: 1298–1305
193 Gafafer WM, Doull JA (1933) A note on the stability of resistance to colds. *Science* 78: 314–315
194 Wilson EB, Worcester J (1944) Note on stability of incidence of the "Common Cold". *Science* 99: 468–469
195 Ball TM, Holberg CJ, Martinez FD, Wright AL (2002) Is there a common cold constitution? *Ambul Pediatr* 2: 261–267
196 Doyle WJ, Winther B, Alper CM (2008) Daily tympanometry for high-resolution measurement of the time between onset of cold-like illness and middle ear effusion. *Laryngoscope* 118: 1066–1071
197 Cedzynski M, Szemraj J, Swierzko AS, Bak-Romaniszyn L, Banasik M, Zeman K, Kilpatrick DC (2004) Mannan-binding lectin insufficiency in children with recurrent infections of the respiratory system. *Clin Exp Immunol* 136: 304–311
198 Heine H, Lien E (2003) Toll-like receptors and their function in innate and adaptive immunity. *Int Arch Allergy Immunol* 130: 180–192
199 Tamura S, Kurata T (2004) Defense mechanisms against influenza virus infection in the respiratory tract mucosa. *Jpn J Infect Dis* 57: 236–247
200 Message SD, Johnston SL (2004) Host defense function of the airway epithelium in health and disease: clinical background. *J Leukoc Biol* 75: 5–17
201 Isaacs D, Clarke JR, Tyrrell DA, Webster AD, Valman HB (1981) Deficient production of leucocyte interferon (interferon-alpha) in vitro and in vivo in children with recurrent respiratory tract infections. *Lancet* 2: 950–952

202 Pitkaranta A, Karma P, Hovi T (1993) Deficiency in interferon production by leukocytes from children with recurrent respiratory infections. *Clin Diagn Virol* 1: 101–108

203 Pitkaranta A, Nokso-Koivisto J, Jantti V, Takala A, Kilpi T, Hovi T (1999) Lowered yields of virus-induced interferon production in leukocyte cultures and risk of recurrent respiratory infections in children. *J Clin Virol* 14: 199–205

204 Bella J, Rossmann MG (2000) ICAM-1 receptors and cold viruses. *Pharm Acta Helv* 74: 291–297

205 Becker N, Abel U, Stiepak C, Meuer SC (1992) Frequency of common colds and serum levels of sICAM-1 (CD54), sLFA-3 (CD58) and sIL-2R (CD25). *Eur Cytokine Netw* 3: 545–551

206 Infante-Duarte C, Kamradt T (1999) Th1/Th2 balance in infection. *Springer Semin Immunopathol* 21: 317–338

207 Skoner DP, Doyle WJ, Tanner EP, Kiss J, Fireman P (1995) Effect of rhinovirus 39 (RV-39) infection on immune and inflammatory parameters in allergic and non-allergic subjects. *Clin Exp Allergy* 25: 561–567

208 Gentile DA, Doyle WJ, Fireman P, Skoner DP (2001) Effect of experimental influenza A infection on systemic immune and inflammatory parameters in allergic and nonallergic adult subjects. *Ann Allergy Asthma Immunol* 87: 496–500

209 Fleming HE, Little FF, Schnurr D, Avila PC, Wong H, Liu J, Yagi S, Boushey HA (1999) Rhinovirus – 16 colds in healthy and in asthmatic subjects: similar changes in upper and lower airways. *Am J Respir Crit Care Med* 160: 100–108

210 Avila PC, Abisheganaden JA, Wong H, Liu J, Yagi S, Schnurr D, Kishiyama JL, Boushey HA (2000) Effects of allergic inflammation of the nasal mucosa on the severity of rhinovirus 16 cold. *J Allergy Clin Immunol* 105: 923–932

211 Corne JM, Marshall C, Smith S, Schreiber J, Sanderson G, Holgate ST, Johnston SL (2002) Frequency, severity, and duration of rhinovirus infections in asthmatic and non-asthmatic individuals: a longitudinal cohort study. *Lancet* 359: 831–834

212 Kimman TG, Vandebriel RJ, Hoebee B (2007) Genetic variation in the response to vaccination. *Community Genet* 10: 201–217

213 Singh N, Agrawal S, Rastogi AK (1997) Infectious diseases and immunity: special reference to major histocompatibility complex. *Emerg Infect Dis* 3: 41–49

214 Nieters A, Brems S, Becker N (2001) Cross-sectional study on cytokine polymorphisms, cytokine production after T-cell stimulation and clinical parameters in a random sample of a German population. *Hum Genet* 108: 241–248

215 Sumiya M, Summerfield JA (1997) The role of collectins in host defense. *Semin Liver Dis* 17: 311–318

216 Ruskamp JM, Hoekstra MO, Rovers MM, Schilder AG, Sanders EA (2006) Mannose-binding lectin and upper respiratory tract infections in children and adolescents: a review. *Arch Otolaryngol Head Neck Surg* 132: 482–486

217 Koch A, Melbye M, Sorensen P, Homoe P, Madsen HO, Molbak K, Hansen CH, Andersen LH, Hahn GW, Garred P (2001) Acute respiratory tract infections and mannose-binding lectin insufficiency during early childhood. *JAMA* 285: 1316–1321

218 Woo P (2000) Cytokine polymorphisms and inflammation. *Clin Exp Rheumatol* 18: 767–771
219 Gentile DA, Doyle WJ, Zeevi A, Piltcher O, Skoner DP (2003) Cytokine gene polymorphisms moderate responses to respiratory syncytial virus in adults. *Hum Immunol* 64: 93–98
220 Doyle WJ, Gentile DA, Cohen S (2006) Emotional style, nasal cytokines, and illness expression after experimental rhinovirus exposure. *Brain Behav Immun* 20: 175–181
221 Gentile DA, Doyle WJ, Zeevi A, Howe-Adams J, Kapadia S, Trecki J, Skoner DP (2003) Cytokine gene polymorphisms moderate illness severity in infants with respiratory syncytial virus infection. *Hum Immunol* 64: 338–344
222 Alper CM, Winther B, Owen Hendley J, Doyle WJ (2008) Cytokine polymorphisms predict the frequency of otitis media as a complication of rhinovirus and RSV infections in children. *Eur Arch Otorhinolaryngol* 266: 199–205
223 Miller GE, Cohen S, Rabin BS, Skoner DP, Doyle WJ (1999) Personality and tonic cardiovascular, neuroendocrine, and immune parameters. *Brain Behav Immun* 13: 109–123
224 Jang KL, Livesley WJ, Vernon PA (1996) Heritability of the big five personality dimensions and their facets: a twin study. *J Pers* 64: 577–591
225 Bratko D, Butkovic A (2007) Stability of genetic and environmental effects from adolescence to young adulthood: results of Croatian longitudinal twin study of personality. *Twin Res Hum Genet* 10: 151–157
226 Hampson SE, Goldberg LR (2006) A first large cohort study of personality trait stability over the 40 years between elementary school and midlife. *J Pers Soc Psychol* 91: 763–779
227 Broadbent DE, Broadbent MH, Phillpotts RJ, Wallace J (1984) Some further studies on the prediction of experimental colds in volunteers by psychological factors. *J Psychosom Res* 28: 511–523
228 Cohen S, Doyle WJ, Skoner DP, Fireman P, Gwaltney JM, Jr., Newsom JT (1995) State and trait negative affect as predictors of objective and subjective symptoms of respiratory viral infections. *J Pers Soc Psychol* 68: 159–169
229 Cohen S, Doyle WJ, Turner RB, Alper CM, Skoner DP (2003) Emotional style and susceptibility to the common cold. *Psychosom Med* 65: 652–657
230 Stone AA, Cox DS, Valdimarsdottir H, Jandorf L, Neale JM (1987) Evidence that secretory IgA antibody is associated with daily mood. *J Pers Soc Psychol* 52: 988–993
231 Hall S, Smith A (1996) Investigation of the effects and aftereffects of naturally occurring upper respiratory tract illnesses on mood and performance. *Physiol Behav* 59: 569–577
232 Smith A, Thomas M, Kent J, Nicholson K (1998) Effects of the common cold on mood and performance. *Psychoneuroendocrinology* 23: 733–739
233 Smith A, Thomas M, Whitney H (2000) Effects of upper respiratory tract illnesses on mood and performance over the working day. *Ergonomics* 43: 752–763

Common Cold
ed. by R. Eccles and O. Weber

Host defenses

Sherif Beniameen Mossad

Department of Infectious Diseases, Section of Transplant Infectious Diseases, Medicine Institute, Cleveland Clinic, 9500 Euclid Avenue, S-32. Cleveland, OH 44195, USA

Abstract

Repeated episodes of viral upper respiratory tract infections occur anywhere from four to eight times per year in healthy individuals. Local and systemic defense mechanisms exist to battle respiratory tract pathogens. Clinical manifestations are mainly due to host inflammatory response. Unfortunately, the host defense mechanisms are very often not sufficient to prevent subsequent/repeated episodes of infection(s). Further insight into the interaction of infectious agent and host immune response, genetic factors, and environmental factors is needed for a better understanding of why humans repeatedly and frequently suffer from infections with respiratory agents and develop a disease syndrome known as common cold.

Introduction

Human beings have come to accept common colds as a 'fact of life'. A cold is mostly a self-limited illness. However, when considered cumulatively, about 1 year of one's life span may be spent confined to bed, or at least at home, recovering from colds. More importantly, our responses to this infection vary significantly, both intra- and inter-individually. One explanation is that many viruses – over 100 serotypes of rhinovirus alone – cause this illness, thus manifesting disease in different manners. Nevertheless, even the same virus may be asymptomatic, or cause a mild illness in one person, while another person may develop a life-threatening illness. The exact mechanisms for these variations have yet to be elucidated, but interplay between the viral virulence factors, host immune response, and viral immune evasion strategies are likely involved. Viral infections may precede secondary infection by other pathogens, precipitate asthma exacerbations, cause severe disease in the lower respiratory tract, and even induce autoimmunity [1]. It is also important to acknowledge that uncomplicated common cold symptoms including sneezing, coughing, hypersecretion resulting in runny nose and local inflammation itself may be interpreted as a complex host defense mechanism with the goal to eliminate the pathogen.

Local defense mechanisms

Nasal vestibule temperature regulation

Temperature of the nasal vestibule is the first host defense mechanism that a virus that causes common cold encounters. Increased incidence of colds during the cold winter months, and in those exposed to extreme cold weather gives us some insight into this defense mechanism [2]. A factor that contributes to the seasonality pattern of common cold may be cooling of the nasal mucosal epithelium, which inhibits mucociliary clearance as well as leukocyte phagocytic activity. On the other hand inhalation of warm vapor may alleviate nasal congestion associated with a cold. Nasal resistance as measured by a rhinomanometer increases with reducing room temperature [3], and that increase is more pronounced in summer than in winter. The latter may be due to cold adaptation of the nasal mucosa in winter.

Mucociliary clearance

Nasal airflow decreases and mucociliary clearance time is prolonged during colds. These changes correlate with abnormalities on sinus CT, and tend to be more common in allergic subjects [4]. Mucociliary clearance transport rate is markedly reduced during acute illness, and slight impairment may persist for about a month [5]. In addition, the number of ciliated nasal epithelial cells decreases, their regeneration slows down, and their beating frequency and intracellular synchrony are changed. Impaired nasal mucosal function in patients with rhinitis correlates with the rheological characteristics (viscosity, elasticity, adhesiveness, spinability, and pourability) of nasal mucus [6].

Nitric oxide (NO) regulates mucociliary activity, and has antiviral and bacteriostatic effects [7]. Increased production of exhaled NO in nasal and lower airways may play a beneficial role in clearance of rhinovirus infection [8].

Local/mucosal immune response

Approximately 90% of microorganisms infecting humans use the mucosae as entry portal. Thus, mucosal epithelia represent an important surface barrier for agents causing respiratory diseases like common cold. The mucosa is protected by numerous effectors of the innate immune system that closely work together with those of the adaptive immune system. Induction of mucosal immune responses occurs in the respiratory tract in Waldeyer's ring, which includes nasopharynx-associated lymphoid tissue like adenoids and the tonsils, although the major part of organized mucosa-associated lymphoid tissue (MALT) is located in the gut (gut-associated lymphoid tissue, GALT, e.g., aggregated Peyer's patches and isolated B-cell follicles). At least 80% of all immunoglobulin (Ig)-producing plasma cells and blasts are located in intestinal lamina propria. Approximately 90% of terminally differentiated B cells produce dimers or large polymers of IgA, which are transported externally as secretory IgA (SIgA) by an epithelial component (membrane secretory component, SC) [9]. The bronchus-associated lymphoid tissue (BALT) is thought to represent a major site in which IgA isotype switch and differentiation of B cells occur [10]. Since this is not a constitutive feature of normal human lung, other parts of the human respiratory tract like the airway epithelium are believed to fulfill supporter functions, e.g., by constitutively producing interleukin (IL)-5, a cytokine with functions for the growth and differentiation of IgA-producing plasma cells [10].

IgA and IgM share the same transport mechanisms because both components contain a similar joining (J) chain [9]. SIgA is able to inhibit invasion and colonization of pathogens, and polymeric forms of Ig may even inactivate viruses inside of secretory epithelial cells and transport them back to the luminal side [11].

Nasal mucosal IgA production is activated during common cold. Salivary Ig secretion rate is reduced in patients with recurrent respiratory infections [12, 13]. Rhinovirus infection induces respiratory epithelial expression of human beta defensin (HBD), a potent stimulant of dendritic cells, suggesting that HBD may play a role in host response to this infection [14]. Influenza virus and respiratory syncytial virus (RSV) mobilize different proportions of immune cells to the nasal respiratory mucosa [15]. Larger numbers of myeloid dendritic cells, plasmacytoid dendritic cells, and monocytes, as well as higher concentrations of monocyte chemoattractant protein-1 concentrations are present in nasal wash samples of patients with influenza [15] (Fig. 1).

Breastfeeding

Common cold is of particular importance for infants. Therefore, when discussing local or mucosal immunology of common cold, it is necessary to briefly review the role of breastfeeding. The interaction between the innate and the adaptive immune system is a prerequisite for the successful defense against respiratory pathogens. This cooperation is of particular interest for newborns because of the immediate exposure to a broad variety of microorganisms after birth. In this context, breast feeding is important for two main reasons, (i) the transfer of antibodies, and (ii) the provision of immune-modulating properties. Lactating mammary glands reflect the status of the

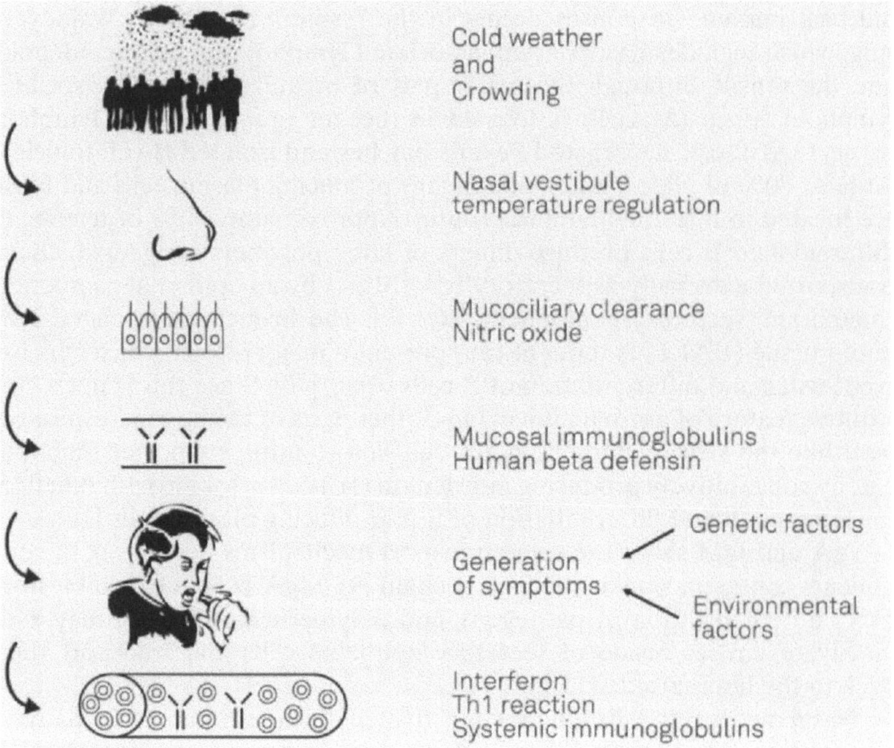

Figure 1. Stages of host defenses.

integrated mucosal immune system of the mother [9, 16] in both gut and airways. Secretory antibodies are targeted against infectious agents in the mother's environment (which are likely to be encountered by the infant during its first weeks of life). SIgA from breast milk has been shown to exhibit specificity to a variety of common intestinal and respiratory pathogens [9, 16]. Interestingly, the protection is not only demonstrable in populations living in poor sanitary conditions. The beneficial effect has also been demonstrated in developed countries [17]. In a recent analysis of approximately 400 observational studies, it was shown that a history of breastfeeding was associated with a reduction in the risk of acute otitis media, nonspecific gastroenteritis, severe lower respiratory tract infections, atopic dermatitis and asthma in young children [18]. In addition to the antibodies in the milk, numerous other factors are thought to protect the breastfed newborn. These are innate defense factors including lysozyme, lactoferrin, peroxidase, and complex oligosaccharides that may serve as receptor analogues as well as fatty acids and mucins. In addition, colostral leukocytes (~4×10^6/ml) play an important role in the protection of the suckling newborn. Macrophages constitute 55–60%, neutrophilic granulocytes 30–40% and lymphocytes (mainly T cells) 5–10% of the cells in colostrums [9, 16, 17].

Systemic immune response/symptoms

The systemic immune response may be influenced by a variety of factors such as general condition, socioeconomic status, levels of maternal antibodies, gender or ethnic group. Because of the multiple interactions between the pathogen and the host's immune system, how local and systemic immune responses are distinguished depends on definitions. In the general population, adaptive immune response in the form of neutralizing antibodies develops in only about 50% of rhinovirus infections [19]. Immunocompromised individuals, including infants, the elderly, and those who are immunosuppressed either by underlying disease or iatrogenically, may suffer severe illness following a common cold [20, 21].

Type-I IFN represent the early, innate antiviral immune response [19, 22]. Even though this response may occur in only a third of patients, experimental administration of IFN reduces the severity of symptoms of the common cold [23]. T cell response to rhinovirus infection is serotype-cross-reactive, with Th1 reaction predominating [24, 25]. In patients with asthma, bronchial epithelial cells have a deficient innate immune response to rhinovirus infections [26]. In these individuals, impaired expression of IFN results in increased viral replication and impaired apoptotic response to rhinoviral infections.

Several weeks following rhinovirus infection, neutralizing antibodies develop in serum and secretions, representing an adaptive immune response [27]. High levels of rhinovirus homotypic serum neutralizing antibodies are associated with fewer and less severe infections [28]. This is not likely to be a reliable protective mechanism for an acute situation – recovery from illness usually occurs within 7–10 days, clearly before the development of these antibodies, and only about half of those infected actually develop them. Even though these antibodies may persist for up to 1 year, they are so specific that infection with other serotypes is possible.

For RSV infections, however, neutralizing antibodies have been found to contribute to viral clearance from the respiratory tract [29]. Also for RSV infections, a Th2 type immune response (favoring the humoral instead of the classical cytotoxic response) has been suggested to play a role in the pathogenesis of asthma [30].

For many viruses, the cytotoxic or cellular immune response is important for viral clearance. Systemic mediators but also epithelial-derived pro-inflammatory cytokines create a Th1-type cytokine environment within the infected tissue, necessary to eradicate the virus infection [31]. The lack of cytopathic effects in the respiratory epithelium contributes to the rapid recovery from common cold, when compared to other infections such as influenza.

Fever as a manifestation of the systemic immune response occurs during the course of an infection. For instance, 30–40% of RSV-infected individuals develop fever. Fever is also commonly observed during parainfluenza virus infection, adenovirus infection [32] but less frequently during rhinovirus infection.

As already mentioned above under systemic immune response, a variety of factors may influence the clinical outcome and the disease severity of a common cold. Genetic factors have been described to play a role in the immune response since infants under 6 months of age with bronchiolitis associated with rhinovirus are more often IL-10 -1082 allele G non-carriers, i.e., homozygous for allele A (AA) [33].

There is ample evidence demonstrating an association between common cold symptoms and various inflammatory mediators. However, the role of specific mediators might be speculative until specific inhibitors have been studied in clinical trials. After rhinovirus infection, the proportion of infected nasal epithelial cells is low and there is not much support for direct viral cytopathic effects on the nasal epithelium [34]. Therefore, the pathogenesis of rhinovirus-induced disease is more likely due to inflammatory responses of the host, than to direct effect of the virus [34]. Although the link between the host's immune response to the clinical symptoms might be generally true for a variety of respiratory tract pathogens, it is safe to say that differences with respect to the interactions of individual pathogens with the host's immune system exist, resulting in a variety of clinical manifestations. For example, rhinoviruses are seen as typical pathogens causing common cold [34], RSV is known to cause common cold, but RSV is also a major producer of bronchiolitis, pneumonia and lower respiratory tract infection [35]. Adenoviruses may play a role in the pathogenesis of chronic obstructive pulmonary disease [36] and a respiratory coronavirus, the SARS-coronavirus is able to cause a severe acute respiratory syndrome resulting in high mortality [37, 38].

Rhinovirus infections of the nasal mucosa results in a number of symptoms including local vasodilatation and increased vascular permeability, due to cholinergic stimulation, manifesting in rhinorrhea, nasal obstruction and sneezing [20]. The host's response is mediated by pro-inflammatory cytokines, including IL-1β, IL-6, IL-8, IL-11 and TNF, and chemokines, such as RANTES (regulated on activation, normally T cell expressed and secreted), which in turn attract leukocytes and dendritic cells [21]. Increased concentrations of IL-1, IL-6 and IL-8 have been reported in nasal secretions of symptomatic subjects with rhinovirus. The concentrations of IL-6 and IL-8 appear to correlate with the severity of common cold symptoms [34]. In addition to IL-1, IL-6 and IL-8, other pro-inflammatory mediators such as the kinins bradykinin and lysylbradykinin have been detected in nasal secretions of volunteers with rhinovirus-induced colds [34]. However, the role of these kinins in the pathogenesis of common cold symptoms is not clear. Although intranasal challenge of uninfected volunteers with bradykinin resulted in symptoms of nasal obstruction, rhinorrhea and sore throat, bradykinin antagonists failed to moderate common cold symptoms [34]. The reasons for this finding remain speculative at this point.

In summary, the picture of systemic host defense mechanisms is complex. Neutralizing antibodies are known to be generated against a variety of respiratory viruses. However, protective immunity appears generally weak and repeated infections are frequently observed.

Environmental factors, exercise, co-infections

People with more diverse social networks are less susceptible to common cold, produce less mucus, have more effective nasal ciliary clearance, and shed fewer viruses [39]. Possible explanations include increased motivation to care for oneself, manifesting in increased health-promoting behaviors and reduced psychological distress. The latter is associated with lower levels of epinephrine, norepinephrine, and cortisol, which affect cellular and humoral immune responses to infection.

Exercise may reduce the risk of upper respiratory tract infections by transiently increasing the leukocyte count or salivary IgA [40]. On the other hand, elite athletes suffer a higher rate of colds during intense training and competition season than recreationally competitive athletes [41].

Viral co-infection may occur in about 5% of cases of common cold [42]. Viral and bacterial co-infection is uncommon, occurring in <1% of cases [42]. The impact of these co-infections on the host defenses and the resolution of illness are not well understood.

References

1 Kirchberger S, Majdic O, Stockl J (2007) Modulation of the immune system by human rhinoviruses. *Int Arch Allergy Immunol* 142: 1–10

2 Eccles R (2002) An explanation for the seasonality of acute upper respiratory tract viral infections. *Acta Otolaryngol* 122: 183–191

3 Sano H (1992) Influence of environmental temperature (cold exposure) on nasal resistance. *Nippon Jibiinkoka Gakkai Kaiho [Journal of the Oto-Rhino-Laryngological Society of Japan]* 95: 1785–1799

4 Alho OP (2004) Nasal airflow, mucociliary clearance, and sinus functioning during viral colds: Effects of allergic rhinitis and susceptibility to recurrent sinusitis. *Am J Rhinol* 18: 349–355

5 Pedersen M, Sakakura Y, Winther B, Brofeldt S, Mygind N (1983) Nasal mucociliary transport, number of ciliated cells, and beating pattern in naturally acquired common colds. *Eur J Respir Dis* S128: 355–365

6 Passali D, Bellussi L, Lauriello M (1995) The rheological characteristics of nasal mucus in patients with rhinitis. *Eur Arch Otorhinolaryngol* 252: 348–352

7 Lindberg S, Cervin A, Runer T (1997) Nitric oxide (NO) production in the upper airways is decreased in chronic sinusitis. *Acta Oto-Laryngol* 117: 113–117

8 Sanders SP, Proud D, Permutt S, Siekierski ES, Yachechko R, Liu MC (2004)

Role of nasal nitric oxide in the resolution of experimental rhinovirus infection. *J Allergy Clin Immunol* 113: 697–702
9 Brandtzaeg P (2003) Mucosal immunity: Integration between mother and the breast-fed infant. *Vaccine* 21: 3382–3388
10 Salvi S, Holgate ST (1999) Could the airway epithelium play an important role in mucosal immunoglobulin A production? *Clin Exp Allergy* 12:1597–1605
11 Brandtzaeg P, Farstad IN, Johansen FE, Morton HC, Norderhaug IN, Yamanaka T (1999) The B-cell system of human mucosae and exocrine glands. *Immunol Rev* 171: 45–87
12 Lenander-Lumikari M, Puhakka T, Makela MJ, Vilja P, Ruuskanen O, Tenovuo J (1999) Effects of the common cold and intranasal fluticasone propionate treatment on mucosal host defense assessed by human saliva. *Oral Surg Oral Med Oral Pathol Oral Radiol Endod* 87: 695–699
13 Chaushu S, Yefenof E, Becker A, Shapira J, Chaushu G (2002) A link between parotid salivary Ig level and recurrent respiratory infections in young Down's syndrome patients. *Oral Microbiol Immunol* 17:172–176
14 Proud D, Sanders SP, Wiehler S (2004) Human rhinovirus infection induces airway epithelial cell production of human beta-defensin 2 both *In vitro* and *in vivo*. *J Immunol* 172: 4637–4645
15 Gill MA, Long K, Kwon T, Muniz L, Mejias A, Connolly J, Roy L, Banchereau J, Ramilo O (2008) Differential recruitment of dendritic cells and monocytes to respiratory mucosal sites in children with influenza virus or respiratory syncytial virus infection. *J Infect Dis* 198: 1667–1675
16 Goldman AS (1993) The immune system of human milk: Antimicrobial antiinflammatory and immunomodulating properties. *Pediatr Infect Dis J* 12: 664–671
17 Wold AE, Hanson LA (1994) Defense factors in human milk. *Curr Opin Gastroenterol* 10: 652–658
18 Ip S, Chung M, Raman G, Chew P, Magula N, DeVine D, Trikalinos T, Lau J (2007) Breastfeeding and maternal and infant health outcomes in developed countries. *Evid Rep Technol Assess (Full Report)* 153:1–186
19 Couch RB (1996) Rhinoviruses. In: BN Fields, DM Knipe, PM Howley et al. (eds): *Fields Virology*, 3rd edn. Lippincott-Raven, New York, 713–734
20 Heikkinen T, Jarvinen A (2003) The common cold. *Lancet* 361: 51–59
21 van Cauwenberge PB, van Kempen MJ, Bachert C (2000) The common cold at the turn of the millennium. *Am J Rhinol* 14: 339–343
22 Katze MG, He Y, Gale M Jr (2002) Viruses and interferon: A fight for supremacy. *Nat Rev Immunol* 2: 675–687
23 Gwaltney JM Jr, Winther B, Patrie JT, Hendley JO (2002) Combined antiviral-antimediator treatment for the common cold. *J Infect Dis* 186: 147–154
24 Pitkaranta A, Hayden FG (1998) Rhinoviruses: Important respiratory pathogens. *Ann Med* 30: 529–537
25 Wimalasundera SS, Katz DR, Chain BM (1997) Characterization of the T cell response to human rhinovirus in children: Implications for understanding the immunopathology of the common cold. *J Infect Dis* 176: 755–759
26 Wark PA, Johnston SL, Bucchieri F, Powell R, Puddicombe S, Laza-Stanca V, Holgate ST, Davies DE (2005) Asthmatic bronchial epithelial cells have a

deficient innate immune response to infection with rhinovirus. *J Exp Med* 201: 937–947
27 Hewat EA, Marlovits TC, Blaas D (1998) Structure of a neutralizing antibody bound monovalently to human rhinovirus 2. *J Virol* 72: 4396–4402
28 Alper CM, Doyle WJ, Skoner DP, Buchman CA, Seroky JT, Gwaltney JM, Cohen SA (1996) Prechallenge antibodies: Moderators of infection rate, signs, and symptoms in adults experimentally challenged with rhinovirus type 39. *Laryngoscope* 106: 1298–1305
29 Collins PL, Crowe JEJ (2007) Respiratory syncytial virus and metapneumovirus. In: Knipe DM, Howley PM, Griffin DE, Lamb RA, Martin MA, Roizman B, Straus SE (eds): *Fields Virology*, 5th edn. Lippincott Williams & Wilkins, Philadelphia, 1601–1646
30 Kim CK, Kim SW, Park CS, Kim BI, Kang H, Koh YY (2003) Bronchoalveolar lavage cytokine profiles in acute asthma and acute bronchiolitis. *J Allergy Clin Immunol* 112:64–71
31 van Kempen M, Bachert C, van Cauwenberge P (1999) An update on the pathophysiology of rhinovirus upper respiratory tract infections. *Rhinology* 37: 97–103
32 Eccles R (2005) Understanding the symptoms of the common cold and influenza. *Lancet Infect Dis* 5: 718–725
33 Helminen M, Nuolivirta K, Virta M, Halkosalo A, Korppi M, Vesikari T, Hurme M (2008) IL-10 gene polymorphism at -1082 A/G is associated with severe rhinovirus bronchiolitis in infants. *Pediatr Pulmonol* 43: 391–395
34 Turner RB, Hayden FG (2003) Rhinovirus. In: H Ruebsamen-Waigmann, K Deres, G Hewlett, R Welker (eds): *Viral infections and treatment.* Marcel Dekker, New York, 139–164
35 Wyde PR, Piedra PA (2003) Respiratory syncytial virus. In: H Ruebsamen-Waigmann, K Deres, G Hewlett, R Welker (eds): *Viral infections and treatment.* Marcel Dekker, New York, 91–137
36 Ginsberg HS, Gold E, Jordan WS Jr, Katz S, Badger GF, Dingle JH (1955) Relations of the new respiratory agents to acute respiratory diseases. *Am J Public Health* 45:915–922
37 Drosten C, Gunther S, Preiser W, van der Werf S, Brodt HR, Becker S, Rabenau H, Panning M, Kolesnikova L, Fouchier RA et al. (2003) Identification of a novel coronavirus in patients with acute respiratory syndrome. *N Engl J Med* 348: 1967–1976
38 Ksiazek TG, Erdman D, Goldsmith CS, Zaki SR, Peret T, Emery S, Tong S, Urbani C, Comer JA, Lim W et al. (2003) A novel coronavirus associated with severe acute respiratory syndrome. *N Engl J Med* 348: 1953–1966
39 Cohen S, Doyle WJ, Skoner DP, Rabin BS, Gwaltney JM Jr (1997) Social ties and susceptibility to the common cold. *JAMA* 277: 1940–1944
40 Chubak J, McTiernan A, Sorensen B, Wener MH, Yasui Y, Velasquez M, Wood B, Rajan KB, Wetmore CM, Potter JD, Ulrich CM (2006) Moderate-intensity exercise reduces the incidence of colds among postmenopausal women. *Am J Med* 119:937–942
41 Spence L, Brown WJ, Pyne DB, Nissen MD, Sloots TP, McCormack JG, Locke

AS, Fricker PA (2007) Incidence, etiology, and symptomatology of upper respiratory illness in elite athletes. *Med Sci Sports Exerc* 39: 577–586
42 Makela MJ, Puhakka T, Ruuskanen O, Leinonen M, Saikku P, Kimpimäki M, Blomqvist S, Hyypiä T, Arstila P (1998) Viruses and bacteria in the etiology of the common cold. *J Clin Microbiol* 36: 539–542

Common Cold
ed. by R. Eccles and O. Weber

Transmission of colds

Diane E. Pappas and J. Owen Hendley

University of Virginia Department of Pediatrics, Charlottesville, VA 22908, USA

Abstract

Rhinorrhea, nasal congestion, and sore throat herald the beginning of the cold season for both children and adults. Although the common cold is a self-limited infection, there are no effective treatments presently available and complications, missed time from work and school, and overall discomfort are not insignificant. Understanding how infections are transmitted may lead to interventions to reduce rates of infection. In order to establish a route of transmission, certain conditions must be met. The virus must be produced and shed at the site of infection. The virus must be deposited in the environment and be able to survive there. The virus must then be able to reach the portal of entry. Finally, interruption of the proposed route of transmission must reduce the incidence of infection under natural conditions. Applying this framework, there is clear evidence in both experimental and home settings that colds can be transmitted *via* self-inoculation. A small amount of evidence is available relating to large and small particle aerosol transmission. Because rhinovirus is responsible for half of all colds, it has been used as the model to understand how virus is transmitted from one person to another in experimental settings. Rhinovirus has been shown to infect *via* self-inoculation following hand-to-hand contact with contaminated hands or hand-to-surface contact with contaminated objects in the environment. Similarly, there is convincing evidence that the self-inoculation method of cold virus transmission occurs in the home environment, where colds are most often transmitted. Aerosol transmission has been studied in the experimental setting and may provide another, albeit less common, method for transmission of rhinovirus infection. As more is understood about the transmission of cold viruses, effective methods to interrupt transmission may be devised.

Introduction

Rhinorrhea, nasal congestion, and a sore or scratchy throat are the unmistakable hallmarks that herald the onset of the common cold. This viral, self-limited upper respiratory tract infection affects both children and adults. Although a number of viruses may produce the symptoms of the common cold, the majority of colds (50% of those in children and adults) are caused by human rhinovirus. Rhinovirus is not normally found in the upper respiratory tract but is acquired by transmission from one person to another. Viral transmission commonly occurs in the home, and children are the primary reservoir [1].

Because rhinoviruses are the most frequent cause of colds, they have been used to study the mechanisms involved in transmission of the common cold. Rhinovirus deposited in the nose, either directly or by way of the nasolacrimal duct from the eye, is carried by mucociliary clearance to the nasopharynx, which is the initial site of rhinovirus infection [2]. Subsequently, rhinovirus infection may spread anteriorly to infect the nasal mucosa [3]. Rhinovirus replication occurs in only a small number of nasal epithelial cells, as demonstrated by studies using *in situ* hybridization of nasal biopsy specimens [4, 5]. Rhinovirus can be recovered from nasal secretions of infected individuals for 5–7 days, but viral shedding in the nasopharynx may persist for 2–3 weeks [3]. In addition, rhinovirus has also been shown to replicate in the lower respiratory tract [6].

It is clear that rhinovirus is shed from the site of infection in the nose, but the means of transmission of rhinovirus from one person to another have been more difficult to determine. Transmissions *via* small particle aerosol, large particle aerosol, and self-inoculation have all been proposed. Virus in a small particle aerosol, produced from the lungs by coughing, would have to be inhaled and reach the lungs in order to transmit infection (Fig. 1). Large particle aerosols, such as the large droplets of saliva expelled during a sneeze, would have to land directly on the eyes or nose, or on a surface to be picked up on the hands for self-inoculation to transmit infection (Fig. 2).

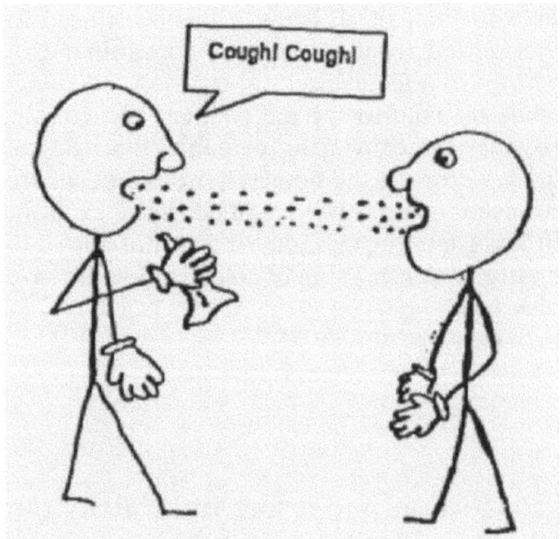

Figure 1. Small particle aerosol transmission (drawings Figures 1–3: With friendly permission of Elizabeth L. Pappas).

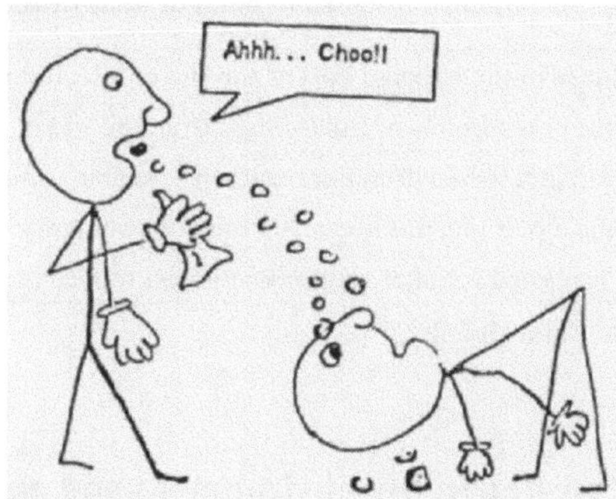
Ahhh... Choo!!

Figure 2. Large particle aerosol transmission.

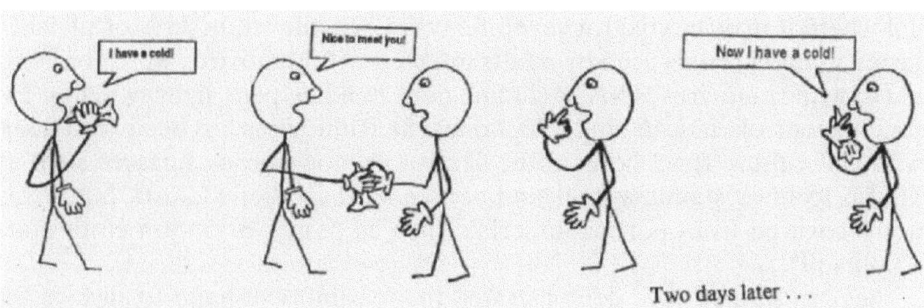
I have a cold!
Nice to meet you!
Now I have a cold!
Two days later . . .

Figure 3. Hand-to-hand with self-inoculation.

Hand-to-hand or hand-to-surface-to-hand transfer with self-inoculation would deposit rhinovirus directly into the nose or eyes from which infection of the nasopharynx could result (Fig. 3).

In order to understand viral transmission, a series of postulates have been developed that must be met to establish that viral transmission occurs *via* the proposed route (Tab. 1). According to this algorithm, the virus must be produced and shed at the site of infection, it must be deposited in the environment and able to survive there, and it must be able to reach the portal of entry, namely the eyes or nose for rhinovirus. Finally, to establish that viral transmission actually occurs *via* a route, interruption of the proposed route must reduce the incidence of infection. This review focuses on deposition of virus in the environment, transfer of virus to the portal of entry, and interruption of transmission.

Table 1. Framework for establishing transmission routes of rhinovirus*

1.	Virus must be produced in the infected host at the site of infection
2.	Virus must be present in secretions or tissues shed from the site of infection
3.	Virus must be deposited in the environment and must be able to survive there
4.	Virus deposited in the environment must reach the portal of entry
5.	Interruption of the proposed route of transmission must reduce the incidence of infection

*Adapted from Gwaltney and Hendley [7]

Virus must be deposited in the environment and able to survive (Tab. 2)

Rhinovirus has been found on the hands of about 40% of naturally infected individuals [7]. From the hands, rhinovirus may be transmitted directly to another person's hand or be deposited on a surface by an infected individual where it may survive for several days [8]. In one study, 35% of surfaces tested in hotel rooms used by adults infected with rhinovirus were contaminated with rhinovirus RNA, including door handles, pens, light switches, TV remote controls, faucets, and telephones [8]. Rhinovirus has been recovered with cell culture for 3 hours after deposit on non-porous surfaces such as plastic, formica, stainless steel, and certain hard synthetic fabrics, but it was not recovered from porous materials such as tissues or cotton cloth after 3 hours [9].

Several studies have demonstrated the feasibility of hand-to-surface-to-hand transfer of rhinovirus. In one study, touching surfaces and objects contaminated with rhinovirus RNA during the course of normal daily activities effectively transferred viral RNA to the fingertips in 47% (28/60) of trials [8]. Transfer was more efficient for surfaces contaminated for only 1 hour, where 60% (18/30) of the trials had positive virus transfer. After 18 hours, transfer decreased to 33% (10/30) [8]. In another experiment, infectious rhinovirus was effectively transferred from contaminated smooth surfaces after normal handling to the hands of 64% (14/22) of volunteers; the contaminated surfaces included table tops and pens [10]. Hand-to-surface-to-hand transfer seems to be a feasible method for transfer of rhinovirus during normal daily activities.

Hand-to-hand contact is one effective method of transferring rhinovirus. Rhinovirus can survive on human skin for 1–2 hours during normal use while studying or eating [9]. In one study, rhinovirus was recovered from the hands of 40% (10/25) of volunteers who had hand-to-hand contact with the contaminated hands of infected donors [11]. In another study, rubbing of inoculated skin resulted in transfer of rhinovirus to the fingers of 42% (16/38) of volunteers [10]. In married couples, the likelihood of rhinovirus infection in the susceptible spouse was directly related to the presence of

Table 2. Virus must be deposited in the environment and be able to survive there

Deposited in the environment:
• Rhinovirus can be recovered for up to 3 hours on non-porous surfaces; rhinovirus survives on human skin for 1–3 hours [9]
• Rhinovirus is found on about 40% of hands of adults with natural rhinovirus infection [7]
• Rhinovirus is found on 35% of surfaces of hotel rooms used by adults infected with rhinovirus [8]
Hand-to-surface-to-hand transfer:
• Rhinovirus transferred to the fingertips used to touch hotel objects contaminated with rhinovirus in 47% of trials; 60% of transfers were positive for surfaces contaminated only 1 hour earlier, and 33% for surfaces contaminated 18 hours earlier [8]
• Rhinovirus was recovered from the hands of 64% of volunteers who handled contaminated objects [10]
• Respiratory syncytial virus (RSV) could be recovered from an average of 2.4 surfaces tested per hospital room that had been occupied by an infant infected with RSV. Nine volunteers became infected, 5 cuddlers and 4 touchers (self-inoculation); none of the sitters (small particle aerosol) became infected [18]
Hand-to-hand transfer:
• Rhinovirus can be recovered from 40% of volunteers who had hand-to-hand contact with the contaminated hands of infected donors [11]
• Rhinovirus was recovered from the fingers of 42% of volunteers who rubbed skin contaminated with rhinovirus [10]
• In married couples, the likelihood of rhinovirus transmission is directly related to the presence of rhinovirus on the nose/hands of the infected spouse [12]
Aerosol transmission:
• Airborne rhinovirus was not detected when experimentally infected volunteers were housed in a room with an air sampler capable of testing 82% of the air in the room [13]
• Picornavirus RNA detected in 32% of air sampling filters from three office buildings; frequency of viral detection correlated with amount of outside ventilation [14]
• Recirculation of air on airline flights did not increase the risk for cold symptoms in passengers [15]
• Rhinoviruses do not circulate well among adults at work at an insurance company [16]
• Rhinovirus can be recovered from only 1/13 sneezes and 0/8 coughs [9]
• Rhinovirus can be detected in a mask after talking, coughing, breathing [17]

rhinovirus on the hands and in the nose of the infected spouse [12]. It is clear that rhinovirus can be effectively transferred from hand to hand.

Other studies have examined deposition and survival of rhinovirus in the air. Experimentally, rhinovirus can remain infectious in small particle aerosols and volunteers can be infected by exposure to them [7], but this has not been shown to occur commonly in natural settings. In one air sample study, experimentally infected volunteers were housed in a room with an air sampler capable of testing 82% of the air in the room, but no rhinovirus was detected [13]. In another air sample study, picornavirus RNA was detected in 32% of air sampling filters from three office buildings, and the frequency of viral detection correlated with the amount of outside ventilation employed [14]. In a natural setting, there was no evidence that recirculation of air during commercial plane flights increased the risk for cold symptoms in passengers [15]. In a study of rhinovirus infection in insurance company employees working in a large room, it was found that rhinoviruses did not circulate well at work [16]. Finally, evaluation of simulated sneezes and coughs of adults with natural rhinovirus colds showed that rhinovirus could be recovered from only 1/13 sneezes and 0/8 coughs [9]; neither of these aerosol-producing behaviors were effective in producing rhinovirus-laden aerosols. A more recent study, using a mask placed closely over the nose and mouth, demonstrated the presence of rhinovirus RNA by PCR analysis after coughing, talking, and breathing, but this may have been due to close contact with the mask and not necessarily due to aerosolization [17].

In a study of another common cold virus, respiratory syncytial virus (RSV), transmission *via* close contact with large droplets or self-inoculation after touching contaminated surfaces has been demonstrated. In this study, volunteers were assigned to be "cuddlers" and care for infants with RSV, "touchers" who touched surfaces in the infant's room while the infant was out of the room, and sitters who sat in the room with an infected infant. When surfaces in the environment were tested, RSV could be recovered from an average of 2.4 surfaces tested per room. Nine volunteers became infected, 5 cuddlers and 4 touchers; none of the sitters became infected. This provides evidence that RSV can be transmitted by self-inoculation (touchers) and not by small particle aerosols (sitters). It is unclear what role large particle aerosol may play in transmission of RSV [18].

Other factors may also influence the survival and transmissibility of cold viruses, including climate and human behavior. Cold viruses in temperate climates move through the community in a predictable and orderly fashion. It begins with an increase in rhinovirus in September after the children return to school. Late October and November herald the onset of parainfluenza, followed by RSV and coronaviruses in the winter months. Influenza peaks in late winter, and rhinovirus has a secondary peak thereafter, while adenovirus remains constant throughout. Because these cold viruses occur in the community at different times, environmental conditions and population characteristics (school attendance, crowding indoors) may affect the survival of these viruses in the environment and their subsequent transmission [19]. In summary, rhinovirus is commonly present on the hands of infected individuals and on the objects that they use in daily activities and can be readily transferred from hands and objects to the hands of susceptible hosts, thus providing a readily available method of rhinovirus transfer from one person to another. Rhinovirus may be present in aerosols, but the frequency of expulsion of viable virus into the air with coughs and sneezes is not clear. Likewise, RSV may be present on surfaces and transmit infection to susceptible individuals following deliberate self-inoculation, but not *via* small particle aerosol. Other factors, such as human behavior and climate, may also play a role in cold virus survival and transmission.

Virus deposited in the environment must reach the portal of entry (Tab. 3)

For infection to occur, rhinovirus must be deposited on the nasal epithelium. This may occur by inoculation of the conjunctiva followed by transfer *via* the nasolacrimal duct or direct inoculation of the nose [3]. Oral inoculation through prolonged kissing [20] or direct inoculation under experimental conditions transmitted infection infrequently [9, 10]. Rhinovirus on hands (fingertips) of a susceptible individual can be transferred to his/her own nose or eyes *via* self-inoculation. Humans are known to frequently touch their own eyes and nose [9], making transfer of rhinovirus from an individual's hands to his/her own eyes and nose a likely possibility, while oral inoculation is not sufficient.

Studies have demonstrated that rhinovirus deposited on the hands can successfully transmit infection. In one study, rhinovirus dried on the fingers was self-inoculated by volunteers onto their own nasal or conjunctival mucosa, resulting in infection in 36% (4/11) of volunteers [9]. In another study, 73% (11/15) of volunteers who had brief, 15-second hand-to-hand contact with the contaminated hands of infected donors followed by touching their own eyes and nose became infected [7]. Finally, in a study of hand-to-hand contact between volunteers and infected donors, 60% (6/10) of the recipient volunteers became infected after touching their own eyes and

Table 3. Virus deposited in the environment must reach the portal of entry

- Oral inoculation through prolonged kissing [20] or direct inoculation transmitted infection infrequently [9, 10]
- Humans frequently touch their eyes and nose [9]
- Rhinovirus dried on the fingers which are then placed in the eyes or nose results in infection in 36% of volunteers [9]
- In volunteers who had brief hand-to-hand contact with contaminated hands and then touched their own eyes and nose, 73% became infected [7]
- Hand-to-hand contact between volunteers and infected donors resulted in infection in 60% of volunteers after they touched their own eyes and nose [11]
- Handling coffee cup handles contaminated with rhinovirus transmitted infection to 50% of recipients; handling plastic tiles contaminated with rhinovirus transmitted infection to 56% of recipients [21]
- None of the volunteers playing poker with objects used by rhinovirus-infected volunteers became infected [22]

nose [11]. These experimental studies provide evidence for the feasibility of hand-to-hand with self-inoculation transmission of rhinovirus.

Other studies have evaluated whether rhinovirus deposited on surfaces can effectively transmit infection. In one study, handling coffee cup handles contaminated with rhinovirus by infected donors followed by self-inoculation resulted in infection of 50% (5/10) of recipients; handling plastic tiles contaminated with rhinovirus transmitted infection to 56% (9/16) of recipients [21]. In contrast, volunteers who played poker with the chips and other objects previously used by individuals infected with rhinovirus did not become infected [22]. It is unclear why infection did not occur in this situation in the same way that it did in the experiment with the tiles and the coffee cups. Because transfer to fingertips is more efficient if the objects or surfaces are touched and handled soon after rhinovirus deposit, hand-to-surface-to-hand transmission may not be as efficient a method of transfer as hand-to-hand transfer.

In summary, in experimental settings rhinovirus is frequently deposited in the environment (on hands or on objects used by infected individuals) and can be transferred to susceptible hosts with resultant infection following deliberate self-inoculation. Transfer appears to be more efficient if the objects have been recently contaminated. Rhinovirus is not transmitted from person to person *via* oral inoculation.

Interruption of the proposed route of transmission must reduce the incidence of infection (Tab. 4)

To establish that transmission of rhinovirus has occurred *via* any particular route, one must be able to demonstrate that disruption of the route can reduce the incidence of infection. In one study in which the hand self-inoculation route was interrupted, volunteers wearing gloves were exposed to infected individuals across a small table while the infected individuals sang, coughed, sneezed, and talked loudly (large and/or small particle aerosol exposure); infection occurred in 8% of the volunteers [23]. Separation of susceptible volunteers from infected individuals across a greater distance while being housed together for 3 days across a double-wire mesh (small particle aerosol exposure) resulted in no infections [23]. These results suggest that small particle aerosol transmission is an infrequent method of rhinovirus transmission.

In different experiments using the poker transmission model, Dick et al. [22] devised methods to interrupt hand self-inoculation transmission using restraints to allow comparison of rates of transmission *via* aerosol alone or by any route. In this study, volunteers wore collar restraints designed to interrupt transmission *via* self-inoculation because the collar prevented them from touching their eyes or nose. They were exposed to infected individuals while playing poker. Five of six restrained players were infected, compared

Table 4. Interruption of the proposed route of transmission must reduce the incidence of infection

- Only 8% of uninfected volunteers became infected after exposure across a small table to rhinovirus-infected individuals who were singing, coughing, sneezing, and talking loudly; when separated by a greater distance, none became infected [23]
- In volunteers playing poker with rhinovirus infected individuals, 67% of those volunteers with restraints to prevent self-touching of the eyes and nose became infected, compared to 56% of unrestrained volunteers [22]
- In volunteers whose hands were pretreated with iodine who had hand-to-hand contact with the contaminated hands of rhinovirus-infected donors and who then touched their own eyes and nose, 60% of the untreated volunteers became infected while only 10% of the iodine treated volunteers became infected; furthermore, rhinovirus could be recovered from the hands of only 11% of the iodine-treated group, compared with 40% of the untreated group [11]
- Rhinovirus suspended in cell culture media passed through commercial tissues 26/27 times, but passed through only 1/18 times when the tissues were treated with a combination of malic acid, citric acid, and lauryl sulfate [24]
- 83% of those who blew their nose without a tissue had rhinovirus recovered from their hands, compared with 42% of those using commercial tissues, and only 3% of those using treated tissues (malic acid, citric acid, and lauryl sulfate) [25]
- Rhinovirus was transferred to fingertips of recipients after brief contact with donor fingers which were contaminated with virus from 95% of donors who used no tissue to blow their nose, from 27% of those who used commercial tissues and from 0% of those who used treated tissues; likewise, 50% of the recipients in the no-tissue group became infected after touching their own eyes and nose, compared with 13% of those in the commercial tissue group and 0% of those in the treated tissue group [25]

to 6/6 control volunteers who were unrestrained [22]. They then placed arm-braces on volunteers as another method of interrupting transmission *via* self-inoculation and found that only 1/6 of the restrained volunteers became infected, compared with 5/6 of the unrestrained volunteers. In a second group of arm-braced volunteers, they found that 4/6 of the restrained volunteers became infected, compared with 1/6 of the unrestrained volunteers. Taken all together, 67% (12/18) of the unrestrained players became infected, as compared with 56% (10/18) of the restrained players, suggesting that infection can occur *via* aerosol transmission [22].

In order to examine transmission *via* self-inoculation, practical interruption strategies to block the self-inoculation process were examined. A study using iodine was carried out to assess transmission by self-inoculation [7]. In this study, donors contaminated their hands and then had hand contact with susceptible volunteers who wore masks. The susceptible volunteers were divided into two groups; the hands in the treatment group were treated with iodine, while the control group received no hand treatment. Both groups then tried to self-inoculate their own eyes and nose. In the no treatment group, 60% (6/10) of the susceptible volunteers became infected; only 10% (1/10) in the iodine-treated group became infected [7]. Additionally, rhinovirus was recovered from 10/25 (40%) of the hand rinses from the control group and from only 3/27 (11%) of hand rinses from the iodine-treated group. In this experimental model, the interruption of the self-inoculation method of transfer clearly resulted in a decreased incidence of infection, consistent with the effectiveness of this method of transmission for rhinovirus.

In other studies, infected donor volunteers have used antiviral tissues in the attempt to interrupt transmission. In one study, rhinovirus suspended in cell culture medium passed through commercial tissues 26/27 times, but virus passed through only 1/18 times when the tissues contained a combination of malic acid, citric acid, and lauryl sulfate [24]. In another study, use of these treated tissues by experimentally infected adults reduced viral contamination of the fingers; 83% of those who blew their nose without a tissue had rhinovirus recovered from their fingers, as compared to 42% of those using commercial tissues and only 3% of those using the treated tissues [25]. Transmission of rhinovirus after brief finger-to-finger contact, when the donor fingers were contaminated with virus, demonstrated viral transfer from 95% of those who used no tissues, 27% from those who used commercial tissues, and 0% from those who used the treated tissues. Finally, recipients rubbed their fingers into their own eyes and noses; 50% of the recipients in the no-tissue group became infected, as compared to only 13% of recipients in the commercial tissue group and 0% of those in the antiviral tissue group. Taken together, these studies demonstrate that transmission can be interrupted by interrupting hand-to-hand transfer of rhinovirus with use of virucidal tissues by infected subjects. The effectiveness of virucidal tissue use may be limited by improper use and disposal, especially when tissues are used by young children.

Interruption of cold transmission in the home environment (Tab. 5)

Although studies in the experimental setting suggest that hand-to-hand, hand-to-surface-to-hand, and aerosol transmission of rhinovirus may occur, less information is available about cold transmission in the home where rhinovirus and other cold viruses are usually acquired. In the experimental setting, interruption of self-inoculation by treatment of the hands of the recipient with iodine to impair the infectivity of rhinovirus is effective in decreasing both transfer from hand to hand and infection after deliberate self-inoculation [11]. Determining how to interrupt transmission in the home setting is a more difficult proposition. In the best evaluation to date [7], careful definitions of exposure, respiratory infection, and secondary infection were employed to evaluate transmission in the home. Application of 2% aqueous iodine to the fingertips of mothers was tested as a means of interrupting transmission to reduce secondary infection in the mothers in the home. Mothers were instructed to apply 2% aqueous iodine or brown

Table 5. Cold transmission in the home/school

- No decrease in absenteeism due to respiratory illness in the classrooms using alcohol-based hand sanitizers and quaternary ammonium wipes compared with classrooms utilizing normal cleaning practices [27]
- No decrease in the incidence of secondary respiratory illness in families using alcohol-based hand sanitizers [28]
- Use of virucidal tissues in the home reduced secondary transmission in the home by 32% compared to placebo tissues [29]
- Use of 2% aqueous iodine applied every 3–4 hours to the fingertips of mothers after the onset of respiratory symptoms in a family member significantly reduced secondary respiratory illness in the home [7]

placebo to their fingertips upon awakening and every 3–4 hours thereafter at the onset of respiratory symptoms in a family member. A respiratory infection was defined as either two respiratory symptoms occurring on the same day or one symptom occurring on two consecutive days. A secondary case (in the mother) was defined as respiratory symptoms beginning at least 2 days and not more than 7 days after onset of respiratory symptoms in the index case. The study was conducted in the fall over 4 years; in the iodine-treated mothers, 6–8% of exposures resulted in secondary illness, compared with 15–26% in the control group. When the results from all 4 years were combined, only 4/58 (7%) of exposures in the iodine-treated group resulted in infection, compared with 16/79 (20%) in the control group [7]. When the results were adjusted for maternal immunity to rhinovirus, only 4/32 (12.5%) of the iodine-treated mothers experienced secondary infection, compared to 16/44 (36%) of the control group. This small study provides convincing evidence that the interruption of self-inoculation can decrease transmission in the home environment. The practical application of this method of interruption of transmission is limited, however, as iodine applied to the hands is drying and stains the hands brown.

Other studies in the natural environment have evaluated the use of alcohol-based hand sanitizers and gels as a method to decrease transmission of the common cold. One study based on a self-report of illness and frequency of hand sanitizer use suggested that use of alcohol-based hand gels may decrease secondary transmission of respiratory infections in families [26]. In a study of school children by the same investigators, classrooms using alcohol-based hand sanitizer and quaternary ammonium wipes to disinfect school surfaces were compared to classrooms using normal hand washing and cleaning procedures. There was a decrease in absenteeism due to gastrointestinal illness in the intervention group, but there was no difference in absenteeism due to respiratory illness [27]. In a third study of the effect of hand sanitizer use in the home [28], the overall rate of secondary respiratory illness did not decrease with hand-sanitizer use. The lack of effect of alcohol-based hand sanitizers on the rate of secondary illness in the home may be due to the fact that alcohol does not impair rhinovirus infectivity, or that aerosol transmission occurs commonly [28]. Under any circumstances, the use of alcohol-based hand gels does not appear to be an effective mechanism for reducing cold transmission in the natural environment.

The use of virucidal tissues as a method to interrupt cold virus transmission in the home environment has shown a modest effect. Use of virucidal tissues reduced secondary transmission in the home by 32% compared to placebo tissues [29]. Unfortunately, the effectiveness of virucidal tissues for interrupting transmission is dependent on proper use and disposal of such tissues by the family member who already is infected, something which young children may not be able to do effectively and routinely.

In summary, the home studies available provide a small but significant body of evidence demonstrating that interrupting the self-inoculation route reduces the transmission of colds in the home. The use of aqueous iodine and of virucidal tissues has been shown to reduce secondary illness when used in the home environment. The use of alcohol-based hand gels did not reduce the rate of secondary respiratory illness in the home. Because alcohol does not inactivate rhinovirus (responsible for up to 50% of colds) this result does not disprove self-inoculation as the predominant method of transmission; aerosol transmission provides an alternative explanation. Interruption of aerosol transmission has not been attempted either in experimental settings or in the home environment.

Conclusion

From the currently available evidence analyzed within a framework [7] for establishing viral transmission, in the experimental setting rhinovirus can be transmitted from person to person through self-inoculation after contact with the contaminated hands of others or with contaminated objects. Interruption studies in the home environment utilizing iodine and virucidal tissues have demonstrated a decrease in secondary transmission consistent with self-inoculation as a method of cold virus transmission in the home. Interruption of transmission *via* aerosols has not been studied. Prevention of secondary transmission may be the most effective means of reducing the misery of the common cold. It seems likely that effective and practical methods of interruption of transmission of colds in the home can be developed.

References

1 Peltola V, Waris M, Osterback R et al. (2008) Rhinovirus transmission within families with children: Incidence of symptomatic and asymptomatic infections. *J Infect Dis* 197: 382–389

2 Hendley JO (1999) Clinical virology of rhinoviruses. *Adv Virus Res* 54: 453–466

3 Winther B, Gwaltney, JM, Mygind, N et al. (1986) Sites of rhinovirus recovery after point inoculation of the upper airway. *JAMA* 256: 1763
4 Arruda E, Boyle TR, Winther B et al. (1995) Localization of human rhinovirus replication in the upper respiratory tract by *in situ* hybridization. *J Infect Dis* 171: 1329–1333
5 Bardin PG, Johnston SL, Sanderson G et al. (1994) Detection of rhinovirus infection of the nasal mucosa by oligonucleotide *in situ* hybridization. *Am J Respir Cell Mol Biol* 10: 207–213
6 Papadopoulos, NG, Bates, PJ, Bardin, PG et al. (2000) Rhinoviruses infect the lower airways. *J Infect Dis* 181: 1875–1884
7 Gwaltney JM Jr, Hendley JO (1988) Mechanisms of transmission of rhinovirus infections. *Epidemiol Rev* 10: 242–258
8 Winther B, McCue K, Ashe K et al. (2007) Environmental contamination with rhinovirus and transfer to fingers of healthy individuals by daily life activity. *J Med Virol* 79: 1606–1610
9 Hendley JO, Wenzel RP, Gwaltney JM Jr (1973) Transmission of rhinovirus colds by self-inoculation. *N Engl J Med* 288: 1361–1364
10 Reed SE (1975) An investigation of the possible transmission of rhinovirus colds through indirect contact. *J Hyg (Camb)* 75: 249–258
11 Gwaltney JM Jr, Moskalski PB, Hendley JO. (1980) Interruption of experimental rhinovirus transmission. *J Infect Dis* 142: 811–815
12 D'Alessio DJ, Peterson JA, Dick CR, Dick EC. (1976) Transmission of experimental rhinovirus colds in volunteer married couples. *J Infect Dis* 133: 28–36
13 Gwaltney JM Jr (1980) Epidemiology of the common cold. *Ann NY Acad Sci* 353: 54–60
14 Myatt TA, Johnston SL, Zuo Z et al. (2004) Detection of airborne rhinovirus and its relation to outdoor air supply in office environments. *Am J Respir Crit Care Med* 169: 1187–1190
15 Zitter JN, Mazonson PD, Miller DP et al. (2002) Aircraft cabin air recirculation and symptoms of the common cold. *JAMA* 288: 483–486
16 Gwaltney JM Jr, Hendley JO (1978) Rhinovirus transmission: One if by air, two if by hand. *Am J Epidemiol* 107: 357–361
17 Huynh KN, Oliver BG, Stelzer S et al. (2008) A new method for sampling and detection of exhaled respiratory virus aerosols. *Clin Infect Dis* 46: 93–95
18 Hall CB, Douglas RG (1981) Modes of transmission of respiratory syncytial virus. *J Pediatr* 99: 100–103
19 Hendley JO (2000) The common cold. In: RL Cecil, JC Bennett, L Boldman (eds): *Cecil Textbook of Medicine*, 21st edn. WB Saunders, Philadlphia, 1790–1793
20 D'Alessio DJ, Meschievitz CK, Peterson JA et al. (1984) Short-duration exposure and the transmission of rhinoviral colds. *J Infect Dis* 150: 189–194
21 Gwaltney JM Jr, Hendley JO (1982) Transmission of experimental rhinovirus infection by contaminated surfaces. *Am J Epidemiol* 116: 828–832
22 Dick EC, Jennings LC, Mink KA et al. (1987) Aerosol transmission of rhinovirus colds. *J Infect Dis* 156: 442–448
23 Gwaltney JM Jr, Moskalski PB, Hendley JO (1978) Hand-to-hand transmission of rhinovirus colds. *Ann Intern Med* 88: 463–467

24 Hayden GF, Gwaltney JM Jr, Thacker DF, Hendley JO (1985) Rhinovirus inactivation by nasal tissues treated with virucide. *Antiviral Res* 5: 103–109
25 Hayden GF, Hendley JO, Gwaltney JM Jr (1985) The effect of placebo and virucidal paper handkerchiefs on viral contamination of the hand and transmission of experimental rhinoviral infection. *J Infect Dis* 152: 403–407
26 Lee GM, Salomon JA, Friedman JF, Hibberd PL et al. (2004) Illness transmission in the home: a possible role for alcohol-based hand gels. *Pediatrics* 115: 852–860
27 Sandora TJ, Shih, M, Goldmann DA (2008) Reducing absenteeism from gastrointestinal and respiratory illness in elementary school students: A randomized, controlled trial of an infection-control intervention. *Pediatrics* 121: e1555-e1562
28 Sandora TJ, Taveras EM, Shih M et al. (2005) A randomized controlled trial of a multifaceted intervention including alcohol-based hand sanitizer and hand-hygiene education to reduce illness transmission in the home. *Pediatrics* 116: 587–594
29 Farr BM, Hendley JO, Kaiser DL, Gwaltney JM (1988) Two randomized, controlled trials of virucidal nasal tissues in the prevention of natural upper respiratory infections. *Am J Epidemiol* 128: 1162–1172

Common Cold
ed. by R. Eccles and O. Weber

Interventions to prevent transmission of the common cold

Mieke van Driel and Chris Del Mar

Faculty of Health Sciences and Medicine, Bond University, Gold Coast, Australia

Abstract

Theoretically, there are several ways of preventing the common cold: quarantine, immunisation (or vaccination); early treatment of effected individuals; or physical barriers to reduce transmission. All these methods can be dismissed after considering the epidemiology of the common cold, apart from the last. Evidence for effectiveness for physical barriers (which include masks to reduce aerosol transmission; handwashing; and gloves and gowns) come from a variety of empirical studies. The chance of bias for these studies is variable, but we can conclude that all of these barrier methods have important potential for preventing transmission of the common cold, although some methods will not be acceptable to the community currently.

Introduction

The burden of disease of the common cold is enormous, not so much because it is a severe disease (it usually is not, although it may act as a precursor for more serious secondary infections), but because it is so common. No-one escapes infection with colds (see the chapter by Ian M. Mackay et al.). It is an endemic disease hardly amenable to treatment (see the chapter by Ian M. Mackay et al.). This leads us to consider prevention.

The most immediately obvious opportunity is the interruption of the transmission.

The model of the phenomenon – Theoretical considerations

Infectious diseases are critically influenced by how many other people are infected by an infected person. If the number is less than one on average, the disease will die out and disappear. If the number is more than one, it will infect more and more of the population in an explosive manner – an

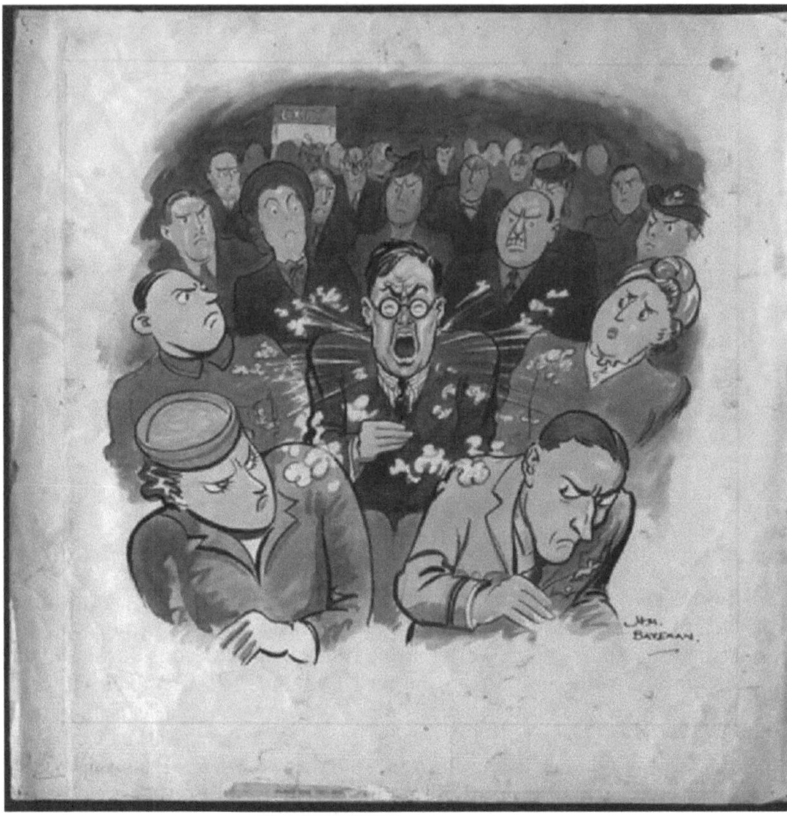

Figure 1. "Coughs and sneezes spread diseases" [1]. Propaganda cartoon from the Ministry of Health and Ministry of Information, UK, 1942, designed to reduce person-to-person transmission of virus infections, here by the use of handkerchiefs.

epidemic. If the number is exactly one (on average) the infection is endemic, meaning it remains always with us (with fluctuations).

This means that preventive interventions are directed at reducing the number of people susceptible to catching the infection.

There are several directions this could take;

1 Quarantine

The term is derived from a practice in the Middle Ages in Italy during the plague, meaning '40 days', during which ships had to stand off port before disembarking. It assured the port population that no-one was infected or incubating infection.

It now involves isolating people who are infected (or could be infected), to prevent their infecting a susceptible population.

This is not a suitable method for the common cold because

a) the common cold is so common;

b) the symptoms are non-specific (colds can easily be confused with allergic phenomena, and a myriad of other respiratory infections);
c) such isolation is not (currently) culturally acceptable (people expect to still be able to work and study – or, indeed they are expected to – or congregate in sporting and entertainment crowds);
d) virus infections causing colds are often asymptomatic [2];
e) such a policy would be impractical to implement.

2 Immunisation or vaccination

Many infectious diseases have been managed by immunisation or vaccination. Indeed, smallpox is no longer an epidemic disease because of vaccination programs against it in the past.

The method depends on vaccinating a sufficient proportion of the population to reduce the person-to-person infection rate to <1.

However designing a vaccination strategy for the common cold presents challenges.

a) The common cold consists of several different viruses (see the chapter by Olaf Weber) [3]. A successful program would have to pick off each of these in turn – and no population benefit would be discernable until a large proportion had been addressed;
b) Many of the viruses mutate easily (see the chapter by Olaf Weber). They are so unstable that the antigens quickly change, making them a quickly moving target for any vaccination program;
c) Common colds are seen by the population as sufficiently trivial, and vaccines, viewed with some suspicion in the past, pose a difficulty in establishing a cost-harm benefit.

3 Early treatment of infected people

This method depends on treating people who are recently infected – or potentially infected by being in contact with an infected person – so that the infection is aborted. It is a method used to protect health workers potentially infected with the HIV virus, or contacts of children with suspected meningococcal disease, for example.

However for the common cold, no effective and available treatment is yet widely available.

4 Physical methods of prevention of transmission

This is left as the main opportunity for prevention of the common cold. It exploits the need for the virus to travel from person to person to spread infection. If we can interfere with that, we can reduce the number of people infected by any infected individual, and hence the total number of people infected. If we reduced the number infected to zero, the common cold would die out.

An intensive investigation of such methods has been undertaken over the years.

There are a number of ways virus can transmit from an infected to an uninfected person. They include two principal modes:

a) aerosol from coughing and sneezing;
   This is the traditional means for the spread of virus particles (and the basis of the caution in the adage *Coughs and sneezes spread diseases* referred to above).
b) fomites* from virus left on contact surfaces in which virus is deposited by an infected person and then picked up by an uninfected one. This is less obvious, and has been the subject of considerable research.
   (* the word 'fomite' derives from the Latin '*fomites*', meaning the tinder or lighting taper for starting fires).

Studies have investigated the relative importance of these two means of common cold transmission.

Sharing an office increased the risk of catching more colds in a Norwegian office study of nearly 900 office workers [4]. However, this did not settle the question of which mode of transmission was the more important [4]. An experiment in which 18 volunteers (playing cards) were prevented from touching common property or not (that is, restricting transmission of cold virus to aerosol or not), suggested that aerosol was the most common method [5].

Evidence for a fomite route comes from artificial studies of rhinovirus inoculation on the fingers of volunteers and then detecting it later [6], or actually transmitting infection to family members [7] or other volunteers [8, 9], although the evidence is conflicting [10]. Certainly inoculation titres picked up by recipients can be high enough to cause fomite spread of colds [11].

In summary, it seems that both methods are important in spreading infection through the community. There seems to be no consensus on the relative importance of either one, but nevertheless it might be reasonable to suppose that both are important, and worth exploiting in any preventive intervention.

Empirical evidence for ways of interrupting the transmission of respiratory virus infections

Theories about the way viruses are spread are important. However, we can decide whether exploiting them is of any use more directly by examining studies that have empirically tested the interruption of these modes of transmission.

The literature is confusing. There are many studies, of different study designs, and reaching different conclusions. For the clinician interested in deriving a useful clinical conclusion from the literature, this can be unsatisfactory. Happily, a method of undertaking such a literature review has been developed which is as explicit, transparent, and objective as possible. It is called "systematic review", and includes its quantitative methods, "meta-analysis".

Some of the best are Cochrane reviews, that is, systematic reviews that are designed in full open view for the world to examine and criticise.

One includes studies of relevance to the question of whether the common cold can be prevented by interfering with physical modes of transmission [12, 13]. The next section summarises that review.

The Cochrane review: Physical methods of interrupting the spread of respiratory viruses

Sources of evidence

The Cochrane review systematically reviewed the empirical evidence for the effectiveness of physical methods aimed at preventing viral animal-to-human or human-to-human transmission of respiratory viruses (isolation, quarantine, social distancing, barriers, personal protection and hygiene) compared with do-nothing or with another intervention. It considered experimental studies (randomised or quasi-randomised trials), observational studies (cohort and case-control designs), and any other comparative design provided some attempt had been made to control for confounding.

The review reports on 49 reports of 51 studies with variable risk of bias, such as could be introduced by incomplete reporting; ignoring the impact of several potential biases such as the impact of viral incidence variability over time. Some studies also used inappropriate comparison interventions, impractical interventions (such as using, as a virucidal agent, iodine which causes unacceptable cosmetic staining), and interventions with low compliance (especially in educational interventions).

The settings of the studies, conducted over four decades, were highly heterogeneous (meaning very variable in terms of their settings and design). Settings ranged from suburban schools to military barracks, intensive care units, and paediatric wards in industrialised countries, slums in developing ones, and to special needs day care centres with a very high teacher to pupil ratio. There were few studies from developing countries, where the vast majority of the burden lies and where cheap interventions are most needed.

What is effective?

Handwashing

The most impressive effects came from cluster-randomised trials of low risk of bias in preventing respiratory virus spread from 'hygienic measures in younger children'. Roberts et al. [14] reported a significant decrease in respiratory illness in children up to 24 months (RR 0.90, 95% CI 0.83–0.97), although the decrease was not significant in older children (RR 0.95, 95% CI 0.89–1.01). Luby et al. [15] reported a 50% (95% CI 65–34%) lower incidence of pneumonia in children aged under 5 years of age in a developing country. Additional benefit from reduced transmission from them to other household members is broadly supported from the results of other study designs, although their potential for confounding is greater.

Physical barriers: Hand washing, gloves, masks and gowns

Six case-control studies assessed the impact of public health measures to curb the spread of the SARS epidemic in 2003 in China, Singapore and Vietnam. The data suggest implementing barriers to transmission, isolation and hygienic measures are effective and relatively cheap interventions to contain epidemics of respiratory viruses such as SARS, with estimates of effect ranging from 55% to 91%: hand washing >10 times daily [odds ratio (OR) 0.45; 95% CI 0.36–0.57, number need to treat (NNT) 4], mask wearing (OR 0.32; 95% CI 0.25–0.40, NNT 6), glove wearing (OR 0.43; 95% CI 0.29–0.65, NNT 7), wearing gowns (OR 0.23; 95% CI 0.14–0.37, NNT 5), and handwashing, masks, gloves and gowns combined (OR 0.09; 95% CI 0.02–0.35 NNT 3). All studies selected cases from hospitals, except one [16] in which the cases were people with probable SARS who reported to the Department of Health in the territory of Hong Kong up to 16 May 2003. There was limited evidence of the superior effectiveness of droplet barrier devices such as the N95 masks (respirators with 95% filtration capability against non-oily particulate aerosols [17]) over simple surgical masks. There was an incremental effect of decreased respiratory disease burden by adding virucidals or antiseptics to normal handwashing in somewhat atypical settings, but the extra benefit may have been, partly at least, from confounding additional routines.

Few studies reported resource consumption for the physical intervention they evaluated. The case control by Lau et al. [12, 13] concluded that handwashing needs to be carried out more than ten times daily to be effective. Ryan (in a military training setting) reported a need to wash hands more than four times daily [18]. Hall and colleagues reported that during 1 month of the RSV 'season' on a ward containing 22 cribs, 5350 gowns and 4850 masks were used [19]. It seems reasonable to advise as frequent handwashing and change of barriers as is possible during an epidemic and at least one complete change per patient seen.

Isolation of cases

The evidence for isolating cases is inconclusive. One study found that isolating together children of less than 3 years of age with suspected RSV reduced transmission by "up to 60%" [20]; however, the statement that nosocomial transmission "was minimised" was not supported by data in a similar study [21].

Isolation of cases during the 2003 epidemic of SARS in China was reported to limit transmission to only those contacts who had actually had home or hospital contact with a symptomatic SARS patient (attack rate 31.1%, 95% CI 20.2–44.4 for carers; 8.9%, 95% CI 2.9–22.1 for visitors; 4.6%, 95% CI 2.3–8.9 for those living with a SARS case) but not to contacts living in the same building, working with cases, or without contact with SARS cases during the incubation period. This suggests that quarantine only needs to be extended for contacts of symptomatic SARS cases [22, 23]. Another brief report carried out in 2003 during the SARS epidemic in a military hospital in Taiwan and 86 control hospitals, compared an integrated infection-control policy to protect healthcare workers against infection; only two from the military hospital were infected with SARS compared to 43 suspected and 50 probable cases in the control hospitals [24].

Quarantine

An ecological study analysed the effects of quarantine and port of entry screening on the SARS epidemic in early 2003 in Beijing, China, from data collected centrally. Hospitals were the initial sources of transmission of the SARS virus. The shape of the epidemic suggests these measures may have reduced SARS transmission, although only 12 cases identified out of over 13 million people screened puts in doubt the direct effectiveness of entry port checks at airports and railway stations, and screening was probably more important [25]. An Israeli study of 186 094 children aged 6–12 years reported that school closure was temporally associated with a 42% decreased morbidity from respiratory tract infections, a consequent 28% decrease in visits to physicians and to emergency departments, and a 35% reduction in purchase of medications [26].

The lack of proper evaluation of global and highly resource-intensive measures such as screening at entry ports and social distancing was disappointing. The handful of studies do not allow us to reach any firm conclusions, although a recent analysis of historical and archival US data from the 1918–1919 influenza pandemic suggests an effect of social distancing measures such as school closures and public gathering bans [27].

Implications for practice

Simple public health measures appear to be highly effective, especially when they are part of a structured programme including instruction and education, and when they are delivered together. There is a clear mandate

to carry out further large pragmatic trials to evaluate the best combinations. In the meantime we recommend implementing the following interventions in a combined fashion to diminish transmission of viral respiratory disease:
- frequent handwashing with or without adjunct antiseptics;
- barrier measures such as gloves, gowns, and masks with filtration apparatus; and
- suspicion diagnosis, with isolation of likely cases.

Most effort should be concentrated on reducing transmission from young children.

References

1 Bateman HM (1942) Coughs and sneezes spread diseases. Ministry of Health and Ministry of Information, UK. www.nationalarchives.gov.uk/theartofwar/prop/home_front/INF3_0407J.htm. Accessed on: 26 December 2008, London, propaganda, The National Archives

2 Peltola V, Waris M, Osterback R, Susi P, Ruuskanen O, Hyypia T (2008) Rhinovirus transmission within families with children: incidence of symptomatic and asymptomatic infections. *J Infect Dis* 197: 382–389

3 Jackson GG, Dowling HF (1959) Transmission of the common cold to volunteers under controlled conditions. IV. Specific immunity to the common cold. *J Clin Invest* 38: 762–769

4 Jaakkola JJ, Heinonen OP (1995) Shared office space and the risk of the common cold. *Eur J Epidemiol* 11: 213–216

5 Dick EC, Jennings LC, Mink KA, Wartgow CD, Inhorn SL (1987) Aerosol transmission of rhinovirus colds. *J Infect Dis* 156: 442–448

6 Ansari SA, Springthorpe VS, Sattar SA, Rivard S, Rahman M (1991) Potential role of hands in the spread of respiratory viral infections: studies with human parainfluenza virus 3 and rhinovirus 14. *J Clin Microbiol* 29: 2115–2119

7 D'Alessio DJ, Peterson JA, Dick CR, Dick EC (1976) Transmission of experimental rhinovirus colds in volunteer married couples. *J Infect Dis* 133: 28–36

8 Gwaltney JM Jr, Moskalski PB, Hendley JO (1978) Hand-to-hand transmission of rhinovirus colds. *Ann Intern Med* 88: 463–467

9 Gwaltney JM Jr, Hendley JO (1982) Transmission of experimental rhinovirus infection by contaminated surfaces. *Am J Epidemiol* 116: 828–833

10 Reed SE (1975) An investigation of the possible transmission of Rhinovirus colds through indirect contact. *J Hyg (Lond)* 75: 249–258

11 Pancic F, Carpentier DC, Came PE (1980) Role of infectious secretions in the transmission of rhinovirus. *J Clin Microbiol* 12: 567–571

12 Jefferson T, Foxlee R, Del Mar C, Dooley L, Ferroni E, Hewak B, Prabhala A, Nair S, Rivetti A (2007) Interventions for the interruption or reduction of the spread of respiratory viruses. *Cochrane Database Syst Rev*: CD006207

13 Jefferson T, Foxlee R, Del Mar C, Dooley L, Ferroni E, Hewak B, Prabhala A, Nair S, Rivetti A (2008) Physical interventions to interrupt or reduce the spread of respiratory viruses: systematic review. *BMJ* 336: 77–80

14 Roberts L, Jorm L, Patel M, Smith W, Douglas RM, McGilchrist C (2000) Effect

of infection control measures on the frequency of diarrheal episodes in child care: A randomized, controlled trial. *Pediatrics* 105: 743–746
15 Luby SP, Agboatwalla M, Feikin DR, Painter J, Billhimer W, Altaf A, Hoekstra RM (2005) Effect of handwashing on child health: A randomised controlled trial. *Lancet* 366: 225–233
16 Lau JT, Tsui H, Lau M, Yang X (2004) SARS transmission, risk factors, and prevention in Hong Kong. *Emerg Infect Dis* 10: 587–592
17 Teleman MD, Boudville IC, Heng BH, Zhu D, Leo YS (2004) Factors associated with transmission of severe acute respiratory syndrome among health-care workers in Singapore. *Epidemiol Infect* 135: 797–803
18 Ryan MA, Christian RS, Wohlrabe J (2001) Handwashing and respiratory illness among young adults in military training. *Am J Prevent Med* 21: 79–83
19 Hall CB, Douglas RG Jr (1981) Nosocomial respiratory syncytial viral infections. Should gowns and masks be used? *Am J Dis Child* 135: 512–515
20 Isaacs D, Dickson H, O'Callaghan C, Sheaves R, Winter A, Moxon ER (1991) Handwashing and cohorting in prevention of hospital acquired infections with respiratory syncytial virus. *Arch Dis Child* 66: 227–231
21 Doherty JA, Brookfield DS, Gray J, McEwan RA (1998) Cohorting of infants with respiratory syncytial virus. *J Hosp Infect* 38: 203–206
22 Centers for Disease Control and Prevention (CDC) (2003) Efficiency of quarantine during an epidemic of severe acute respiratory syndrome – Beijing, China, 2003. *MMWR Morb Mortal Wkly Rep* 52: 1037–1040
23 Ou JM, Dun Z, Li Q, Qin AL, Zeng G (2003) Efficiency of the quarantine system during the epidemic of severe acute respiratory syndrome in Beijing, 2003. *Chung-Hua Liu Hsing Ping Hsueh Tsa Chih [Chin J Epidemiol]* 24: 1093–1095
24 Yen MY, Lin YE, Su IJ, Huang FY, Huang FY, Ho MS, Chang SC, Tan KH, Chen KT, Chang H et al. (2006) Using an integrated infection control strategy during outbreak control to minimize nosocomial infection of severe acute respiratory syndrome among healthcare workers. *J Hosp Infect* 62: 195–199
25 Pang X, Zhu Z, Xu F, Guo J, Gong X, Liu D, Liu Z, Chin DP, Feikin DR (2003) Evaluation of control measures implemented in the severe acute respiratory syndrome outbreak in Beijing, 2003. *JAMA* 290: 3215–3212
26 Heymann A, Chodick G, Reichman B, Kokia E, Laufer J (2004) Influence of school closure on the incidence of viral respiratory diseases among children and on health care utilization. *Pediatr Infect Dis J* 23: 675–677
27 Markel H, Lipman HB, Navarro JA, Sloan A, Michalsen JR, Stern AM, Cetron MS (2007) Nonpharmaceutical interventions implemented by US cities during the 1918–1919 influenza pandemic. *JAMA* 298: 644–654

Antivirals for the common cold

Tom Jefferson

Cochrane Acute Respiratory Infections Group, Via Adige 28a, Anguillara Sabazia, 00061 Roma, Italy

This chapter is dedicated to the memory of Dr. David Tyrrell

Abstract

Despite a 60-year history of discovery, trial and evaluation of scores of different compounds, there are no currently licensed effective antivirals for the common cold. The history of the development and abandonment of all potential compounds so far teaches us some important lessons for the continuation of our fight against colds. First, the common cold is a benign self-limiting condition, making the consumption of 'harmless' antivirals a requisite of prime importance for regulators. Second, the common cold is a syndrome caused by a myriad of known and unknown agents, which reduces the effectiveness of compounds that interfere with single specific agents or types of agents. The multifactorial nature of the genesis of colds makes it difficult for compounds showing *in vitro* efficacy to 'make the jump' to field effectiveness. Last, despite the heavy burden that the cold imposes on society, the vagueness and shortness of symptoms make it difficult for sufferers to present in time for physicians to prescribe antivirals, which are only effective if taken within a short time frame. Attention should be paid to the development of compounds with a non-virus-specific action.

Background

Modern attempts at identifying causal agents of the common cold started in the 1920s, in the aftermath of the great 1918–19 influenza pandemic [1, 2]. After Smith, Andrewes and Laidlaw identified the influenza A virus in 1936, research was conducted in specialised facilities such as the UK's Medical Research Council's Common Cold Research Unit (CCU), the Australian Department of Community Medicine at the University of Adelaide and by Gwaltney and Hayden, at the Department of Medicine, University of Virginia, Charlottesville, USA [3–5]. Eventually more than 200 different agents, types and subtypes have been associated with the common cold.

An early historical trial carried out during the Second World War by the MRC on patulin (a metabolic product of the mould *Penicillium patulum*) testifies to the interest in reducing the burden of the common cold especially among troops and munitions workers [6, 7].

Despite its ubiquitous nature, the high incidence and relatively high morbidity, several problems remain in our understanding of common cold epidemiology and, most of all, in the use of effective and simple preventive or therapeutics tools.

This chapter focuses on antiviral compounds for the prevention or early treatment of the common cold using available evidence from randomised controlled trials carried out on human volunteers or in naturally occurring colds in a community. Antiviral drugs may be defined as natural or synthetic compounds that interfere with different stages of the cycle of the agent. I have stretched this definition to include both substances that act against specific viruses and those that work by building up our immune response.

The chapter is based on an earlier Cochrane review that I co-authored with the late Dr. David Tyrrell, the last director of the MRC Common Cold Unit (CCU). Our original dataset included correspondence records about the trials between CCU staff and manufacturers and other researchers active in the field. The Cochrane review identified 129 trials of antivirals and 63 of interferons carried out in the CCU between 1949 and 1989, the year of its closure (Tab. 1). Because of the difficulty in reconciling the raw data of the trials carried out in the CCU with those published in international journals at the time, we privileged the raw records, referring to them by the prefix "CCU" followed by the original trial serial number (e.g. CCU 362). In most cases no leading investigator's name was recognisable from existing records. In addition, several trials were run in 1 year making the use of the year identifier impossible. The final number of trials from CCU and all other sources included in our Cochrane review was 89. The review has since been withdrawn because of lack of funds for its maintenance. I hope

Table 1. Number of identified MRC Common Cold Unit trials of interventions for the common cold

Intervention	Number of CCU trials
Antivirals (other than IFN)	129
Interferon (IFN)	63
Environmental	13
Zinc	11
Nedocromil	8
Vaccines	7
Vitamin C	6
Antibiotics	5
Promethazine Hydrochloride	1
GRAND TOTAL	243

this chapter will serve as a memorial to the huge amount of work carried out on antivirals for the common cold in past decades and help direct the work ahead.

I was asked to update the content of the original review for this chapter. I have done this with the help of my Trial Search Coordinator Alessandro Rivetti who conducted searches of six different databases. As of today there are no antivirals registered for the common cold anywhere in the world, so the evidence is grouped according to type of compound, rather than its commercial name. Each compound is presented firstly by its pharmaceutical manufacturer (if known) and then its route of administration but readers should be aware that some of the reports contained data from several sub-studies. The sub-studies have been subdivided using alphabetical suffixes.

Interferons

After its discovery in 1957, the interest in the use of interferon for its marked *in vitro* antiviral properties grew rapidly. Early methods of preparation of interferon were bedevilled by problems of impurity (leading to high incidence of harm to recipients) and availability. By the early 1970s, purity and availability of interferon had considerably improved and a new set of trials could be conducted [8]. As knowledge of interferon grew, several types of interferons were synthesised. These are indicated by a Greek alphabet suffix.

The early trials (from 1962) had multiple arms, only two of which were concerned with assessing interferon against a control intervention (such as tissue culture fluids) and the potential harm of its use. In these early experiments volunteers were exposed to artificial challenge with mainly rhinoviruses (RV). Quarantine periods ranged from 2 to 3 days (necessary to minimise the chances of volunteers being exposed to viruses circulating in the community) and isolation periods from 9 to 10 days. Later interferon trials were carried out between 1972 and the closure of the CCU in the summer of 1989. Some of the earliest trials are reported in Merigan 1973 [9].

With advances in biology and genetics the recombinant interferons entered the scene. For example, trials CCU 843–853 [10] are reports of a double-blind, placebo-controlled study, self-administered intranasal human interferon alpha A produced by Hoffman LaRoche Ltd and Schering Plough Ltd by recombinant DNA technology. This was administered both before and after viral challenge with respiratory coronavirus and RV9 and RV14.

Four separate comparisons can be constructed from available data.

The first comparison assessed the effects of intranasal interferon in the prevention of experimental colds caused by a variety of common cold viral types (rhino, corona, parainfluenza, influenza and coxsackie) and subtypes. In addition, we included data on different commonly reported adverse events, ranging from nasal stuffiness to blood-tinged mucus. Data on adverse events (in all comparisons) must be read singly and not cumulatively as one participant could have reported more than one adverse event at a time. Results show that, overall, interferon is significantly more efficacious than placebo in preventing experimental colds (protective efficacy: mean 46%, range 37–54%). The effect is significant in larger trials and against RV and coronavirus. Interferon does not appear to prevent middle ear and Eustachian tube pressure dysfunction, although denominators are very small. Administration of intranasal interferon is significantly associated with nasal stuffiness [odds ratio (OR) 2.22, 1.33–3.70] and increased sneezing. Blood-tinged nasal mucus was not statistically significantly associated with exposure to interferon (OR 1.71, 1.00–2.94) but there is a clear tendency favouring the control intervention.

The second comparison assessed the effects of intranasal interferon in the prevention of naturally occurring colds. Results show that when the denominator considered are the number of participants, interferon is, overall, significantly more efficacious than placebo in all age groups in preventing naturally occurring colds (preventive efficacy 26%, 23–29%) and those caused by RV (preventive efficacy 35%, 17–49%), despite the negative outcome of the study by Douglas et al. [11]. Readers should note that age categories (adults, children and families) are not mutually exclusive and there are overlaps in years and grouping. Interferon, however, is no better than placebo when the denominator considered are the number of courses administered (preventive efficacy 11%, 4%–26%). Blood-tinged nasal mucus was observed with statistically significant increased frequency in the interferon arm of trials of naturally occurring common colds (OR 4.52, 3.78–5.41), as well as nasal erosion (OR 2.58, 1.71–3.91), sneezing and nasal irritation (OR 2.58, 1.88–3.52) and nasal stuffiness (OR 3.07, 2.09–4.51) (see Figs 1 and 2).

The third comparison assessed the effects of intranasal interferon in combination with the synthetic antiviral enviroxime in the prevention of experimental colds. The single small trial by Higgins et al. [12] shows no statistically significant difference between placebo and interferon with eviroxime (efficacy 43%, 0–78%), probably a reflection of the small denominator.

Finally, the fourth comparison assessed the effects of intranasal interferon alone or in combination with naproxen and ipatropium in the treatment of experimental colds caused by RV.

The combination appeared significantly more effective than placebo in attenuating the course of colds by reducing the amount of nasal secretion [weighted mean difference (WMD) 7.40, 2.98–11.82] and appears safe, although this observation is based on a single study [13]. Interferon alone is also significantly more effective than placebo in attenuating the course of experimental colds (WMD 15.90, 13.42–18.38) [14–16].

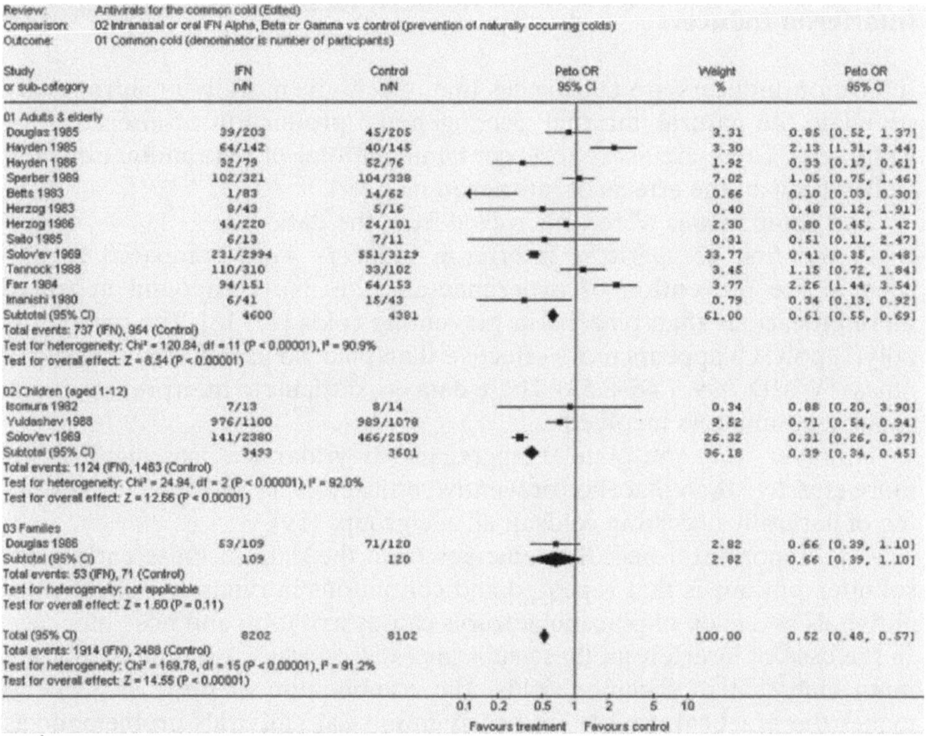

Figure 1. Effectiveness of intranasal interferon alpha, beta or gamma in preventing the onset of the common cold in the community by age group of participants. Comparators were a mixture of do-nothing or placebo recipients. The forest plot of the meta analysis is based on over 16 000 observations.

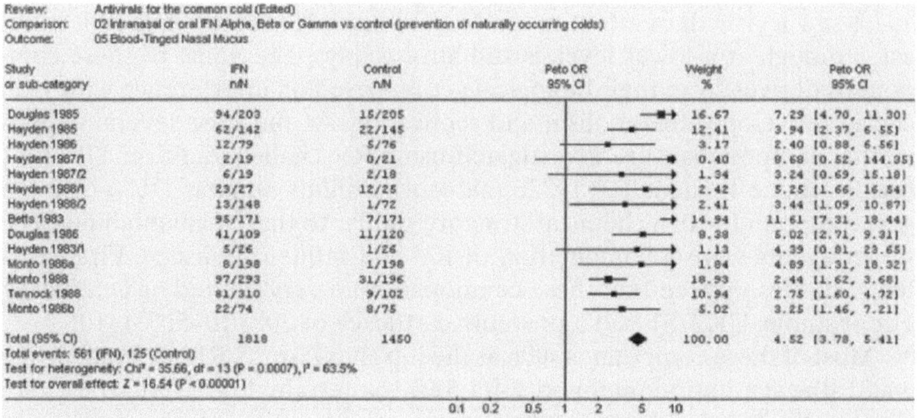

Figure 2. Harm (nasal discharge of blood tinged mucus) induced by the intranasal administration of interferon alpha, beta or gamma in preventing the onset of the common cold in the community by age group of participants. Comparators were a mixture of do-nothing or placebo recipients. The forest plot of the meta analysis is based on over 3200 observations.

Interferon inducers

Interferon inducers are substances that, when given orally or intranasally, stimulate the natural 'internal' (endogenous) production of interferon by white cells. There are six reports containing a total of ten randomised controlled trials of the effects of interferon inducers.

Two comparisons were constructed from the data.

In the first comparison, interferon inducers were compared to placebo in the prevention of experimental colds. No compound appeared more efficacious than placebo in preventing colds [17, 18]. The compound poly(I)·poly(C) appears more effective than placebo in reducing severity of illness (WMD 7.99, 7.45–8.53). These data are difficult to interpret, given the small denominators involved.

However, the anti-platelet aggregant dipyridamole was significantly more effective than placebo (preventive efficacy 49%, 30–62%) in preventing of naturally occurring colds in all age groups [19].

One important aspect that emerges from the data of these early aerosol interventions is that repeated and continuous intranasal application of antivirals and even of placebo aerosols causes irritation and nose blockage. In the case of interferons, these substances also induce systemic symptoms mimicking that of common colds. The combination of these side effects makes the practical use of these early intranasal antivirals problematic as, although effective, their application led to dubious benefits.

Capsid-binding compounds

Alongside assessment of interferon and its inducers, the late 1960s and early 1970s saw a growth of attention on "capsid-binding" compounds (this interest, although at a lower level, is still alive today). The name of these compounds derives from their biological action based on interference with viral capsid (envelope) metabolism and replication. At the time several experimental compounds were investigated using RV challenge: Pfizer UK 2731 (oral), Rhone-Poulenc RP 19326 (aerosol), Phillips Duphar DU 34796 (an oral compound with a chemical structure similar to that of amantadine). The target agents were a combination of RV and influenza viruses. Viral challenge studies showed that these compounds had very limited or no efficacy. For example, UK2731 had a preventive efficacy of 20% (0–51%) [10].

Most of these compounds such as the intranasal spray Rhone Poulenc RP 44081 {the synthetic compound, 2-[(1,5,10,10a-tetrahydro-3H-thiazolo[3,4b] isoquinolin-3-ylidene) amino]-4-thiazoleacetic acid (S)} (which was assessed in a small trial in 1983) inhibited the multiplication of RV in cell cultures but had no effect in preventing infection and symptoms after challenge [19].

Other compounds equally failed to live up to their *in vitro* performance promise.

The CCU carried out three trials between February and November 1973 to assess the effects of the oral antiviral M&B 15497. The target agents were a combination of influenza viruses. Quarantine was applied for 3 days and isolation for 10 days. The nasal spray and oral Eli Lilly compound Enviroxime was then assessed by five trials carried out between 1980 and 1981. The target agents were RV9. Quarantine was applied for 3 days and isolation for 10 days. Surviving CCU enviroxime records appear to contain data from a larger volunteer population than the corresponding publications [20]. RP 19326 (preventive efficacy 0%, 0–33%), Enviroxime (preventive efficacy 0%, 0%–36%), RP 44081 (preventive efficacy 31%, 0–81%), CGP 19635 (preventive efficacy 0%, 0–63%) do not appear to be more effective than placebo in preventing experimentally induced colds due to RV or influenza virus. This was another dead end for common cold antiviral research.

Other experimental molecules were developed from existing registered antivirals. Between 1983 and 1985 the oral compound ICI 130, 685 (a cyclononane compound, related to amantadine but thought to have superior preventive and therapeutic effects) was tested in 13 trials against influenza A viruses. Both the resulting publication [21] and surviving CCU records show a good preventive efficacy (58%, 35–74%) compared to placebo in preventing and providing early treatment for influenza-related common colds. However, because of concerns over side effects (mainly CNS effects, similar to those caused by the other adamantanes: amantadine and rimantadine) the compound was not developed further.

Some capsid-binding compounds were mixed with other substances, as in the case of the intranasal spray Janssen Pharmaceuticals Ltd R61837 (a pyridazine mixed with a cyclodextrin). However, R61837 was no more effective than placebo in preventing experimental colds caused by RV (0.49, 0.22–1.07) [10].

In the case of the bradykinin antagonist Nova Pharmaceuticals Ltd NPC 567 ([22] integrated with CCU data) this compound also did not work and as always with intranasally administered substances, worsened the clinical course of colds.

Testing of oral Eli Lilly LY 217896 was reported in a trial carried out in the USA [23]. The compound appeared to be no more effective than placebo in the prevention of colds due to influenza A virus (preventive efficacy 0%, 0–32%).

One unexpected finding concerned the performance of SPOFA Pharmaceutical Works oral Impulsin (*N*-2-hydroxyethyl palmitamide). Impulsin was tested in three controlled clinical trials reported in [24]. The field trials were carried out on 1864 male volunteers in Czechoslovakian army units in January 1973, 1974 and 1975. Impulsin appears to be more effective than placebo in preventing acute respiratory infections and colds from all causes (preventive efficacy 44%, 35–52%), but its therapeutic effect is less marked.

Pirodavir spray (Janssen Ltd) (formerly known as R 77975) is a synthetic antiviral (phenoxy-pyridazinamine) with potent *in vitro* activity against RV. The trials were carried out in Virginia, USA. Pirodavir appears to be no more effective than placebo in preventing RV-induced colds if used at least six times a day (preventive efficacy 85%, 0–98%), although this observation is based on a very small denominator (25 individuals). Its therapeutic effect is no better than that of placebo. Adverse effects such as nasal dryness may affect compliance [25].

The compound WIN 54954 Sterling Winthrop Inc (oral) was no more effective than placebo in the prevention of colds due to RV (preventive efficacy 7%, 0–49%) [26].

Isoquinoline derivatives

These are compounds that showed antiviral activity in cell culture and in animals. The class includes Hoffmann-La Roche oral 3, 4-dihydro-1-isoquinolineacetamide hydrochloride (DIQA) [27] and Newport Pharmaceuticals oral Inosiplex (Isoprinosine, formerly NPT 10381) [28, 29]. Of the isoquinoline derivatives, both DIQA (preventive efficacy 1%, 0–75%) and Inosiplex (preventive efficacy 38%, 0–64%) may have been assessed with insufficient denominator size, but the latter appears to have promising preventive efficacy. Few data on the safety profile of these compounds are available.

Chalcones

Hoffmann-La Roche Ltd Ro-09-0410 (liquid chalcone) inactivated RV particles in suspension. Trials CCU 875, CCU 876, CCU 920, and CCU 927–9 assessed the preventive effects of liquid Ro-09-0410, against RV2 and RV9. The trials were carried out in the winter of 1983/84. CCU 875 and CCU 876 are interruption-of-transmission trials, in which volunteers self-inoculated RV9 into the nose with fingers pre-treated with either drug or placebo. Ro 09-9415 chalcone either by oral or intranasal routes appears to be no more effective than placebo in the prevention of colds due to RV, a conclusion in agreement with that reported in the two published versions [30, 31] (preventive efficacy 9%, 0–36%).

Several other miscellaneous antivirals were assessed in the CCU. This grouping includes compounds tested in few trials or for which few CCU data are available because of lack of allocation schedules.

Lederle Guanidine (liquid), [1-phenyl-3-(4 phenyl-2-thiazolyl) guanidine (CL 88,277)], was tested in a CCU trial 369 [10] and in a trial carried out in the USA [32].

Lederle Guanidine appears to be no more effective than placebo in the prevention of colds due to RV or coxsackie A21 virus (preventive efficacy 0%, 0–58% and 20%, 0–68%, respectively).

Ciba-Geigy CGP 19635 (nasal liquid) is an immunomodulatory compound that had been shown to have anti-influenza A properties in rodents. CCU trials 955–960 assessed the prophylactic effects of CGP 19635 against influenza A/Eng/40/83 virus. The trials were carried out in the spring of 1987 and volunteers completed psychological profiles and performance tests before and after viral challenge. No description of allocation methods is made.

In the CCU archives we identified evidence of testing of other miscellaneous antivirals comprising the following compounds: CP-196J aerosol (Janssen Ltd), RO5-3369 (Roche Ltd) capsules, AH 1581 (oral) and ICI 73602. Evidence is thin, comprising either single small trials of two to three participants for which allocation codes are missing. No data are reported for these compounds.

Finally, the effects of intranasal 7-thia-8-oxoguanosine (NARI 10146), a nucleoside analogue with proven immunomodulatory activity against coronavirus 229E were tested in the summer of 1989, shortly before the closure of the CCU. It was no more effective than placebo in the prevention of colds due to coronavirus (preventive efficacy 33%, 0–64%). Possible reasons for the failure to confirm successful rodent experiments in man include an inadequate dosage, a different concentration of the viral challenge and differences in rodent and human immune systems.

Recent antivirals and a look to the future

An interesting (and ongoing) story is that of Pleconaril, an oral capsid-binding antiviral developed jointly by ViroPharma Inc. and Sanofi-Synthelabo.

Pleconaril (formally known as WIN 63843) effectively interferes with capsid function of picornaviruses, especially RV, both *in vitro* and *in vivo* by inhibiting viral docking to the intercellular adhesion receptor molecule-1 (ICAM-1) of which the respiratory epithelium is particularly rich. Pleconaril administration within 24 hours of symptoms onset shortens the duration of colds by up to 24 hours. In a preventive role Pleconaril prevented 71% (15–90%) of RV-related colds. Despite notable media hype and these promising Phase II trial results, the oral formulation of Pleconaril was refused registration by the FDA in August 2002 chiefly on the basis of side effects (menstrual irregularities and pregnancy in women already on oral contraceptives) [33–36].

In 2007, Schering-Plough, under license of ViroPharma, completed a Phase II clinical trial of an aerosol formulation of Pleconaril on common cold symptoms and asthma exacerbations but its results have not been published yet (Study P04295AM2).

At present, Pleconaril is used on a compassionate basis for serious cases of picornavirus infections (such as acute pancreatitis).

However, efforts to develop an effective antiviral against picornavirus-associated diseases are ongoing.

Rupintrivir (AG 7088), an RV protease inhibitor developed by the Pfizer subsidiary Agouron Pharmaceuticals, reached clinical trials but its development was stopped. Finally, the anti-RV drug BTA-798 developed by the Australian company Biota started Phase II prevention challenge studies trials in August 2008 [37]. The full results are expected by the end of April 2009 [38].

Other efforts have been directed at interfering with viral functions that are mediated by antigens with high level of conservation across viral serotypes (i.e. in the case of RV all or most of the 100-odd serotypes present the same antigenic structure). On the basis of advances in the understanding of viral docking and uncoating, it is possible to design potential antiviral compounds (a recent example are di-substituted and tri-substituted benzamides) that show good *in vitro* promise [39].

No other antiviral compounds appear to be under development despite perusal of eight trial registers and one meta-register of trials.

Methodological quality of studies mentioned in the chapter

Most of the published reports and surviving records from the CCU do not allow a systematic evaluation of the four key design aspects of antiviral testing in humans: randomisation schedule generation, allocation concealment, blinding and completeness of follow-up. However, it was possible to reconstruct some of the methodology by looking at existing documentation and interviewing scientists. Here is how one scientist described early CCU viral challenge studies (carried out in the 1940s and 1950s): "volunteers' names were listed and also the number of experimental groups defined. Then they were allocated usually using a table of random numbers (Yates). The group, usually indicated as A, B, C, was written on the list and was also used for the server capped bottles in which the inoculum was carried round to the flats. The list and the bottles could not easily be seen by the volunteers and the clinician and the nurse made their rounds separately and so did not see them at all. The list was kept in a laboratory drawer and rarely visited by the clinical team members. The scientist who performed the inoculum and often administered it had little contact with the volunteers in the early trials. He/she might collect nasal secretions if a cold developed. After 1960 there were influenza trials. Blood rhinovirus antibodies could be often measured, but we could not pre-screen our volunteers as they did in the USA. Antiviral treatments at this stage might have been 'wasted' on volunteers who could have been shown to be immune. Thus, two researchers would bleed volunteers on arrival, do a rapid antibody assay and arrange volunteers in groups with similar antibody titres, usually nil or low, and the high-titre individuals might be allocated to experiments with an alternative virus or placebo (we always included volunteers with dummy inocula to motivate clinicians and volunteers – they were firmly told that some of them would be given inert drops and dummy drops and so they would be, we believe, discouraged from reporting symptoms if they fell into these placebo groups). Ordinarily, the groups would be allocated to treatments by a random method. Things became more formalised in the last phase with trials of interferons and capsid-binding drugs. Many of these trials were set up by Dr. Peter Higgins. The blinding methods remained virtually the same, though they were enhanced during the 1980s by distributing the inoculum into trials with the volunteers' names on the labels, so that the allocation information never left the lab and there was an extra safeguard against the volunteer being given the wrong material by mistake in the volunteer accommodation. It is difficult to document all these points, or to be precise about the dates on which practices were changed, but it should be possible to work out to some extent by using the date and clues supplied by the descriptions in the reports and papers. It is a generalisation that we never did open trials. Even when we were testing the effect of hot humid air we used a comparison or "control" in which the machine was adapted to generate warm but not too hot (43°C) air. In the zinc lozenge experiment we used a very strong washing flavour, and in the lab we thought the active and placebo preparations tasted the same on a direct comparison and by volunteers reorganising the active preps. I would want to be able to go back and do more experiments to contest that challenge. We did have some evidence that in the vitamin C experiments there was a fault of this sort. We had the practice of telling the volunteers at the end of the trial that they had been given active or placebo material. It then appeared that vitamin C was reducing symptoms after the end of the trial – the system then included the volunteers sending back a postcard with a report of symptoms they had after they got home. But we wondered whether this was an error, and only told the volunteers their treatment after they had sent their postcard. There were reports of apparent 'late' cures of symptoms."

One of the critical aspects that scientists had to decide on was: how do you define a cold?

Here is more evidence: "The diagnosis of colds within the unit of course included a number of the symptoms reported by volunteers. In the early days they looked for an 'objective' means of detecting a response, and concluded that the best was the 'handkerchief' count – any record of an increase of five or more used per day signified a cold. Nevertheless, a number of symptoms could be used and indeed the opinion of the volunteer that they had a cold seemed very reliable and was supported by a direct comparison organised with the MRC Epidemiology unit in Glasgow. In order to document the time course and to measure the response quantitatively, we added the handkerchief weight and found that with non-parametric statistics we could analyse the results in more detail. However, from the very first years it was clear that the very mildest cold could occur in those given non-infectious material and, although they were summarised as for example an "abortive cold", they did not represent a significant response. When there was a recognisable excess of nasal secretions this was considered a mild cold, more severe symptoms signified a moderate cold and a systemic response meant a severe cold. When we started working with influenza viruses these criteria did not quite meet the case. It was possible to have a definite systemic response with very little in the way of respiratory symptoms, so for these trials we added a separate assessment of systemic reactions. In general I think our threshold for a significant cold is very similar to that of the Virginia group and the Australians".

Because of small numbers, the problem of volunteer susceptibility was ever present and we have received criticism from fellow researchers. Here is how two surviving CCU staff remember how they dealt with the problem: "Volunteers were divided into two groups, which were balanced for age and sex. Rapid antibody assays were done using serum collected when they arrived at the unit and the antibody assay results were available by the end of the quarantine period. So the groups were balanced for antibody levels also. On the day of the beginning of the experiment the excluded volunteers were notified, and the volunteers with highest antibody were usually allocated to receive saline placebo. The groups were then allocated to either drug or placebo as described above – there was no particular system or method in this, e.g. no particular flat was used for drug treatment and because of the construction of groups the flats were allocated differently in each trial. After the trial volunteer's questionnaires were also scored for psychological susceptibility and it usually turned out that these were allocated in a balanced way too. Drugs and virus were sent out labelled with the volunteer's name. For drug trials, volunteers were allocated to groups balanced by age, sex and antibody titre against the virus to be given. There were always a few given no virus. Volunteers were not divided by flats but by individual characteristics. No particular method was used to decide which group had which treatment. When trials against two different viruses were running, volunteers with high titres against one virus would be put into a group to be given the other one. They were very strict about ensuring that the volunteer allocation record was shut away in the laboratory and not seen by either clinical staff or volunteers (it would be passed to the clinician after the final schedule of the volunteer clinical records had been written)".

To sum up, the outcome "cold" is defined in early CCU trials as volunteers presenting with the symptom "coryza" plus one other constitutional symptom (such as malaise, sore throat or fever). From 1973 the definition of a cold relied on a clinical score based on the 9-day average of daily handkerchief counts, presence and grading from 1 to 4 of a list of signs and symptoms (nasal discharge, nasal obstruction, postnasal discharge, sinus pain, red throat, cervical adenitis, hoarseness, cough, sputum, headache, malaise, myalgia and chills), presence of pyrexia, retirement to bed and other supplementary signs and symptoms (e.g. earache). Throughout our review of CCU data we considered volunteers as presenting with a "cold" if they suffered from a "mild", "moderate" or "severe" cold as defined in CCU records. "Very mild" and "doubtful" colds were classified by us as "no colds". Other routinely assessed outcomes, such as a rise in antibody titres and nasal shedding of viruses, were not included in the review as their clinical significance is doubtful.

It would appear that CCU trials did not have a standard method of allocating participants but were a mixture of individual randomisation, cluster randomisation (by accommodation block) and non randomised allocation depending on the compound being tested, volunteer numbers and profile and scientists involved. When reading this, one must remember that standardised methods, huge resources and clinical registries were not available at the time.

What history and evidence tell us

Interferons are effective in preventing colds caused by RV, respiratory syncytial virus, coronavirus and influenza viruses. Their ease of application is counterbalanced by their effects on the nasal mucosa. Adverse events due to the use of interferons became more evident as more potent and purer interferons became available in the 1970s and 1980s. The reversible infiltrate and inflammation caused by intranasal administration led to the symptoms and signs of the very syndrome interferon use was trying to prevent. This caused poor compliance and ultimately poor effectiveness. The effects were more marked after prolonged intranasal administration. Little can be said about interferon effectiveness in treating ongoing colds, given the small denominators of the relevant studies and the difficulty in distinguishing between prevention and early treatment. These observations confirm what is known on the effects of interferons and confirm the rationale for their failure to achieve further development and registration.

The best interferon inducer appears to by dipyridamole but for reasons which are not clear this widely used, cheap and potentially effective drug has not been further studied for this indication.

Pleconaril appears to be the most promising (or at least the best tested so far) compound. However, results of the trials of its aerosol formulation need to be available before reaching a more definite verdict.

As we have seen, the history of antiviral development is littered with promising compounds that failed to live up to expectations. Either because of their lack of *in vivo* efficacy (in viral challenge studies) or effectiveness (in field trials), or because of their side effects (which are of prime importance when dealing with a benign and self-limiting syndrome like the common cold). In addition, the apparent effectiveness of non-specific interventions such as interferons and dypiridamole teaches us an important lesson. When you are dealing with what is to all effects and purposes a syndrome caused by scores of different known and unknown agents, your best bet of success lies in introducing interventions or administering compounds that have a non-specific action like erecting physical barriers (social distancing), removing agents by physical attrition (hand washing), or building up your immune defences (immunomodulators). Until we understand more of the aetiopathogenesis of the common cold this is where our efforts should lie.

Acknowledgements

The late Dr David Tyrrell and Drs Peter Higgins and Sylvia Reed provided many hours of their time and expertise to reconstruct the history of antiviral testing. Iain Chalmers, Carlo Dipietrantonj, Bob Douglas, Ron Turner, Jack Gwaltney Jr, Fred Hayden, Arnold Monto, Vasiliy Vlassov, Alan Cassels, Stefano Jefferson, Melanie Rudin, Anne Lusher, Amy E Zelmer, Ruth Chadwick, Garrath Williams and Reidar Lie assisted in the preparation of the original Cochrane review.

References

1 Tyrrell DAJ (1988) Discovery of influenza viruses. In: Nicholson, Hay and Webster (eds): *Textbook of Influenza*. Blackwell, London, 19–26
2 Ferguson FR, Davey AFC, Topley WWC (1933) The value of mixed vaccines in the prevention of the common cold. *JAMA* 101: 2042–49
3 Thompson KR (1991) Harvard Hospital and its volunteers. In: *The story of the Common Cold Research Unit*. Danny Howell Books, Warminster
4 Tyrrell DAJ (1990) The origins of the Common Cold Unit. *J R Coll Physicians Lond* 24: 137–140
5 Tyrrell DAJ (1992) Acute respiratory virus infections. *Indoor Environ* 1: 16–18
6 Clarke M, The 1944 patulin trial of the British Medical Research Council: An example of how concerted common purpose can get reliable answers to important questions very quickly. The James Lind Library (www.jameslindlibrary.org) (accessed 17 December 2008)
7 Chalmers I, Clarke M (2004) The 1944 patulin trial: The first properly controlled multicentre trial conducted under the aegis of the British Medical Research Council. *Int J Epidemiol* 32: 253–260
8 Tyrrell DAJ (1992) A view from the common cold unit. Mini review. *Antiviral Res* 18: 102–125
9 Merigan TC, Reed SE, Hall TS, Tyrrell DA (1973) Inhibition of respiratory virus infection by locally applied interferon. *Lancet* 1: 563–7
10 CCU unpublished trials records numbers 1001b/4b/5b, 362, 363, 380, 364, 365, 366, 369, 369a, 370, 371, 372, 375, 430, 487, 495, 499, 500, 501, 502, 503, 524, 525,

526, 527, 530, 531, 584, 585, 587, 558, 623, 626, 641a 645, 653, 654, 781, 784, 787, 800, 802, 804, 813, 814, 843, 844, 845, 847, 849, 851, 852, 853, 856, 857, 858, 859, 866, 867, 868, 869, 872b, 875, 876, 877, 879, 881, 883, 884, 885, 886, 887, 889, 890, 902, 903, 904, 905, 920, 927, 928, 929, 955a, 956, 957, 958, 959, 960, 993, 994, 995, 996

11 Douglas RM, Moore BW, Miles HB et al. (1986) Prophylactic efficacy of intranasal alpha 2-interferon against rhinovirus infections in the family setting. *N Engl J Med* 314: 65–70

12 Higgins PG, Barrow GI, Al-Nakib W et al. (1988) Failure to demonstrate synergy between alpha-interferon and a synthetic antiviral, enviroxime, in rhinovirus infections in volunteers. *Antiviral Res* 10: 141–49

13 Gwaltney JM (1992) Combined antiviral and antimediator treatment of rhinovirus colds. *J Infect Dis* 166: 776–82

14 Dolin R, Betts RF, Treanor J et al. (1983) Intranasally administered interferon as prophylaxis against experimentally induced influenza A infection in humans. In: *Proceedings of 13th International congress of Chemotherapy*, Vol. 60. Vienna, 20–23

15 Samo TC, Greenberg SB, Couch RB et al. (1983) Efficacy and tolerance of intranasally applied recombinant leukocyte A interferon in normal volunteers. *J Infect Dis* 148: 535–42

16 Turner RB, Felton A, Kosak K et al. (1986) Prevention of experimental coronavirus colds with intranasal alpha-2b interferon. *J Infect Dis* 154: 443–47

17 Panusarn C, Stanley ED, Dirda V (1974) Prevention of illness from rhinovirus infection by a topical interferon inducer. *N Engl J Med* 291: 57–61

18 Gatmaitan BC, Stanley ED, Jackson GG (1973) The limited effect of nasal interferon induced by rhinovirus and a topical chemical inducer on the course of infection. *J Infect Dis* 127: 401–7

19 Zerial A, Werner GH, Phillpotts RJ et (1985) Studies on 44 081 R.P., a new antirhinovirus compound, in cell cultures and in volunteers. *Antimicrob Agents Chemother* 27: 846–50

20 Phillpotts RJ, Scott GM, Higgins PG et al. (1983) An effective dosage regimen for prophylaxis against rhinovirus infection by intranasal administration of HuINTERFERON-Alpha2. *Antiviral Res* 3: 121–36

21 Al-Nakib W, Higgins PG, Willman J et al. (1986) Prevention and treatment of experimental influenza A virus infection in volunteers with a new antiviral ICI 130,685. *J Antimicrob Chemother* 18: 119–29

22 Higgins PG, Barrow GI, Tyrrell DAJ (1990) A study of the efficacy of the bradykinin antagonist NPC 567 in rhinovirus infection in human volunteers. *Antiviral Res* 14: 339–44

23 Hayden FG, Tunkel AR, Treanor JJ et al. (1994) Oral LY217896 for prevention of experimental influenza A virus infection and illness in humans. *Antimicrob Agents Chemother* 38s: 1178–81

24 Kahlich R, Klima J, Cihla F et al. (1979) Studies on efficacy of *N*-2-hydroxyethyl palmitamide (Impulsin) in acute respiratory infections. Serologically controlled field trials. *J Hyg Epidemiol Microbiol Immunol* 23: 11–24

25 Hayden FG, Andries K, Janssen PAJ (1992) Safety and efficacy of intranasal

Pirodavir (R 77975) in experimentally induced rhinovirus infection. *Antimicrob Agents Chemother* 36: 727–32

26 Turner RB, Dutko FJ, Goldstein NH et al. (1993) Efficacy of oral WIN 54954 for prophylaxis of experimental rhinovirus infection. *Antimicrob Agents Chemother* 37: 297–300

27 Togo Y, Schwartz AR, Hornick-RB (1973) Antiviral effect of 3, 4-dihydro-1-isoquinolineacetamide hydrochloride in experimental human rhinovirus infection. *Antimicrob Agents Chemother* 4: 612–6

28 Soto AJ, Hall TS, Reed-SE (1973) Trial of the antiviral action of isoprinosine against rhinovirus infection of volunteers. *Antimicrob Agents Chemother* 3: 332–4

29 Waldman RH, Ganguly R (1977) Therapeutic efficacy of inosiplex (Isoprinosine) in rhinovirus infection. *Ann N Y Acad Sci* 284: 153–60

30 Phillpotts RJ, Higgins PG, Willman JS, et al. (1984) Intranasal lymphoblastoid interferon ('wellferon') prophylaxis against rhinovirus and influenza virus in volunteers. *J Interferon Res* 4: 535–41

31 Al-Nakib W, Higgins PG, Barrow I, Tyrrell DA, Lenox-Smith I, Ishitsuka H (1987) Intranasal chalcone, Ro 09-0410, as prophylaxis against rhinovirus infection in human volunteers. *J Antimicrob Chemother* 20: 887–92

32 Togo Y, Durr FE, Laurenzana DA (1977) Clinical evaluation of prophylactic intranasal 1-phenyl-3-(4-phenyl-2-thiazolyl) guanidine (CL 88,277) medication against rhinovirus 44 challenge. *Med Microbiol Immunol (Berl)* 163: 37–44

33 Schiff GM, Sherwood JR (2000) Clinical activity of pleconaril in an experimentally induced coxsackievirus A21 respiratory infection. *J Infect Dis* 181: 20–6

34 Hayden FG, Hassman HA, Coats T et al. (1999) Pleconaril treatment shortens duration of picornavirus respiratory illness in adults. 39th ICAAC September, Abstract LB–3

35 Switzer G (2003) How the media left the evidence out in the cold. *BMJ* 326: 1403–4

36 Pevear DC, Hayden FG, Demenczuk TM, Barone LR, McKinlay MA, Collett MS (2005) Relationship of pleconaril susceptibility and clinical outcomes in treatment of common cold caused by rhinoviruses. *Antimicrob Agents Chemother* 49: 4492–9

37 http: //www.ausbiotech.org/data/downloads/Biota%20-%20human%20rhino virus%20Phase%20IIa%20clinical%20trial%20commences,%2011%20 August%202008.pdf (accessed 11 November 2008)

38 De Palma AM, Vliegen I, De Clercq E, Neyts J (2008) Selective inhibitors of picornavirus replication. *Med Res Rev* 28: 823–84

39 Maugeri C, Alisi MA, Apicella C et al. (2008) New anti-viral drugs for the treatment of the common cold. *Bioorg Med Chem* 16: 3091–107

Antibiotic use for common cold

Timothy W. Kenealy and Bruce Arroll

Department of General Practice and Primary Health Care, Tamaki Campus, University of Auckland, Private Bag 92019, Auckland, New Zealand

'Do something, *anything*!' is a universal cry for help at the onset ... of illness.

William Silverman (1917–2004) [1]

Abstract

Antibiotics do not help patients with an uncomplicated common cold. Antibiotics can have side effects for the individual taking them that range from unpleasant to serious, even lethal. Antibiotic use also contributes to communal harm by encouraging antibiotic resistance. If there can be no benefit, but there can be harm, why is the common cold the commonest reason for doctors to prescribe antibiotics? We note that antibiotics are also overused in other conditions and other medical disciplines, as well as in agriculture and the food industry. The harm caused by antibiotics ranges from mild gastrointestinal disturbance to death. Reasons for overuse of antibiotics to treat the common cold include patient expectations, patient and doctor uncertainty around diagnosing complications of the common cold, and the pressure on the doctor to 'do something doctor – anything'. Strategies to limit inappropriate antibiotic use are explored, particularly the use of 'delayed prescriptions', and evidence is presented that with education of doctors and patients the overuse can be reduced.

Antibiotics do not help patients with a common cold

We have previously undertaken a Cochrane systematic review and meta-analysis on the effectiveness of antibiotics for the common cold [2]. We included randomised controlled trials that compared antibiotic with placebo in patients who had symptoms of the common cold for less than 7 days. Trials were excluded if they compared antibiotic to an active substance such as analgesic or cough suppressant; however, trials were included if they allowed patients in both antibiotic and control groups to use other symptom-relief medication. Trials were excluded if more than 5% of patients had throat swabs positive for beta haemolytic streptococcus, or if patients were diagnosed as having 'bronchitis' or a history of serious illness that might require antibiotics, such as chronic obstructive pulmonary disease.

The six included trials varied considerably in quality. All studies included a statement that medication was given in a double-blind manner, although no formal description of blinding was included in any of the papers and none reported assessment of unblinding. The method of randomisation was marginally satisfactory for some of the studies – with one study reporting 'haphazard' randomisation! Loss to follow up was also variable and none reported an intention-to-treat analysis.

Antibiotics used included tetracycline, penicillin, ampicillin, amoxycillin, amoxicillin-clavulanic acid, erythromycin and co-trimoxazole. Studies reported different outcome measures but all those with analysable data reported some general measure of improvement. This was defined in a variety of combinations of persistent symptoms or signs at 24 hours, 3 days, 5 days or 7 days.

People receiving antibiotics did no better in terms of persistence of symptoms at day 1–7 than those on placebo [relative risk (RR) 0.89, 95% confidence interval (CI) 0.77 to 1.04, fixed effects model], based on a pooled analysis with 1147 patients.

Are there patients for whom an antibiotic is reasonable, or is needed?

Are there 'complications' of a common cold, associated infections, or conditions that are difficult to distinguish from common cold, that do benefit from or even require an antibiotic? The symptoms that may occur as part of the common cold overlap with those of bacterial infections, viral infections and allergies. The differential diagnosis is, therefore, relatively wide and includes streptococcal tonsillitis, otitis media, purulent rhinitis, sinusitis, laryngitis, allergic rhinitis, bronchitis and asthma. Ideally, one makes a precise diagnosis and decides on whether an antibiotic might help the patient. The clinical reality can be more blurred. We consider in turn a series of conditions that are commonly treated with antibiotics.

Streptococcal pharyngitis

Unfortunately, patients present with a sore throat or tonsillitis rather than a proven streptococcal infection. Whether or not to treat with an antibiotic has been a long-standing dilemma in primary care [3]. Rapid antigen tests are now available, although costs limits their use; throat swabs can be taken but take 24–48 hours to return a result. Clinical assessment is notoriously inaccurate, although accuracy can be improved modestly using scoring systems [4]. Current advice in most regions is to opt for symptomatic control without using antibiotics, subject to clinical judgement and excluding the very young and the very old [5]. The most important concern is the risk of rheumatic fever. A current draft guideline for primary prevention of rheumatic fever in New Zealand recommends antibiotic treatment for children with a sore throat if the local rate of rheumatic fever exceeds 20 per year per 100 000 children aged 5–14. This would include Maori and Pacific Island children in many areas of New Zealand and children in many developing countries.

Bronchitis

Two systematic reviews conclude that antibiotic use does not significantly affect the resolution of acute cough nor change the course of illness and any modest benefits may be outweighed by the side effects [6, 7]. Some doubt whether 'bronchitis' even exists as a real entity, and we have suggested that variation in diagnostic criteria and subsequent variation in participants included in studies contribute to conflicting results in the literature regarding treatment of bronchitis with antibiotics [8]. We also wonder if ambiguity of symptoms allows 'diagnostic flexibility' by doctors – and in cynical moments one of us calls bronchitis 'the diagnostic label you are given immediately before a doctor gives you an antibiotic'.

Purulent rhinitis or sputum

Guidelines for acute rhinosinusitis in adults advise against antibiotic treatment for all but severe or prolonged cases [9]. We have previously shown that antibiotics may give a modest benefit for patients with acute purulent rhinitis, with a number needed to treat of about 8 [2, 10]. Nevertheless, we have also argued that a modest benefit for a relatively minor condition may not warrant antibiotic use [11]. The same is true with purulent sputum. Nevertheless, Tables 1 and 2 show that purulent sputum is considered by the majority of patients and general practitioners (GPs) to be a reason for prescribing antibiotics.

Important caveats

It is important to note that the trials we have cited do not include the elderly, the very young, the very sick (as indicated by fever or clinical judgement), those with a past history of serious conditions such as chronic obstructive pulmonary disease or bronchiectasis or those who are immunosuppressed; and some trials exclude smokers. In all of these patient groups, doctors are more likely to use antibiotics, and it is more likely to be appropriate. Although in general such treatment has not been tested in randomised controlled trials, such trials would likely be considered unethical and guidance specific to those conditions or groups of people should be followed [12, 13].

Table 1. Reasons general practitioners (GPs) in New Zealand would prescribe antibiotics for a common cold in 2002–2003 ($n = 65$) [46]

Reason	Percent GPs who would prescribe antibiotic
Planning overseas trips in near future	82
Productive cough all day	78
Green-coloured sputum	75
Purulent nasal discharge	71
Patient older	68
Patient expected and asked for antibiotics	63
Patient young, previous recurrent otitis media	58
Patient sick and febrile	58
Patient a smoker	54
Productive cough in morning	40
Patient will go to another doctor for antibiotics if not given	31
Patient tried over-the-counter medications first	28
Persisting dry cough	14
Patient was young	11
Cough at night	11
White productive sputum	6

GPs frequently prescribe antibiotics for upper respiratory tract infections

Large numbers of patients attending GPs with symptoms of upper respiratory tract infections – mostly the common cold – still receive antibiotics [14–16]. Studies have reported rates ranging from 17% in the United Kingdom to more than 60% in United States [17]. In one New Zealand town of about 13000 people, 42% of residents received one or more dispensing of antibiotics in 2002 [18]. Children received antibiotics more often than adults, females more than males and there was a strong relationship between socioeconomic status and antibiotic dispensings. (Not all antibiotic dispensings in this study were for upper respiratory infections.)

There is also a general trend to use broad-spectrum agents for many purposes, including use for upper respiratory infections [19]. Representative national surveys in the US showed that the rate of broad-spectrum antibiotic use increased from 24% to 48% of antibiotic prescriptions in adults, and from 23% to 40% in children from 1991–1992 to 1998-1999 [20]. By 1998–1999, 22% of adult and 14% of paediatric prescriptions for broad-spectrum antibiotics were for the common cold, unspecified upper respiratory tract infections, and acute bronchitis-conditions that are primarily viral [20].

Table 2. Patient behaviours and attitudes in relation to using antibiotics for upper respiratory tract infections (URTI) in New Zealand in 2003 ($n=200$) [24]

	Percent patients
When patients have an URTI they:	
try an over-the-counter medication before seeing doctor	68
have ever consulted doctor about an URTI	45
have been given an "as-needed" prescription at least once	24
went to doctor for last URTI	20
usually see a doctor	15
Patients who consulted the doctor with an URTI did so:	
to relieve symptoms	90
to clarify diagnosis	77
to get an antibiotic	60
to get a note for work	14
When the patient consulted the doctor for an URTI:	
the doctor gave antibiotics	74
the patient collected prescription from chemist	98
the patient took some of the course	93
the patient expected to get antibiotics	63
the patient wanted antibiotics	50
the patient would have gone to another doctor if not given antibiotics	11
the patient asked specifically for antibiotics	8
the doctor asked what patient expected to be given as treatment for URTI	5
Patients taking antibiotics for URTI believe that antibiotics:	
help symptoms	85
shorten the course of URTI	80
Patients perceive that antibiotics are beneficial for:	
tonsillitis	91
coloured phlegm	75
all day phlegm	66
sinusitis	58
morning phlegm	40
coloured nasal discharge	36
fever	28
sore throat	25
clear phlegm	20
night cough	14
preventing complications for planned overseas trip	13
dry cough	5
runny nose	2

Why do GPs prescribe antibiotics for the common cold?

The imperative 'Do something, *anything*', cited from Silverman at the start of this chapter [1], appears to be a visceral urge – felt alike by both doctors and patients – that drives the otherwise-irrational use of antibiotics for the common cold.

When asked why they prescribe antibiotics New Zealand GPs nominated a mixture of medical and social reasons (Tab. 1). Other evidence puts patient expectations – or doctors' perceptions of these expectations – even higher on the list of causes [6, 21, 22].

When comparing recent studies with earlier studies of antibiotic prescribing, it is worth keeping in mind that, if patients are indeed delaying initial consultations while appropriately waiting for natural resolution of symptoms, GPs may be seeing mostly patients with more severe symptoms and hence be more likely to prescribe antibiotics.

Patient attitudes contribute to antibiotic use

A 2001 study interviewed patients across nine countries (UK, France, Belgium, Turkey, Italy, Morocco, Colombia, Spain, and Thailand) [23]. Patients perceived antibiotics as strong, efficient drugs, although they believed antibiotics could undermine their immunity. Interviewees believed that most respiratory infections required antibiotic therapy. Some degree of antibiotic misuse was reported in each country. In all countries it was possible to obtain antibiotics directly from a pharmacy without a prescription, even when this was illegal. Patients exaggerated symptoms to get a prescription for antibiotics or otherwise pressured doctors for a prescription. One patient in four kept some of an antibiotic course for future use. The author concluded that lack of patient knowledge regarding antibiotic use and the consequences of misuse made public education a major priority.

New Zealand patient attitudes and behaviour in relation to antibiotic use for upper respiratory infections are set out in Table 2 [24].

Antibiotics may harm patients – Directly and indirectly

Direct harm, i.e., side-effects, from antibiotics are well known to doctors and patients, but seem surprisingly easy to ignore. We expect that this is at least partly because doctors and patients can often name an antibiotic that was used previously without problems. Ironically, that same antibiotic may have been given to them unnecessarily. Nevertheless, in interviews with 5379 people from nine countries, 27% had experienced side effects during the last course of antibiotics they received [23]. Older patients complained most of dizziness and headaches, whereas diarrhoea and rashes were more common in children [23]. While most adverse events due to antibiotics resolve on stopping the medication, nevertheless fatalities from anaphylaxis, Stevens-Johnson syndrome, hepatic necrosis, renal failure and aplastic anaemia continue to occur occasionally and unpredictably [25].

In addition, prescribing an antibiotic to one patient may later indirectly harm this patient and others by contributing to the major, international and escalating problem of antibiotic resistance. Resistance problems include penicillin-resistant pneumococci, multidrug-resistant *Salmonella typhi*, multidrug-resistant mycobacteria, methicillin (and multidrug)-resistant *Staphylococcus aureus* (MRSA), vancomycin-insensitive *Staphylococcus aureus* (VISA), vancomycin-resistant enterococci (VRE) and penicillin-resistant meningococci [26]. Pseudomembranous colitis is caused by the organism *Clostridium difficile*, usually associated with antibiotic use. It can be difficult to diagnose in the early stages as it initially appears to be 'normal' antibiotic-associated diarrhoea. The diagnosis requires the specific testing for *Clostridium difficile* toxin and in some jurisdictions requires special testing beyond the usual fecal culture. If not treated early the colitis can result in death or colectomy. This is perhaps the most serious immediate harm associated with antibiotic use. In the USA there has been a 203% increase in mortality from *Clostridium difficile* enterocolitis between 1999 and 2003 [27], and an enormous associated economic burden [28].

One US estimate of antibiotic prescriptions in excess of the number expected to treat bacterial infections, estimated at 55% of all antibiotics prescribed for acute respiratory infections, put the cost at about $726 million [29]. It is worth noting that, of the 22.7 million kg (22700 tonnes) of antibiotics that were prescribed in the US in 1997, approximately half were used by human patients and the other half used in animals, agriculture, and aquaculture [30].

The need to identify effective and acceptable alternatives to antibiotics

There seems a strong demand by both patients and doctors to find effective remedies for the misery of the common cold. Presumably if a clearly effective treatment was available, the demand for antibiotics would drop away. Other chapters in this book cover vitamins, over-the-counter, herbal products and antivirals.

Programmes to persuade doctors and patients to reduce antibiotic use

New Zealand's Pharmaceutical Management Agency is responsible for nationwide funding of pharmaceuticals. In 1999 the Agency launched a campaign aimed at reducing antibiotic use by educating the public that antibiotics are ineffective against viruses [31]. The campaign involved posters in general practice waiting rooms and pharmacies, leaflets given to patients in pharmacies and primary health care clinic, plus small group training for GPs. An associated decrease in antibiotic use caused the national drug bill to decrease by 20% from 1996 to 2003. Further, from 1995 to 2002, penicillin resistance among pneumococci decreased nationally from 7% to 3.5% [32].

A nationwide programme in Finland in the 1990s nearly halved the rate of erythromycin prescriptions and was associated with a 50% drop in the frequency of erythromycin resistance among group A streptococci [33]. Pneumococcal resistance to penicillin dropped in Iceland following a programme using radio, television, and newspaper articles; although perhaps the most crucial component was dropping government subsidies for antibiotic prescriptions [34]. A Swedish programme started in 1994 was still considered successful after 10 years [35]. Programmes in US, Canada, Belgium and Australia aimed at controlling antibiotic use and resistance have also reported success [36].

Delayed prescriptions – An intervention specifically with doctors

'Delayed prescriptions' are also known as 'back pocket prescriptions' or 'backup prescriptions' [37]. The term is used when a family physician offers the patient a prescription for an antibiotic to be taken after a time delay. This time delay may be enforced by asking the patient to return to the doctor to pick up a prescription, or the doctor may give the prescription to the patient but advise the patient not to take it yet. In either case, the decision when or if to take the antibiotic is left to the patient. The strategy is intended to meet the needs of both parties when the doctor does not think that a patient medically needs an antibiotic, but the patient wants or expects an antibiotic. Several randomized controlled trials have demonstrated the effectiveness of this strategy in reducing antibiotic use [38–42]. Interestingly, the natural history of this intervention appears to be frequent use by doctors, progressively decreasing, perhaps over several years, as doctors become used to not prescribing antibiotics and patients become used to not taking them (but nevertheless recovering) [43].

Pearls of wisdom offered to our medical colleagues: say No!

As two authors of some of the work on delayed prescriptions, we are concerned that, while delayed prescriptions are effective in decreasing antibiotic use for the common cold, nevertheless some 50% of the population still end up taking antibiotics. We have therefore come to the conclusion in our own practice that the best solution is probably for the doctor to clearly decline to give a prescription for antibiotics, to discuss any issues that arise, and offer symptom control and follow up. Symptom control could include analgesia, nasal sprays such as oxymetazoline and ipratropium nasal and perhaps oral decongestants. However, phenylpropanolamine used as an oral decongestant may increase the risk of stroke in women (odds ratio 3.13), though not in men [44].

We have also developed our own personal ways or mannerisms that make it easier for us to reduce antibiotic prescriptions in our clinics. One of us (BA) promotes his 'Augmentin-free office' (Augmentin is a trade name for amoxicillin-clavulanic acid) [45]. The other (TK) tells patients that 'Bodies are much cleverer than doctors.'

References

1 Silverman W (1998) *Where's the Evidence? Debates in Modern Medicine.* Oxford University Press, Oxford

2 Arroll B, Kenealy T (2005) Antibiotics for the common cold and acute purulent rhinitis. *Cochrane Database of Systematic Reviews*: Art. No.: CD000247

3 McIsaac WJ, Kellner JD, Aufricht P, Vanjaka A, Low DE (2004) Empirical validation of guidelines for the management of pharyngitis in children and adults. *JAMA* 291: 1587–1595

4 McIsaac WJ, Goel V, To T, Low DE (2000) The validity of a sore throat score in family practice. *CMAJ* 163: 811–815

5 Kenealy T (2007) Sore throat. In: F Godlee (ed): *Clinical Evidence.* BMJ Publishing Group, London, 597–599

6 Puhakka T, Pitkaranta A, Ruuskanen O (2000) Common cold and its complications. *Duodecim* 116: 39–45

7 Smucny J, Fahey T, Becker L et al. (2000) Antibiotics for acute bronchitis. *Cochrane Database of Systematic Reviews* CD000245

8 Arroll B, Kenealy T (2001) Antibiotics for acute bronchitis. Four reviews and still no answers: our clinical definitions are at fault. *BMJ* 322: 939–940

9 Hickner J, Bartlett J, Besser R, Gonzales R, Hoffman JR, Sande MA (2001) Principles of appropriate antibiotic use for acute rhinosinusitis in adults: background. *Ann Emerg Med* 37: 703–710

10 Arroll B, Kenealy T (2006) Are antibiotics effective for acute purulent rhinitis? Systematic review and meta-analysis of placebo controlled randomised trials. *BMJ* doi:10.1136/bmj.38891.681215.AE

11 Arroll B, Kenealy T (2002) Antibiotics for acute purulent rhinitis. Probably effective but not routinely recommended (editorial). *BMJ* 325: 1312–1313

12 Baraff LJ, Bass JW, Fleisher GR, Klein JO, McCracken GH Jr, Powell KR, Schriger DL (1993) Practice guideline for the management of infants and children 0 to 36 months of age with fever without source. Agency for Health Care Policy and Research. *Ann Emerg Med* 22: 1198–1210

13 Abramson MJ, Crockett AJ, Frith PA, McDonald CF (2006) COPDX: an update of guidelines for the management of chronic obstructive pulmonary disease with a review of recent evidence. *Med J Aust* 184: 342–345
14 Wang E, Einarson T, Kellner J, Conly J (1999) Antibiotic prescribing for Canadian preschool children: evidence of overprescribing for viral respiratory infections. *Clin Infect Dis* 29: 155–160
15 Marwick J, Grol R, Borgiel A (1992) *Quality Assurance for Family Doctors.* WONCA, Jolimont, Australia
16 Cantrell R, Young A, Martin B (2002) Antibiotic prescribing in ambulatory care settings for adults with colds, upper respiratory tract infections, and bronchitis. *Clin Ther* 24: 170–182
17 Carrie A, Zhanel G (1999) Antibacterial use in community practice: Assessing quantity, indications and appropriateness, and relationship to the development of antibacterial resistance. *Drugs* 57: 871–881
18 Norris P, Becket G, Ecke D (2005) Demographic variation in the use of antibiotics in a New Zealand town. *N Z Med J* 118: U1352
19 Gonzales R, Barrett PJ, Crane L, Steiner J (1998) Factors associated with antibiotic use for acute bronchitis. *J Gen Intern Med* 13: 541–548
20 Steinman M, Gonzales R, Linder J, Landefeld C (2003) Changing use of antibiotics in community-based outpatient practice, 1991–1999. *Ann Intern Med* 138: 525–533
21 Cockburn J, Pit S (1997) Prescribing behaviour in clinical practice: patients' expectations and doctors' perceptions of patients' expectations – a questionnaire study. *BMJ* 315: 520–523
22 Bonn D (2003) Consumers need to change attitude to antibiotic use. *Lancet Infect Dis* 3: 678
23 Pechere JC (2001) Patients' interviews and misuse of antibiotics. *Clin Infect Dis* 33: S170–173
24 Curry M, Sung L, Arroll B, Goodyear-Smith F, Kerse N, Norris P (2006) Public views and use of antibiotics for the common cold before and after an education campaign in New Zealand. *N Z Med J* 119: U1957
25 Cunha B (2001) Antibiotic side effects. *Med Clin North Am* 85: 149–185
26 Hart C (1998) Antibiotic resistance: an increasing problem? *BMJ* 316: 1255–1256
27 Wysowski DK (2007) Surveillance of prescription drug-related mortality using death certificate data. *Drug Safety* 30: 533–540
28 Song X, Bartlett J, Speck K, Naegeli A, KC, Perl T (2008) Rising economic impact of *Clostridium difficile*-associated disease in adult hospitalized patient population. *Infect Control Hosp Epidemiol* 29: 823–828
29 Gonzales R, Malone D, Maselli J, Sande M (2001) Excessive antibiotic use for acute respiratory infections in the United States. *Clin Infect Dis* 33: 757–762
30 Levy S (1997) Antibiotic resistance: origins, evolution, selection and spread. *Ciba Found Symp* 207: 1–14
31 Pharmaceutical Management Agency (2003) Annual Review 2003. Pharmaceutical Management Agency (PHARMAC), Wellington
32 Heffernan H (2002) Annual summaries in bacteriology. *Lablink* 10: 9
33 Seppala H, Klaukka T, Vuopio-Varkila J, Muotiala A, Helenius H, Lager K,

Huovinen P, for The Finnish Study Group for Antimicrobial Resistance (1997) The effect of changes in the consumption of macrolide antibiotics on erythromycin resistance in group A streptococci in Finland. Finnish Study Group for Antimicrobial Resistance. *N Engl J Med* 337: 441–446

34 Stephenson J (1996) Icelandic researchers are showing the way to bring down rates of antibiotic-resistant bacteria (news). *JAMA* 275: 175

35 Mölstad S, Erntell M, Hanberger H, Melander E, Norman C, Skoog G, Lundborg C, Söderström A, Torell E, Cars O (2008) Sustained reduction of antibiotic use and low bacterial resistance: 10-year follow-up of the Swedish Strama programme. *Lancet Infect Dis* 8: 125–132

36 Finch R, Metlay J, Davey P, Baker L, International Forum on Antibiotic Resistance colloquium (2002) Educational interventions to improve antibiotic use in the community: Report from the International Forum on Antibiotic Resistance (IFAR) colloquium, 2002. *Lancet Infect Dis* 4: 44–53

37 Arroll B, Goodyear-Smith F, Thomas D, Kerse N (2002) Delayed prescriptions. What are the experiences and attitudes of doctors and patients? *J Fam Pract* 51: 954–959

38 Arroll B, Kenealy T, Kerse N (2002) Do delayed prescriptions reduce the use of antibiotics in the common cold? A single-blind controlled trial. *J Fam Pract* 51: 324–328

39 Arroll B, Kenealy T, Kerse N (2003) Do delayed prescriptions reduce antibiotic use in respiratory tract infections? A systematic review. *Br J Gen Pract* 53: 871–877

40 Arroll B, Kenealy T, Kerse N, Goodyear-Smith F (2003) Delayed prescriptions: Can reduce antibiotic use in acute respiratory infections. *BMJ* 327: 1361–1362

41 Little P, Gould C, Williamson I, Warner G, Gauntley M, Kinmonth A (1997) Reattendance and complications in a randomised trial of prescribing strategies for sore throat: the medicalising effect of prescribing antibiotics. *BMJ* 315: 350–352

42 Little P, Williamson I, Warner G, Gould C, Gauntley M, Kinmonth A (1997) Open randomised trial of prescribing strategies in managing sore throat. *BMJ* 314: 722–727

43 Arroll B, Goodyear-Smith F (2003) Delayed prescriptions: Evolution of an innovation. *N Z Fam Physician* 30: 30–34

44 Kernan W, Viscoli C, Brass L, JP Broderick, Brott T, Feldman E, Morgenstern L, Wilterdink J, Horwitz R (2000) Phenylpropanolamine and the risk of hemorrhagic stroke. *N Engl J Med* 343:1826–32

45 Arroll B (2007) Upfront: The Augmentin free office. *BPAC*: 6–8

46 Sung L, Arroll J, Arroll B, Goodyear-Smith F, Kerse N, Norris P (2006) Antibiotic use for upper respiratory tract infections before and after a education campaign as reported by general practitioners in New Zealand. *N Z Med J* 119: U1956

Common Cold
ed. by R. Eccles and O. Weber

Over the counter medicines for colds

Ronald Eccles

Common Cold Centre, Cardiff School of Biosciences, Cardiff University, Museum Avenue, Cardiff CF10 3AX, UK

Abstract

Over the counter (OTC) medicines may be defined as medicines that are freely available to the public without a prescription from a doctor. Self-medication for common cold is now encouraged by most government health authorities in order not to overload health resources in winter. This chapter examines the efficacy of the different groups of medicines for the relief of common cold symptoms (analgesics, decongestants, antihistamines, antitussives, menthol, expectorants and mucolytics, throat lozenges and sprays, multi-symptom products, and hot drinks). Safety is the most important factor in any common cold medicine because of the widespread use of the medicines. Because of limitations in dose due to safety concerns many OTC medicines are used at the limits of efficacy and there is often little clinical data to support efficacy, and safety is often supported from a long history of safe use. Aspirin, paracetamol and ibuprofen are the most widely used analgesic treatments to alleviate pain and fever both as monotherapies and in combination with other cold medicines and their efficacy and safety is supported by data from trials on other pain models. The efficacy of nasal decongestants can be supported by clinical trials, and similarly the symptom relief provided by menthol for nasal congestion. The efficacy data for antihistamines, and antitussives is limited and controversial, and there is no real clinical support for the efficacy of expectorants and mucolytics. There is no doubt that all of the OTC common cold medicines are popular with consumers and that they do provide relief from symptoms that in some cases may be more due to a placebo effect than a pharmacological effect of an active ingredient. Multi-symptom medicines provide a safe and convenient way of treating the common cold syndrome of multiple symptoms but their use is sometimes criticised when not all symptoms need to be treated. Hot drinks can provide immediate and sustained relief from symptoms, especially cough and sore throat.

Introduction

Over the counter (OTC) medicines may be defined as medicines that are freely available to the public without a prescription from a doctor. The term OTC is widely used in Europe and the USA, although it is a little confusing, as most medicines are freely available on the pharmacist or supermarket shelf and only certain medicines are kept out of reach at the pharmacist. The OTC common cold market presents a huge business opportunity to the pharmaceutical companies, but there is relatively little research undertaken by the pharmaceutical industry in the development of new medicines for this condition. OTC common cold medicines, with few exceptions, are marketed for the relief of common cold symptoms, and they do not prevent or alter the viral cause of a common cold. Since most colds are acute self-limiting conditions the goal of controlling symptoms is a reasonable goal for OTC medicines, as symptom relief will allow the patient to carry on with their life.

In recent years there has been an increased focus on safety issues associated with OTC common cold medicines. Antitussives such as codeine have always been at risk of increased regulatory control or a ban due to the potential risk of abuse [1] and recently the recreational abuse of dextromethorphan has led to restrictions on sale or a ban in many countries [2, 3]. Nasal decongestants because of their vasoconstrictor activity have the potential to cause cardiovascular side effects and safety concerns led to a ban on the sale of phenylpropanolamine in the USA in 2000. More recently, concerns over the recreational abuse of the nasal decongestant pseudoephedrine have led to the loss of its OTC status in many countries and its substitution in many products with a relatively less-well-characterised decongestant, phenylephrine [4].

The loss or restriction of many popular cold medicines in recent years due to safety issues means there are fewer active ingredients available to the pharmaceutical industry. Each company has access to the same limited pool of active ingredients, and the marketing of these active ingredients is mainly on the brand name or on claims about strength or speed of action. Because of the focus on advertising rather than research, the pharmacology of the OTC common cold active ingredients has been neglected as a review topic in scientific and medical journals, and it is hoped that this chapter will be of use to those doctors, pharmacists and brand managers who need an overall review of the active ingredients commonly used in cold treatments.

This chapter discusses the active ingredients that make up many of the OTC medicines. The OTC medicines are divided into several groups for discussion: analgesics, decongestants, antihistamines, antitussives, expectorants and mucolytics, menthol and other aromatics, sore throat lozenges and sprays.

Analgesics

Analgesics such as aspirin, paracetamol (acetaminophen in the USA) and ibuprofen are the most common treatments for common cold, either as mono-medicines or in combination with other cold medicines such as antihistamines and nasal decongestants. The use of analgesics as treatments for colds and flu has recently been reviewed [5].

Medicines

The analgesics, aspirin, paracetamol and ibuprofen can provide relief for a range of common cold symptoms such as headache, sore throat pain, fever, muscle aches and pains, sinus pain, and earache [5].

Analgesics are usually marketed as combination medicines for treatment of common cold, and these medicines may be formulated as tablets, capsules, hot drinks, effervescent drinks and syrups. Analgesics are often combined with a nasal decongestant or an antihistamine, and in some multi-symptom products the analgesic may be combined with nasal decongestant, antihistamine and antitussive or expectorant.

Pharmacology

Aspirin and ibuprofen are usually classified as non-steroidal anti-inflammatory drugs (NSAIDs) as they have anti-inflammatory actions in high doses, whereas paracetamol (acetaminophen) is not usually classed as an NSAID as it does not have any anti-inflammatory activity. The three analgesics have a similar mode of action in treating the pain and fever symptoms of common cold as they all inhibit the activity of cyclooxygenase (COX) enzymes responsible for the biosynthesis of prostaglandins and related inflammatory mediators [6]. Prostaglandins play an important role in the inflammatory response to infection as they cause local vasodilation and nasal congestion, and also potentiate the local pain effects of bradykinin, to cause sore throat pain, earache and sinus pain [7]. The sensitisation of pain nerve endings in the upper airway by prostaglandins leads to the pain symptoms of common cold and the inhibition of prostaglandin synthesis by the analgesics provides relief from local pain symptoms such as sore throat pain [8, 9].

The generation of common cold symptoms can be divided into two components: a local response to cellular damage that causes the local synthesis of inflammatory mediators such as bradykinin and prostaglandins; and a systemic response caused by cytokines released from macrophages and neutrophil granulocytes [7, 10]. The cytokines circulate in the blood stream to the brain to cause headache and fever and they also initiate muscle aches and pains. These systemic responses are mediated by prostaglandin synthesis [11] and the inhibition of prostaglandin synthesis by the analgesic will therefore relieve the common cold symptoms of headache, fever and muscle aches and pains as well as localised pain symptoms in the upper airway.

Paracetamol is believed to act as an analgesic and antipyretic by inhibiting prostaglandin synthesis in the pain pathways in the central nervous system, whereas aspirin and ibuprofen act to inhibit prostaglandin synthesis both in the brain and in peripheral tissues. It is the peripheral action of aspirin and ibuprofen on prostaglandin synthesis that is responsible for any anti-inflammatory effects.

Efficacy

Considering the widespread use of analgesics in treating common cold symptoms, it is surprising that there is relatively little literature on the efficacy of analgesics in colds, and that most of the efficacy and safety data must be derived from studies on other pain and fever models [5].

Placebo-controlled studies have demonstrated the efficacy of aspirin as a treatment for sore throat pain, fever and muscle aches and pains associated with common cold [9, 12–14]. The effects of a single dose of 800 mg aspirin on sore throat pain associated with common cold are illustrated in Figure 1. The graph shows the differences in pain intensity compared to a baseline score before treatment and the relatively large placebo response is typical

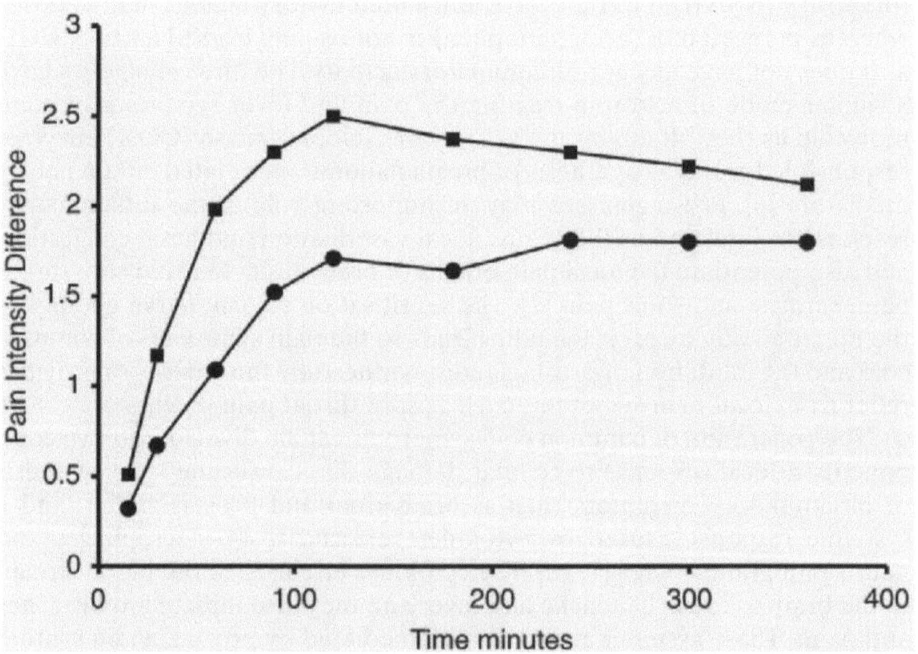

Figure 1. Effects of a single dose of 800 mg aspirin on scores for pain intensity in patients with sore throat pain associated with common cold. The scores represent the mean differences in pain intensity from the baseline scores. Square symbols represent scores for the aspirin treatment group and round symbols for the placebo treatment group. The graph is based on the results of a published clinical trial on the efficacy of aspirin [9].

of most pain studies. Similarly, paracetamol has been shown to be an effective analgesic for pain and fever symptoms associated with common cold [12, 14–16]. Ibuprofen is the most recent analgesic to achieve OTC status for treatment of common cold and, although the efficacy of ibuprofen has been established in various pain and fever models, there is very little information available on its efficacy as a treatment for colds. Clinical trials have shown ibuprofen to be an effective treatment for sore throat pain, headache, fever, earache, sneezing and muscle aches and pains [15, 17].

Although it is generally accepted that aspirin and ibuprofen have anti-inflammatory actions when used in the treatment of rheumatoid arthritis, there is no convincing evidence that they have anti-inflammatory effects in common cold treatment when used in the normal OTC dose range [5]. No convincing case can be made for a difference in efficacy between aspirin, paracetamol and ibuprofen for treatment of pain and fever associated with common cold [5]. However, a combination of paracetamol plus ibuprofen may be superior on some parameters to either drug alone in treatment of fever-associated discomfort in children aged between 6 months and 6 years [18].

Safety

In considering the safety of the analgesics for treatment of symptoms of upper respiratory tract infection (URTI), it is necessary to understand that much of the concern over the use of NSAIDs such as aspirin and ibuprofen is related to long-term therapy with higher doses than available for OTC use, for example in the treatment of chronic rheumatoid arthritis. Similarly, concerns about the safety of paracetamol are often linked to alcohol abuse and overdose. Because of the limited number of trials on the use of analgesics in patients with URTI, it is necessary to rely on safety data gathered from trials on indications other than URTI.

The major concerns about safety are related to liver damage with paracetamol, especially in overdose, and in relation to alcohol ingestion. Aspirin may cause gastric irritation, bleeding and exacerbation of asthma. Ibuprofen may also cause gastric irritation and bleeding. However, all three analgesics are generally recognised as having a good safety profile when used in OTC doses for the treatment of acute pain and fever associated with common cold [5]. There is little evidence for any difference in overall safety between the analgesics, although special cases can be made for contra-indications such as for aspirin in children (Reye's syndrome), and for paracetamol in cases of excess alcohol intake.

The discovery of two different enzymes for prostaglandin synthesis, COX-1 and COX-2, has revolutionised the development of new analgesic anti-inflammatory drugs. COX-1 is the constitutive enzyme found normally in tissues such as the stomach and kidney and inhibition of this enzyme system is responsible for side effects such as gastric irritation. COX-2 is the enzyme that is induced by inflammation and there is interest in developing specific COX-2 inhibitors in order to have a more specific analgesic and anti-inflammatory effect [19, 20]. The development of specific COX-2 inhibitors may eventually provide new analgesics that will gain OTC status in the future for treatment of common cold but at present this is a distant goal and much more information is needed on the side effect profiles of COX-2 inhibitors before they could become freely available without prescription.

Effects on the immune system

High doses of NSAIDs such as ibuprofen and aspirin have a depressant action on the immune response and this is beneficial in diseases such as rheumatoid arthritis where the autoimmune response causes damage to joints. However, a depressant action on the immune system would not be beneficial in the treatment of URTI, and analgesics are sometimes implicated in prolonging the course of infections, especially when the infection is associated with fever [21]. There is no evidence that treatment with analgesics interferes with the natural recovery from URTI but there are reports that aspirin and paracetamol may increase the severity of the symptom of nasal obstruction associated with URTI. A single dose of 900 mg aspirin has been reported to cause an increase in nasal resistance to airflow in healthy volunteers [22] and there is one report that daily doses of 4000 mg aspirin and paracetamol caused nasal congestion when used by volunteers infected *via* rhinovirus challenge [23].

Conclusions

Aspirin, paracetamol and ibuprofen are the most commonly used analgesic treatments for common cold in both adults and children. In OTC doses they are safe and effective, and apart from their specific contraindications, there is little difference between the analgesics as regards safety and efficacy.

Nasal decongestants

The nasal decongestants fall into three groups: topical nasal decongestants administered as a nasal spray or nose drops (oxymetazoline, xylometazoline and phenylephrine); oral decongestants that may be formulated as a tablet or syrup (ephedrine, pseudoephedrine and phenylephrine); and inhaler sticks containing ephedrine (also known as levo-methamphetamine or leveometamfetamine in the USA).

Medicines

The oral decongestants pseudopehedrine and phenylephrine are usually formulated as a combination medicine with an analgesic in tablet formulations, and they may also be combined in multi-symptom treatments with antihistamines and antitussives. The topical nasal decongestants are usually formulated as a mono-therapy nasal spray that may also contain menthol and other aromatics. More recently there has been interest in developing a combination treatment for congestion and runny nose by combining xylometazoline with ipratropium [24].

Pharmacology

The nasal decongestants open up the nose by constricting the large nasal veins in the anterior part of the nose that control nasal airway resistance [25]. The medicines are sympathomimetics in that they mimic the effects of the sympathetic neurotransmitter noradrenaline or facilitate its release from sympathetic nerve endings [26]. Both the topical and oral decongestants achieve nasal decongestion by acting on alpha receptors on nasal veins to cause constriction of vascular smooth muscle [25].

Efficacy

The topical decongestants oxymetazoline and xylometazoline have a rapid onset of action, as they are applied directly to the nasal epithelium and quickly reach the nasal blood vessels to cause vasoconstriction. Decongestion is achieved within 5–10 minutes and sustained for up to 10 hours as shown in Figure 2. The oral decongestants pseudophedrine and phenylephrine have a slow onset of action over 30–60 minutes, as they must first be absorbed from the gut to achieve their action on nasal blood vessels. The efficacy of topical and oral decongestants is compared in Figure 3, which demonstrates that the oral decongestants improve nasal conductance by around 10% compared to a 70% change in nasal conductance associated with topical decongestants. The efficacy of the topical nasal decongestants oxymetazoline and xylometazoline is not in doubt, as large changes in nasal conductance can be easily shown in clinical trials [25, 27], but the efficacy of the oral decongestants pseudoephedrine and phenylephrine is more difficult to show in clinical trials. Published clinical trials on pseudoephedrine have reported significant but small changes in nasal airflow measured by rhinomanometry [16, 28], but there are no good quality published studies on the efficacy of phenylephrine as an oral decongestant, and its efficacy may be limited by first pass metabolism of phenylephrine in the gut [4]. Meta-analysis of studies on phenylephrine

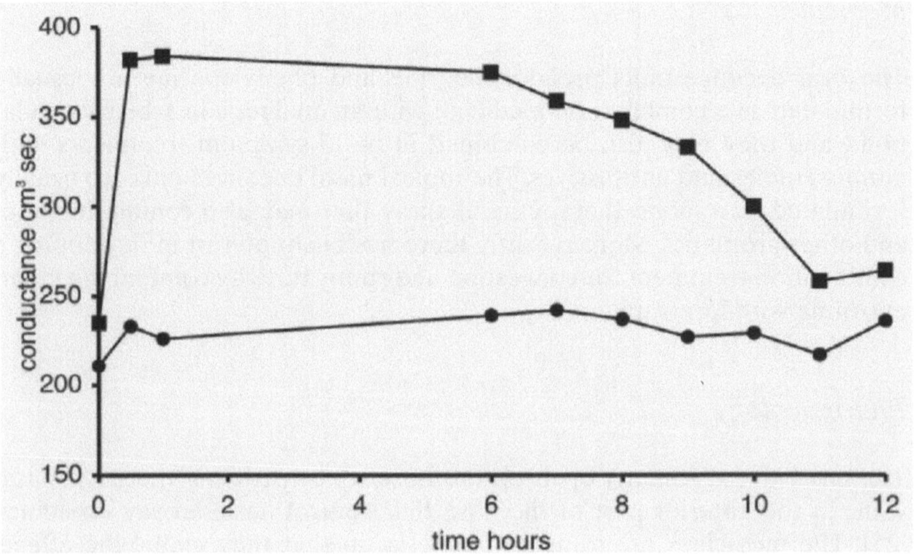

Figure 2. Effects of a single spray of 0.1% xylometazoline topical nasal decongestant on nasal airflow measured by rhinomanometry in patients with nasal congestion associated with common cold. The placebo treatment was a saline nasal spray. Square symbols represent airflow for the xylometazoline treatment group and round symbols for the placebo treatment group. The graph is based on the results of a published clinical trial on the efficacy of xylometazoline as a nasal decongestant [27].

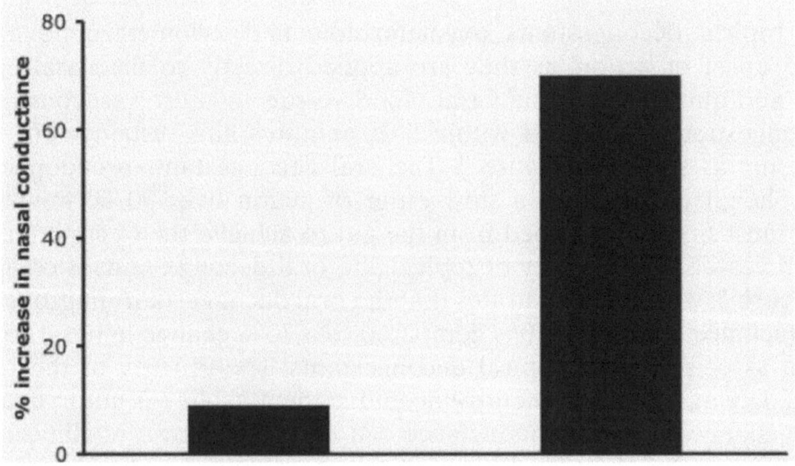

Figure 3. Effects of oral and topical decongestants on nasal airflow. The figure shows the percentage increase in nasal conductance as measured by rhinomanometry for a single oral dose of 60 mg pseudoephedrine or one spray in each nostril of 0.1% xylometazoline, in patients with nasal congestion associated with common cold. The change in conductance was measured at 60 minutes after treatment and is expressed as a mean percentage change relative to the change in conductance observed in the placebo treatment group. The results are calculated from the data reported in clinical trials [27, 28].

held on file by the FDA have provided divergent views on efficacy [29, 30].

Ephedrine is used in wick inhalers to treat nasal congestion but no references have been found to support the efficacy of inhaled ephedrine as a nasal decongestant.

Safety

Safety issues are mainly related to cardiovascular events as the nasal decongestants are sympathomimetics and cause vasoconstriction [25]. Concerns about the conversion of pseudoephedrine to the recreational drug methamphetamine have led to restrictions on the availability of common cold medicines containing pseudoephedrine. This has led to the substitution of pseudoephedrine with phenylephrine in many common cold products despite there being some debate about the efficacy of phenylephrine as a nasal decongestant [4].

Long-term use of topical nasal decongestants (over months or years) may cause nasal irritation and rhinitis medicamentosa [31]. The development of rhinitis medicamentosa is sometimes explained on the basis of nasal rebound congestion after use of topical nasal decongestants, with the patient continuing to use the nasal decongestant to treat congestion caused by use of the decongestant [32]. The nasal irritation and rhinitis induced by topical nasal decongestants may be due to the presence of preservatives such as benzalkonium rather than due to a pharmacological action of the medicine [32].

Conclusions

The topical nasal decongestants oxymetazoline and xylometazoline are safe and effective decongestants, but some caution is needed with any long-term use due to the development of rhinitis medicamentosa. The oral decongestants pseudoephedrine is less effective than the topical decongestants, and the efficacy of phenylephrine as an oral decongestant in OTC doses is debatable.

Antitussives

Cough is a vital reflex to protect the airway from aspiration of food and fluid but cough associated with common cold is disturbing and usually of no benefit. Even in cases of chesty productive cough when cough is important as a means of clearing the airway of mucus, excessive coughing may be debilitating. Antitussives can be used to decrease the frequency and intensity of cough to provide symptom relief without abolishing the protective cough reflex.

Medicines

Almost all cough medicines are formulated as sweet syrups and this maybe related to the powerful placebo effects of a sweet taste on cough [33]. The sweet taste of honey may explain the traditional use of honey to treat cough and its efficacy as an antitussive [34].

Pharmacology

The antitussives may be divided into opiates such as codeine, opiate derivatives such as dextromethorphan and pholcodine, and sedating antihistamines such as diphenhydramine. Antitussives are believed to act by an inhibitory action on the brainstem areas that control cough. The opiates and dextromethorphan may have some specific effects on the brainstem area, whereas the antihistamines may only act as sedatives.

Efficacy

The efficacy of OTC antitussives has proven difficult to determine as there is no generally accepted method of determining efficacy and there is no generally accepted gold-standard antitussive to validate methods [35, 36]. Some authors doubt if any of the antitussive medicines are superior to placebo treatment with a sweet syrup [33, 34, 37, 38]. Meta-analysis of studies provides some limited support for the efficacy of dextromethorphan [39] but other studies demonstrate no superiority above placebo [34, 40]. In all acute cough studies there is a large placebo response and this makes it difficult to determine the efficacy of any pharmacologically active ingredient in an antitussive treatment. The large placebo response and rapid decline in cough severity after treatment with a cough medicine illustrated in Figure 4 is typical of this type of study. Cough associated with common cold may be under voluntary control and related to a sensation of airway irritation [41, 42], and this is another problem in conducting clinical trials as subjects may control cough according to their expectations about the efficacy of any medicine. Any unblinding of the study or side effects of an active treatment may influence voluntary control of cough and complicate the interpretation of cough clinical trials.

An explanation of the variability in antitussive response to dextromethorphan is that differences in the rate of metabolism of the drug between individuals cause much variability on the response to dextromethorphan [43]. There are few studies on the antitussive efficacy of sedating antihistamines,

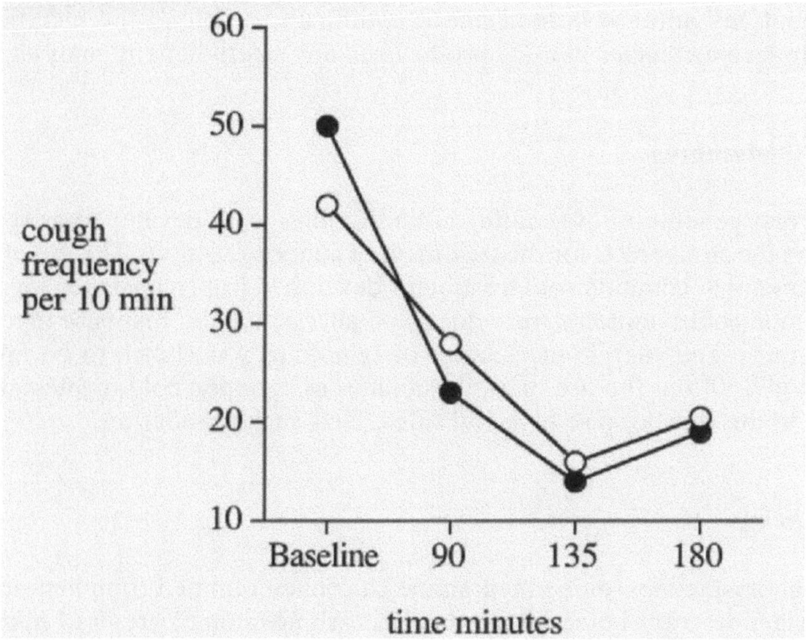

Figure 4. Median cough frequency (per 10 minutes) for patients with cough associated with common cold. Immediately after the baseline measurement (0 minutes) patients were treated with either a single dose of 30 mg dextromethorphan powder in a hard gelatin capsule (filled symbols, $n=21$), or a matched placebo capsule containing lactose powder (open symbols, $n=22$) [40].

pholcodine and codeine, and little support for any efficacy in the treatment of acute cough [36, 38, 44, 45]. Reviews provide no good evidence for the efficacy of OTC cough medicines [46].

Safety

The antitussive medicines, because of their effects on the central nervous system, are dangerous in overdose, especially in children [44, 47] and their central effects may be utilised for recreational abuse [48]. The recreational abuse of dextromethorphan has led to restrictions on the availability of this medicine in several countries [2, 3] and this trend is likely to continue.

Conclusions

There is only very limited support for the efficacy of OTC antitussives, especially in children, and since simple sweet syrups can provide relief of cough without any antitussive medicine it is difficult to defend the inclusion of antitussive medicines in OTC products on any safety-benefit analysis.

Antihistamines

The first generation of sedating antihistamines were developed as specific histamine antagonists for the treatment of allergic reactions. The use of antihistamines as common cold treatments developed from a mistaken idea that common cold symptoms were due to an allergic type of response involving histamine. The allergic mechanism of symptoms was shown to be false in 1950 [49, 50] but the use of antihistamines as common cold medicines persists to this day because of useful side effects such as sedation.

Medicines

The antihistamines (diphenhydramine, chlorpheniramine, brompheniramine, doxylamine, triprolidine, promethazine, carbinoxamine) are used in a very wide range of medicines both as syrups and tablets for multi-symptom relief of cough, runny nose and sneezing, in combination with analgesics, decongestants, antitussives, and expectorants.

Pharmacology

The first generation antihistamines are useful as treatments because of their sedative and anticholinergic properties. The sedative actions make them useful as night-time treatments and antitussives, and the anticholinergic properties may help in the control of nasal secretions and sneezing [51, 52]. There is no support for the efficacy of newer non-sedating antihistamines in the treatment of common cold symptoms and this is probably because of the more specific antihistamine effect and lack of sedation and anticholinergic effects [50, 53].

Efficacy

The antihistamines were introduced as some of the first commercial common cold treatments in the 1940s before the advent of placebo-controlled trials, and although there are a few placebo-controlled studies supporting the efficacy of antihistamines as antitussives and antisecretory medicines, the evidence base is weak [44, 52, 54–56]. There is no doubt that the antihistamines are sedative, and this is a benefit for night-time medicines but an unwanted side effect for day-time use. There is some support for use of antihistamines in controlling runny nose and sneezing [52, 57].

Safety

The central sedative effect of the first generation antihistamines is a problem, especially in overdose, and because of the relative lack of evidence to support efficacy, some authors have proposed that antihistamines should be withdrawn from all OTC products [44]. However, this may be an extreme point of view as the antihistamines are widely used in OTC common cold products with relatively few adverse events when taken as directed.

Conclusions

The antihistamines survive as common cold treatments because of their sedative and anticholinergic effects rather than any effect on histamine. There is some support for their use as treatments for runny nose and sneezing but the sedative actions limit their usefulness. Use in children is difficult to support.

Expectorants

Expectorants are used to aid in the clearance of mucus from the bronchi in the lungs by making the mucus more fluid so that it is easier to clear by coughing. Expectorants such as ipecacuanha, squill and guaicol derivatives are probably the oldest surviving OTC treatments with a long history of various medical uses.

Medicines

Expectorants are usually taken as syrups to treat a ‘chesty’ or ‘productive’ cough. Medicines such as ipecacuhna, squill and guaicol have been used for centuries to treat coughs and colds. Squill was included in the first edition (1618) of the London Pharmacopoeia [58], and the history of guaicol as a medicine originates as an import from the new world in the early 17th century [59].

Pharmacology

The expectorants ipecacuhna, squill, guaicol and guaiphenesin are believed to act as gastric irritants and by means of a gastro-vagal reflex they stimulate airway secretions [60, 61]. The expectorants were first used in medicine as emetics to relieve the body of excess fluid that was believed to be the cause of rhinorrhea and cough. Gunn (1927) [60] states that "A large number of drugs which have no common pharmacological property, other than that of being gastric irritants have in the course of time come to be used empirically as secretory expectorants when given by mouth. Many of these drugs have been used as emetics in larger doses". Ammonium salts may also work by means of gastric irritation and the mode of action of expectorants such as bromohexine is not known. Iodide salts may work *via* gastric irritation or alternatively, iodide may be secreted into airway mucus to alter the properties of the mucus, but the mode of action is unclear [61].

Guaiphenesin is a synthetic derivative of guaicol and is believed to act as a gastric irritant, although the mode of action is not known and there may be other effects of guaiphenisin such as antitussive activity [62].

Efficacy

There is little evidence that expectorants have any effect on cough and mucus composition in common cold. Most studies on expectorants have studied chronic cough rather than acute conditions such as common cold and even here there is little support for any beneficial effect [61, 63]. Some studies report a decrease in the viscosity of airway secretions associated with treatment with guaiphenesin during cough associated with colds [64, 65] but these studies have not yet been confirmed by other investigators.

One major problem in studying the efficacy of an expectorant is that there is no generally agreed method to assess efficacy [66] and that expectoration of saliva can complicate measurement of sputum viscosity and volume. Reviews on efficacy of expectorants in OTC cough medicines do not provide any support for this treatment [46].

Safety

The small number of clinical trials on expectorants do not raise any safety issues and the widespread use of these products over many years does support safety.

Conclusions

Expectorants are widely used in OTC medicines for the treatment of chesty cough associated with common cold but the lack of efficacy data to support this mode of treatment means that their use as a common cold treatment is not clearly proven.

Mucolytics

Mucolytic medicines are believed to alter the composition of mucus and make it more fluid and thus aid expectoration. The most widely used mucolytics are ambroxol, N-acetylcysteine and carbocysteine and, although the mode of action of these medicines is not fully understood, they are believed to alter the physical properties of mucus in this manner. There are only limited data that mucolytics provide any benefit in chronic pulmonary disease, and in this condition their efficacy is assessed over months rather than weeks or days [67, 68]. There is no clinical data to support the efficacy of mucolytics as expectorants in acute respiratory infections such as common cold but one study does indicate that ambroxol may help to prevent colds [69].

Menthol

Because of the popularity of menthol products this ingredient is discussed as a separate section, although it does not form a specific class of ingredients. Menthol and other plant aromatic oils such as eucalyptus and camphor have been used as treatments for colds in traditional remedies for centuries. Menthol has been used in vaporubs since the development of 'Vicks VapoRub' in 1890 [70]. Menthol is probably the most commonly used ingredient in common cold medicines. Menthol is often combined with camphor, eucalyptus and other aromatic oils, especially in vaporubs and inhalants and this sometimes makes it difficult to determine the efficacy and safety of the separate ingredients of the medicine. Only menthol is discussed as there is very little literature on the effects of the other aromatic oils on common cold.

Medicines

Menthol is a very versatile medicine as it is used in vapour rubs, lozenges, cough syrups, decongestant nasal sprays, throat sprays, aromatherapy oils, and even bath oils and shampoos. The typical smell of menthol is so commonly associated with cold medicines that it is often referred to as a 'Vicks' smell. Menthol is not always declared as an active ingredient in cold medicines and this sometimes makes it difficult to conduct a clinical trial to demonstrate efficacy of the declared active ingredient as both the placebo control and active medicine will contain menthol, and the menthol will relieve symptoms of common cold. The popularity of menthol-containing confectionery that may also be used as treatments for cold symptoms may be due to the effects of menthol on thirst and because of its mild stimulant effect [71].

Pharmacology

Menthol acts on temperature receptors in skin and mucosal surfaces to cause a sensation of coolness or warmth [72]. The cooling sensation is believed to be mediated by a transient receptor channel (TRPM8) located on the cell membrane of thermoreceptors on sensory nerve endings [73]. Menthol, cooling agent Icilin and cool temperature have all been shown to activate TRPM8 to cause an increase in intracellular calcium and generation of an action potential in the thermoreceptor sensory nerve ending [73]. The interaction with TRPM8 has some similarity to interaction with a specific pharmacological receptor as there are differences in the efficacy of different menthol isomers in inducing the sensation of coolness [74, 75]. L-Menthol has the greatest cooling activity and the stereo isomer D-menthol has little cooling activity [74, 76].

Menthol is used in vaporubs, lozenges, and nasal sprays to relieve the sensation of nasal stuffiness associated with colds, and this effect is brought about by stimulation of cold receptors in the nose [77, 78]. Menthol lozenges are monographed by the FDA as effective cough drops and menthol may influence cough by acting on airway sensory nerves or smooth muscle [79]. Although menthol is claimed to have a bronchodilator action there is little support for this effect [80].

Efficacy

Inhalation of menthol vapour on sucking a menthol lozenge causes a sensation of improved airflow due to a cool sensation in the nose, without any objective change in nasal airway resistance as illustrated in Figure 5 [78]. Menthol vapour can relieve symptoms of nasal congestion but is not a nasal decongestant. In high concentrations menthol acts as an irritant and may cause nasal congestion [81, 82].

Menthol is a common ingredient in cough medicines but there is little support for efficacy as an antitussive. Studies on citric acid-induced cough in healthy adult subjects provide some support for an antitussive effect [83], but this has not been confirmed in a similar study on children [80].

Menthol is a common ingredient in lozenges for treatment of sore throat and the local anaesthetic action of menthol may be beneficial in this form of treatment [75]. Despite the widespread use of menthol in throat lozenges, no support has been found in the literature for the use of menthol to treat sore throat apart from a recommendation in 1890 [84].

Topical application of menthol in peppermint oil or balm to the forehead has been shown to relieve headache [85, 86].

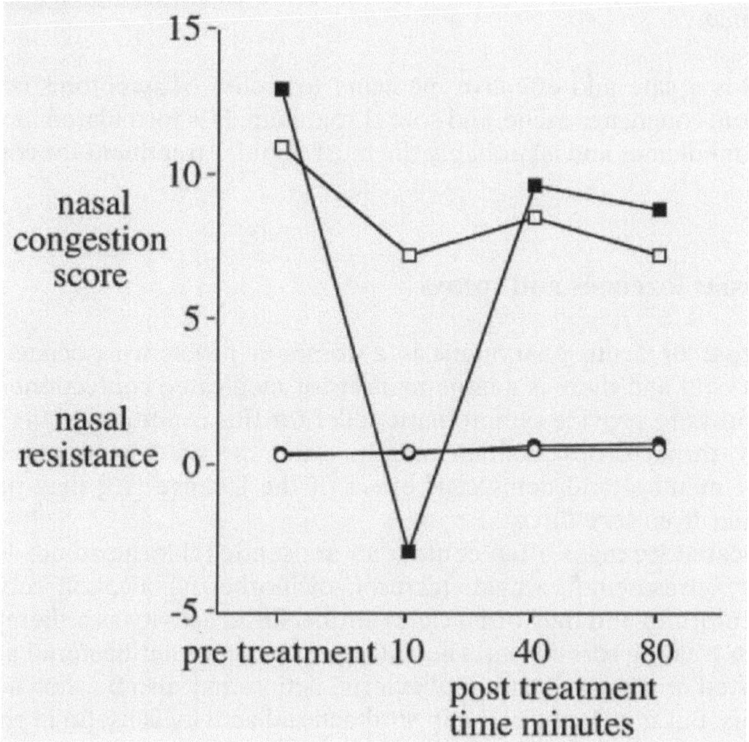

Figure 5. The effects of ingestion of an 11 mg L-menthol lozenge on subjective sensation of nasal congestion and nasal resistance to airflow in human volunteers with common cold. The subjective sensation of nasal congestion, measured on a 100-mm visual analogue scale, was significantly reduced 10 minutes after ingestion of the lozenge but nasal airway resistance as measured by rhinomanometry was unaffected. Shaded symbols represent the values for the menthol-treated group and the open symbols represent the mean values for the placebo-treated group. Results taken from [78].

Safety

Menthol-containing medicines in a wide range of topical and systemic medicines have been used for over a hundred years in the treatment of common cold and there are few reports of any adverse events attributed to menthol. Vaporubs and other menthol-containing medications are used on infants and there are concerns that high concentrations of menthol applied close to the nose may cause apnoea in susceptible infants [87, 88]. However, when used as directed, vaporubs may ease breathing in infants with acute bronchitis associated with common cold [89].

Conclusions

Menthol is a safe and effective medicine for relief of symptoms of nasal congestion, cough, headache, and sore throat pain. It is formulated in a wide range of medicines and is probably the most popular treatment for common cold.

Sore throat lozenges and sprays

Sore throat or acute pharyngitis is a common problem associated with common cold and there is a large market for medicated confectionery and throat sprays to provide symptomatic relief for this condition. Many of the so-called 'throat drops' contain menthol, and the mild local anaesthetic action of menthol and demulcent effect of the lozenge [75] may provide some relief from sore throat.

Medicated lozenges often contain an antiseptic (chlorhexidine, dequalinium, hexylresorcinol, amylmetacresol, bichlorbenzyl alcohol, cetylpyridinium chloride) and they often claim antibacterial activity as a therapeutic benefit in treating sore throat. The antiseptics do have antibacterial activity when tested *in vitro*, and this antibacterial action may also be shown in the oral cavity, but it is doubtful if any antibacterial activity is useful in treating sore throat, as most throat infections are caused by viruses [90]. There is no clinical or scientific support for the use of antiseptics in the treatment of sore throat, but the public perception of the usefulness of antibacterials in this condition persists in much the same way as the demand for antibiotic prescription for sore throat, despite the fact that there is no evidence that antibiotics provide any benefit [91].

Sore throat sprays and lozenges containing a local anaesthetic agent (lidocaine, benzocaine) may provide relief from sore throat pain [92] but they do have a numbing effect on the tongue that affects taste, and this side effect may limit the tolerability of the sprays.

Placebo effect

OTC medicines for the treatment of common cold may provide the greatest benefit to the patient by means of a placebo effect. Because of safety issues in OTC medicines that are freely available to the public, the active pharmacological ingredient in cold medicines is often at the level of the minimal effective dose. In cough medicines it has been proposed that 85% of the benefit of the medicine is due to the placebo effect of the medicine and only 15% is contributed by the antitussive medicine [37]. The placebo effect is related to the patients' belief in the efficacy of the medicine and this may be enhanced by the 'brand' of the medicine and advertising [93]. The placebo effect is not just a psychological effect as placebo treatment may cause physical changes in the body such as effects on the immune system [94]. In this respect, the faith in a medicine and the subsequent placebo effect may influence the course of a common cold illness [95].

Multi-symptom treatments

Multi-symptom treatments that contain several medicines to treat several symptoms simultaneously are popular with consumers but are viewed critically by some pharmacists and clinicians. The consumers like the multi-symptom treatments because they provide a cheap and safe way of treating multiple symptoms with what is viewed as a single treatment. However, the medicines may be criticised as exposing patients to one of the ingredients when they do not have all the symptoms that the multi-symptom medicine is proposed to treat. Common combination medicines are analgesic plus decongestant, and a triple therapy may include a sedating antihistamine to control cough or runny nose and sneezing. In some cases the multi-symptom treatment may contain four active ingredients (paracetamol, dextromethorphan, doxylamine, and ephedrine and there is some support for the efficacy of this mix as an effective and convenient therapy for multiple symptoms [96].

Common cold symptoms usually occur as a complex of multiple symptoms [97] and therefore it is reasonable to develop multi-symptom medicines to conveniently treat the symptom complex, even if on some occasions there may not be a need for all of the medicines in the treatment.

Hot drinks

Despite the widespread folklore that hot drinks are an effective treatment for colds and flu, and the use of hot drink formulations for many current common cold OTC medicines, there is little evidence base in the medical literature supporting the efficacy of a hot drink for common cold and flu. A study investigated the effects of a hot fruit drink on objective and subjective measures of nasal airflow, and on subjective scores for common cold/flu symptoms in 30 subjects suffering from common cold/flu [98]. The results demonstrated that the hot drink had no effect on objective measurement of nasal airflow but it did cause a significant improvement in subjective measures of nasal airflow. The hot drink provided immediate and sustained relief from symptoms of runny nose, cough, sneezing, sore throat, chilliness and tiredness as shown in Figure 6, whereas the same drink at room temperature only provided relief from symptoms of runny nose, cough and sneezing. The effects of the drinks on symptom relief may be explained in terms of a placebo effect and physiological effects on salivation and airway

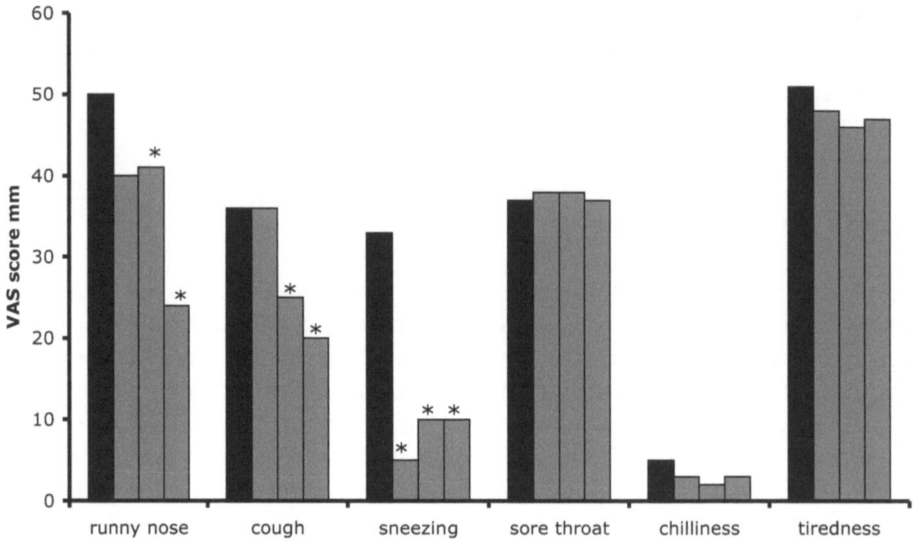

Figure 6. Effects of a hot fruit drink on common cold symptoms scored on visual analogue scales (0 = no symptom, 100 = worst symptom I can imagine). Each bar represents the median value of data from 15 subjects, for baseline (dark), and 10, 15 and 30 minutes after the drink. Statistically significant differences from baseline ($p < 0.05$) are indicated by an asterisk [98].

secretions [33], especially for relief of sore throat and cough symptoms where promotion of salivation will lubricate inflamed mucosal surfaces.

References

1 Sim MG, Hulse GK, Khong E (2004) Cough mixtures: Not always for cough. *Aust Fam Physician* 33: 327–331

2 Levine DA (2007) "Pharming": The abuse of prescription and over-the-counter drugs in teens. *Curr Opin Pediatr* 19: 270–274

3 Bryner JK, Wang UK, Hui JW, Bedodo M, MacDougall C, Anderson IB (2006) Dextromethorphan abuse in adolescence: An increasing trend: 1999–2004. *Arch Pediatr Adolesc Med* 160: 1217–1222

4 Eccles R (2007) Substitution of phenylephrine for pseudoephedrine as a nasal decongeststant. An illogical way to control methamphetamine abuse. *Br J Clin Pharmacol* 63: 10–14

5 Eccles R (2006) Efficacy and safety of over-the-counter analgesics in the treatment of common cold and flu. *J Clin Pharm Ther* 31: 309–319

6 Kantor TG (1993) Pharmacology and mechanisms of some pain relieving drugs. *Headache Q* 4: 57–62

7 Eccles R (2000) Pathophysiology of nasal symptoms. *Am J Rhinol* 14: 335–338

8 Ferreira SH (1986) Prostaglandins, pain, and inflammation. *Agents Actions Suppl* 19: 91–98

9 Eccles R, Loose I, Jawad M, Nyman L (2003) Effects of acetylsalicylic acid on

sore throat pain and other pain symptoms associated with acute upper respiratory tract infection. *Pain Med* 4: 118–124
10 Eccles R (2007) Mechanisms of symptoms of the common cold and influenza. *Br J Hosp Med* 68: 71–75
11 Eccles R (2005) Understanding the symptoms of the common cold and influenza. *Lancet Infect Dis* 5: 718–725
12 Schachtel BP, Fillingim JM, Beiter DJ, Lane AC, Schwartz LA (1984) Rating scales for analgesics in sore throat. *Clin Pharmacol Ther* 36: 151–156
13 Schachtel BP, Fillingim JM, Lane AC, Thoden WR, Baybutt RI (1991) Caffeine as an analgesic adjuvant. A double -blind study comparing aspirin with caffeine to aspirin and placebo in patients with sore throat. *Arch Intern Med* 151: 733–737
14 Bachert C, Chuchalin AG, Eisebitt R, Netayzhenko VZ, Voelker M (2005) Aspirin compared with acetaminophen in the treatment of fever and other symptoms of upper respiratory tract infection in adults: A multicenter, randomized, double-blind, double-dummy, placebo-controlled, parallel-group, single-dose, 6-hour dose-ranging study. *Clin Ther* 27: 993–1003
15 Schachtel BP, Fillingham JM, Thoden WR, Lane AC, Baybutt RI (1988) Sore throat pain in the evaluation of mild analgesics. *Clin Pharmacol Ther* 44: 704–711.
16 Eccles R, Jawad M, Jawad S, Ridge D, North M, Jones E, Burnett I (2006) Efficacy of a paracetamol-pseudoephedrine combination for treatment of nasal congestion and pain-related symptoms in upper respiratory tract infection. *Curr Med Res Opin* 22: 2411–2418
17 Winther B, Mygind N (2001) The therapeutic effectiveness of ibuprofen on the symptoms of naturally acquired common colds. *Am J Rhinol* 15: 239–242
18 Hay AD, Costelloe C, Redmond NM, Montgomery AA, Fletcher M, Hollinghurst S, Peters TJ (2008) Paracetamol plus ibuprofen for the treatment of fever in children (PITCH): Randomised controlled trial. *BMJ* 337: a1302
19 Prescott LF (2000) Paracetamol: Past, present, and future. *Am J Ther* 7: 143–147
20 Hawkey CJ (2001) COX–1 and COX–2 inhibitors. Best Pract Res 15: 801–820
21 Hudgings L, Kelsberg G, Safranek S, Neher JO (2004) Clinical inquiries. Do antipyretics prolong febrile illness? *J Fam Pract* 53: 57–58, 61
22 Jones AS, Lancer JM, Moir AA, Stevens JC (1985) Effect of aspirin on nasal resistance to airflow. *BMJ* 290: 1171–1173
23 Graham NMH, Burrell CJ, Douglas RM, Debelle P, Davies L (1990) Adverse effects of aspirin, acetaminophen and ibuprofen on immune function, viral shedding and clinical status in rhinovirus-infected volunteers. *J Infect Dis* 162: 1277–1282
24 Eccles R, Pedersen A, Regberg D, Tulento H, Borum P, Stjarne P (2007) Efficacy and safety of topical combinations of ipratropium and xylometazoline for the treatment of symptoms of runny nose and nasal congestion associated with acute upper respiratory tract infection. *Am J Rhinol* 21: 40–45
25 Davis SS, Eccles R (2004) Nasal congestion: Mechanisms, measurement and medications. Core information for the clinician. *Clin Otolaryngol* 29: 659–666
26 Eccles R (1999) Nasal airflow and decongestants. In: RM Naclerio, SR Durham,

N Mygind (eds): *Rhinitis Mechanisms and Management.* Marcel Dekker, New York, 291–312

27 Eccles R, Eriksson M, Garreffa S, Chen SC (2008) The nasal decongestant effect of xylometazoline in the common cold. *Am J Rhinol* 22: 491–496

28 Eccles R, Jawad MS, Jawad SS, Angello JT, Druce HM (2005) Efficacy and safety of single and multiple doses of pseudoephedrine in the treatment of nasal congestion associated with common cold. *Am J Rhinol* 19: 25–31

29 Kollar C, Schneider H, Waksman J, Krusinska E (2007) Meta-analysis of the efficacy of a single dose of phenylephrine 10 mg compared with placebo in adults with acute nasal congestion due to the common cold. *Clin Ther* 29: 1057–1070

30 Hatton RC, Winterstein AG, McKelvey RP, Shuster J, Hendeles L (2007) Efficacy and safety of oral phenylephrine: Systematic review and meta-analysis. *Ann Pharmacother* 41: 381–390

31 Scadding GK (1995) Rhinitis medicamentosa. *Clin Exp Allergy* 25: 391–394

32 Graf P (1997) Rhinitis medicamentosa: Aspects of pathophysiology and treatment. *Allergy* 52: 28–34

33 Eccles R (2006) Mechanisms of the placebo effect of sweet cough syrups. *Respir Physiol Neurobiol* 152: 340–348

34 Paul IM, Beiler J, McMonagle A, Shaffer ML, Duda L, Berlin CM Jr (2007) Effect of honey, dextromethorphan, and no treatment on nocturnal cough and sleep quality for coughing children and their parents. *Arch Pediatr Adolesc Med* 161: 1140–1146

35 Chung KF (2006) Measurement of cough. *Respir Physiol Neurobiol* 152: 329–339

36 Bolser DC, Davenport PW (2007) Codeine and cough: An ineffective gold standard. *Curr Opin Allergy Clin Immunol* 7: 32–36

37 Eccles R (2002) The powerful placebo in cough studies. *Pulm Pharmacol Ther* 15: 303–308

38 Schroeder K, Fahey T (2002) Systematic review of randomised controlled trials of over the counter cough medicines for acute cough in adults. *BMJ* 324: 329–331

39 Pavesi L, Subburaj S, Porter-Shaw K (2001) Application and validation of a computerized cough acquisition system for objective monitoring of acute cough – A meta-analysis. *Chest* 120: 1121–1128

40 Lee PCL, Jawad MSM, Eccles R (2000) Antitussive efficacy of dextromethorphan in cough associated with acute upper respiratory tract infection. *J Pharm Pharmacol* 52: 1137–1142

41 Hutchings HA, Eccles R, Smith AP, Jawad M (1993) Voluntary cough suppression as an indication of symptom severity in upper respiratory tract infections. *Eur Respir J* 6: 1449–1454

42 Lee P, Cotterill-Jones C, Eccles R (2002) Voluntary control of cough. *Pulm Pharmacol Ther* 15: 317–320

43 Manap RA, Wright CE, Gregory A, Rostami-Hodjegan A, Meller ST, Kelm GR, Lennard MS, Tucker GT, Morice AH (1999) The antitussive effect of dextromethorphan in relation to CYP2D6 activity. *Br J Clin Pharmacol* 48: 382–387

44 Hendeles L (1993) Efficacy and safety of antihistamines and expectorants in non prescription cough and cold preparations. *Pharmacotherapy* 13: 154–158
45 Eccles R (1996) Codeine, cough and upper respiratory infection. *Pulm Pharmacol Ther* 9: 293–297
46 Smith SM, Schroeder K, Fahey T (2008) Over-the-counter medications for acute cough in children and adults in ambulatory settings. *Cochrane Database of Systematic Reviews* (Online): CD001831
47 Bem JL, Peck R (1992) Dextromethorphan. An overview of safety issues. *Drug Safety* 7: 190–199
48 Schwartz RH (2005) Adolescent abuse of dextromethorphan. *Clin Pediatr* 44: 565–568
49 Fabricant ND (1950) Critical evaluation of antihistaminic drugs in the common cold. *Arch Otolaryngol Head Neck Surg* 52: 888–899
50 Gaffey MJ, Kaiser DL, Hayden FG (1988) Ineffectiveness of oral terfenadine in natural colds: Evidence against histamine as a mediator of common cold symptoms. *Pediatr Infect Dis J* 7: 223–228
51 Woodward JK (1990) Pharmacology of antihistamines. *J Allergy Clin Immunol* 86: 606–612.
52 Eccles R, Vancauwenberge P, Tetzloff W, Borum P (1995) A clinical study to evaluate the efficacy of the antihistamine doxylamine succinate in the relief of runny nose and sneezing associated with upper respiratory-tract infection. *J Pharm Pharmacol* 47: 990–993
53 Muether PS, Gwaltney JM Jr (2001) Variant effect of first- and second-generation antihistamines as clues to their mechanism of action on the sneeze reflex in the common cold. *Clin Infect Dis* 33: 1483–1488
54 West S, Brandon B, Stolley P, Rumrill R (1975) A review of antihistamines and the common cold. *Pediatrics* 56: 100–107
55 Luks D, Anderson MR (1996) Antihistamines and the Common Cold – A review and critique of the literature. *J Gen Intern Med* 11: 240–244
56 Sutter AI, Lemiengre M, Campbell H, Mackinnon HF (2003) Antihistamines for the common cold. *Cochrane Database of Systematic Reviews* (Online): CD001267
57 Howard JC, Kantner TR, Lillenfield LS, Princiotto JV, Krum RE, Crutcher JE, Belman MA, Danzig MR (1979) Effectiveness of antihistamines in the symptomatic management of the common cold. *J Am Med Assoc* 242: 2414–2417
58 Cowen DL (1974) Squill in the 17th and 18th centuries. *Bull N Y Acad Med* 50: 714–722
59 Munger RS (1949) Guaiacum, the holy wood from the New World. *J Hist Med Allied Sci* 4: 196–229
60 Gunn J (1927) The action of expectorants. *BMJ* 2: 972–975
61 Richardson PS, Phipps RJ (1978) The anatomy, physiology, pharmacology and pathology of tracheobronchial mucus secretion and the use of expectorant drugs in human disease. *Pharmacol Ther* 3: 441–479
62 Dicpinigaitis PV, Gayle YE (2003) Effect of guaifenesin on cough reflex sensitivity. *Chest* 124: 2178–2181
63 Schroeder K, Fahey T (2004) Over-the-counter medications for acute cough

in children and adults in ambulatory settings (Cochrane Review). *Cochrane Database of Systematic Reviews* 2004, Issue 4
64 Robinson RE, Cummings WB, Deffenbaugh ER (1977) Effectiveness of guaifenesin as an expectorant: A cooperative double-blind study. *Curr Ther Res* 22: 284–296
65 Kuhn JJ, Hendley O, Adams KF, Clark JW, Gwaltney JM (1982) Antitussive effect of guaifenesin in young adults with natural colds. *Chest* 82: 713–718
66 Lurie A, Mestiri M, Huchon G, Marsac J, Lockhart A, Strauch G (1992) Methods for clinical assessment of expectorants: A critical review. *Int J Clin Pharmacol Res* 12: 47–52
67 Rogers DF (2007) Mucoactive agents for airway mucus hypersecretory diseases. *Respir Care* 52: 1176–1193; discussion 1193–1177
68 Zheng JP, Kang J, Huang SG, Chen P, Yao WZ, Yang L, Bai CX, Wang CZ, Wang C, Chen BY et al. (2008) Effect of carbocisteine on acute exacerbation of chronic obstructive pulmonary disease (PEACE Study): A randomised placebo-controlled study. *Lancet* 371: 2013–2018
69 Nobata K, Fujimura M, Ishiura Y, Myou S, Nakao S (2006) Ambroxol for the prevention of acute upper respiratory disease. *Clin Exp Med* 6: 79–83
70 Poetsch C (1967) Brief history of topical rub therapy. In: FH Dost, B Leiber (eds): *Menthol and Menthol-containing External Remedies: Use, Mode of Effect and Tolerance in Children. International Symposium (Paris 1966)*. George Thieme Verlag, Stuttgart
71 Eccles R (2000) Role of cold receptors and menthol in thirst, the drive to breathe and arousal. *Appetite* 34: 29–35
72 Eccles R (1994) Menthol – A spectrum of efficacy. *Int Pharm J* 8: 17–21
73 Patel T, Ishiuji Y, Yosipovitch G (2007) Menthol: A refreshing look at this ancient compound. *J Am Acad Dermatol* 57: 873–878
74 Eccles R, Griffiths DH, Newton CG, Tolley NS (1988) The effects of D and L isomers of menthol upon nasal sensation of airflow. *J Laryngol Otol* 102: 506–508
75 Eccles R (1994) Menthol and related cooling compounds. *J Pharm Pharmacol* 46: 618–630
76 Eccles R, Griffiths DH, Newton CG, Tolley NS (1988) The effects of menthol isomers on nasal sensation of airflow. *Clin Otolaryngol Allied Sci* 13: 25–29
77 Burrow A, Eccles R, Jones AS (1983) The effects of camphor, eucalyptus and menthol vapour on nasal resistance to airflow and nasal sensation. *Acta Otolaryngol (Stockholm)* 96: 157–161
78 Eccles R, Jawad MS, Morris S (1990) The effects of oral administration of (–)-menthol on nasal resistance to airflow and nasal sensation of airflow in subjects suffering from nasal congestion associated with the common cold. *J Pharm Pharmacol* 42: 652–654
79 Ito S, Kume H, Shiraki A, Kondo M, Makino Y, Kamiya K, Hasegawa Y (2008) Inhibition by the cold receptor agonists menthol and icilin of airway smooth muscle contraction. *Pulm Pharmacol Ther* 21: 812–817
80 Kenia P, Houghton T, Beardsmore C (2008) Does inhaling menthol affect nasal patency or cough? *Pediatr Pulmonol* 43: 532–537

81 Fox N (1927) Effect of camphor, eucalyptol, and menthol on the vascular state of the mucous membrane. *Arch Otolaryngol* 6: 112–122
82 Eccles R, Jones AS (1983) The effect of menthol on nasal resistance to air flow. *J Laryngol Otol* 97: 705–709
83 Morice AH, Marshall AE, Higgins KS, Grattan TJ (1994) Effect of inhaled menthol on citric acid induced cough in normal subjects. *Thorax* 49: 1024–1026
84 Potter F (1890) The use of menthol in diseases of the upper air passages. *JAMA* 14: 147–149
85 Gobel H, Fresenius J, Heinze A, Dworschak M, Soyka D (1996) Effectiveness of peppermint oil and paracetamol in the treatment of tension headache. *Nervenarzt* 67: 672–681
86 Schattner P, Randerson D (1996) Tiger Balm as a treatment of tension headache. A clinical trial in general practice. *Aust Fam Physician* 25: 216, 218, 220 passim
87 Dost FH, Leiber B (eds) (1967) *Menthol and Menthol-containing External Remedies: Use, Mode of Effect and Tolerance in Children.* George Thieme Verlag, Stuttgart
88 Javorka K, Tomori Z, Zavarska L (1980) Protective and defensive airway reflexes in premature infants. *Physiol Bohemoslov* 29: 29–35
89 Berger H, Jarosch E, Madreiter H (1978) Effect of vaporub and petrolatum on frequency and amplitude of breathing in children with acute bronchitis. *J Int Med Res* 6: 483–486
90 Georgitis JW (1993) Nasopharyngitis, pharyngitis, and tonsillitis. *Immunol Allergy Clin North Am* 13: 109–118
91 Little P, Williamson I (1996) Sore throat management in general practice. *Fam Pract* 13: 317–321
92 Wonnemann M, Helm I, Stauss-Grabo M, Rottger-Luer P, Tran CT, Canenbley R, Donath F, Nowak H, Schug BS, Blume HH (2007) Lidocaine 8 mg sore throat lozenges in the treatment of acute pharyngitis. A new therapeutic option investigated in comparison to placebo treatment. *Arzneimittelforschung* 57: 689–697
93 Branthwaite A, Cooper P (1981) Analgesic effects of branding in treatment of headaches. *Br Med J* 282: 1576–1578
94 Eccles R (2007) The power of the placebo. *Curr Allergy Asthma Rep* 7: 100–104
95 Hunter P (2007) A question of faith. Exploiting the placebo effect depends on both the susceptibility of the patient to suggestion and the ability of the doctor to instil trust. *EMBO Rep* 8: 125–128
96 Mizoguchi H, Wilson A, Jerdack GR, Hull JD, Goodale M, Grender JM, Tyler BA (2007) Efficacy of a single evening dose of syrup containing paracetamol, dextromethorphan hydrobromide, doxylamine succinate and ephedrine sulfate in subjects with multiple common cold symptoms. *Int J Clin Pharmacol Ther* 45: 230–236
97 Tyrrell DA, Cohen S, Schlarb JE (1993) Signs and symptoms in common colds. *Epidemiol Infect* 111: 143–156
98 Sanu A, Eccles R (2008) The effects of a hot drink on nasal airflow and symptoms of common cold and flu. *Rhinology* 46: 271–275

Common Cold
ed. by R. Eccles and O. Weber

Vitamins and minerals

Harri Hemilä

Department of Public Health, University of Helsinki, Helsinki, FIN-00014 Finland

Abstract

Taking vitamins and minerals to fight the common cold is popular in western countries and thus it is important to find out whether or not they are effective. A large number of trials have found that regular vitamin C supplementation shortens the duration of colds, and is probably beneficial when administered therapeutically starting soon after the onset of symptoms. Zinc lozenges have reduced the duration of common cold symptoms when the total daily zinc doses were over 70 mg. Consequently, both vitamin C and zinc have the potential to become options for treating the common cold, but more research is needed to determine optimal doses and treatment strategies. The prophylactic effect of vitamins and minerals has also been examined in several trials. Vitamin C has no preventive effect in the general community, but may reduce the incidence of respiratory symptoms in restricted population groups such as people under acute physical stress and people with a particularly low dietary intake of vitamin C. There is no evidence that vitamin E supplementation prevents colds in middle-aged people. Nevertheless, the effects of vitamin E in elderly males have been found to be heterogeneous, and further studies are warranted in elderly people. β-Carotene has been promoted for improving the immune system, but there is no evidence that it is effective against colds. The use of multivitamin and multimineral combinations against respiratory tract infections in elderly people has been studied in a number of trials, but a nearly uniform lack of efficacy has been found. Vitamin D and folic acid have been constituents of multivitamin supplements, and the absence of benefits of these supplements implies that increasing the intake of vitamin D or folic acid in elderly people would not have substantial preventive effects against respiratory infections.

Introduction

The term 'the common cold' does not denote any precisely defined disease, yet the symptoms of this illness are personally familiar to practically everybody. Although the great majority of common cold episodes are caused by the group of respiratory viruses, the symptom-based definition of the 'common cold' also covers some diseases caused by non-respiratory viruses and even some bacterial infections and allergies. The large number of etiological agents, the benign character of the disease, and the high cost of the virological tests (e.g., $ 700 per patient in one study [1]) mean that a functional everyday definition of the 'common cold' cannot be based on laboratory tests, but must be based on symptoms. Furthermore, a chest x-ray has no relevance in excluding pneumonia when the patient is not seriously ill.

The liberal definition of 'the common cold' has implications for research in the general community. First, it is much cheaper to count the number of respiratory-symptom episodes and the days of illness compared with searching for the etiological agent. Second, the general community does not have access to rapid tests that reveal the cause of the disease. Therefore a treatment that is focused on a specific agent cannot be efficiently used in the community anyway. Third, the rationale for vitamin and mineral supplementation is based on the assumption of non-specific effects on the immune system and against diverse infections. Thus, the symptom-based definition is particularly appropriate when examining whether vitamins or minerals have non-specific effects relevant at the public health level.

The primary focus of this chapter is on the common cold type of symptoms; however, the border between upper respiratory infections (URTI) and lower respiratory infections (LRTI) is ambiguous. For example, computer tomography identifies many more cases of pneumonia compared with a chest x-ray [2], and thus a patient may be classed as having an URTI simply because he or she has not been studied with sophisticated methods. In some trials all respiratory infections or all infections were combined. Those trials are not excluded from this chapter, because the great majority of infections in the general community are URTI so that the wide definitions primarily measure the URTI and the common cold.

Taking vitamins to improve health and the immune system is popular in the western countries. About half of the elderly in the USA take some vitamin or mineral supplements [3]. Therefore it is important to find out whether they have effects on respiratory infections. If vitamins or minerals are shown to be effective, their use may be encouraged. If they are ineffective, their use should be discouraged. I focus on the findings of controlled trials and describe the biological rationales only to a minor extent. The p values presented are consistently two-tailed.

Vitamin C

In the early 1970s, Linus Pauling published a meta-analysis of four placebo-controlled trials on vitamin C and the common cold and concluded that there was strong evidence that vitamin C reduced 'integrated morbidity' caused by colds, meaning the combination of incidence and severity [4]. In a second meta-analysis Pauling restricted analysis to the two methodologically best trials, and calculated a combined $p = 0.001$ to reject the hypothesis that vitamin C equals placebo [5–7].

Pauling's proposal that vitamin C might affect infections was not novel. Vitamin C deficiency, scurvy, is associated with a high risk of pneumonia [8, 9], and after vitamin C was identified in the 1930s, there was much interest in its effects on infections [9–11]. In 1942, two trials with schoolchildren found that vitamin C reduced the incidence of colds and pneumonia [6, 12–14]. After the World War, the Sheffield trial examined the effects of vitamin C deprivation and found that the mean duration of colds was 6.4 days in vitamin C-deprived subjects and 3.3 days in non-deprived subjects [15]. Nevertheless, these early studies did not affect the mainstream medicine, which considered that vitamin C was effective only against scurvy.

Methodologically, Pauling's work was novel as his meta-analyses were among the very first in medicine. Furthermore, he was a public figure because of his Nobel prizes in Chemistry (1954) and in Peace (1963) [14, 16] and therefore his message, spread also in popular books [17, 18], received wide audiences. Although Pauling was unable to convince the medical community of the benefits of vitamin C, his activity led to a series of new trials.

Before Pauling's first book was published [17], only one trial had examined the effects of regular high-dose vitamin C, ≥1 g/day, on the common cold [7], whereas a dozen new trials were carried out within a few years after Pauling made the issue popular (Fig. 1). In the mid-1970s, the interest in this issue evaporated, not because of consistently negative results, but for reasons described at the end of this section.

In his analyses, Pauling used 'integrated morbidity' – the combination of incidence and severity. However, the effects of vitamin C on the incidence and severity of colds are different and it is more useful to analyze them separately.

Incidence of the common cold

In our Cochrane review on vitamin C and the common cold, we restricted analysis to placebo-controlled trials that used ≥0.2 g/day vitamin C [24]. We used the number of participants catching a cold as the incidence outcome, and analyzed separately trials in the general community and trials with participants under heavy acute physical stress. In 24 general community trials with 10 708 participants, vitamin C had no effect on common cold incidence: risk ratio (RR) = 0.98 (95% CI: 0.95–1.00). In another meta-analysis restricted to the six largest trials that had used ≥1 g/day vitamin C, the 5480 common cold episodes were divided equally between the vitamin C and placebo groups: RR = 0.99 (0.93–1.04) [22].

Thus, there is strong evidence that vitamin C does not reduce the average incidence of colds in the general western populations. However, the picture is more complex than indicated by the narrow confidence intervals of the above meta-analyses. It is possible that vitamin C affects susceptibility to the common cold under special conditions or in specific subpopulations.

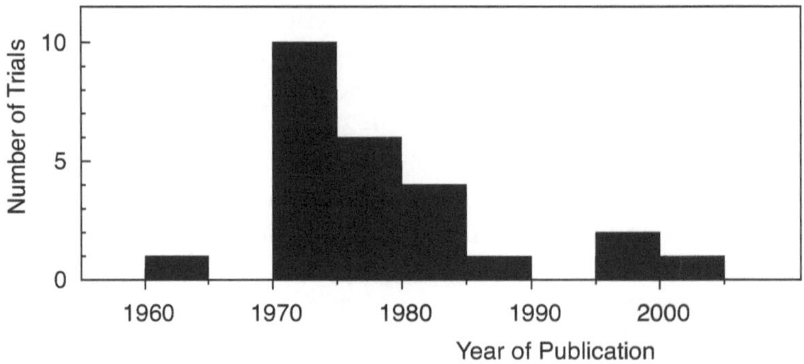

Figure 1. The number of placebo-controlled trials in which ≥1 g/day vitamin C was administered regularly to the participants over the study period.
Regular supplementation means initiating supplementation with healthy people and continuing over the occurring common cold episodes. The number of studies published over the 5-year period is combined. For the list of references up to 1992, see [19]; thereafter, Himmelstein et al. [20] reported two trials with 1 g/day vitamin C and van Straten and Joslin [21] reported one trial with 1 g/day vitamin C. In addition to the large number of trials in the 1970s, the importance of that decade is also reflected by the fact that five out of the six largest trials so far were carried out in the 1970s [22], and the only large trial published after the 1970s was not published in a medical journal but in a book [23].

In 1996, I pooled the results of three trials with participants under heavy acute physical stress and found that vitamin C halved the incidence of colds: RR = 0.50 (95% CI: 0.35–0.69) [25]. Thereafter, three new trials with similar participants reported consistent results [14, 24, 26]. Four of the six trials were with marathon runners [20, 27–29], one with Canadian troops on a short winter exercise [30], and one with Swiss schoolchildren in a skiing camp in the Swiss Alps [7]. Thus, the conditions were extraordinary. Furthermore, even though the authors of the six papers thought that they were measuring the common cold, the etiology of the recorded respiratory symptoms is not evident. Running for hours causes severe physical stress to the airways and can cause exercise-induced bronchoconstriction (EIB) [31]. Thus, cough and sore throat after a marathon run does not necessarily imply a viral cause. Possibly the respiratory symptoms in the six trials were caused by the combination of viral infections and EIB. In three laboratory studies vitamin C prevented EIB [32–34]. Thus, the benefit of vitamin C in the six trials with physically stressed participants may be caused by effects against both viral infections and EIB.

A further subpopulation in which vitamin C supplementation may affect common cold incidence is people who have low dietary vitamin C intake, 'marginal deficiency.' Among the western countries, dietary vitamin C intake has been particularly low in the UK [22]. In four trials with British males, vitamin C supplementation reduced common cold incidence: RR = 0.70 (95% CI: 0.60–0.81), whereas in four trials with females it had no effect: RR=0.95 (0.86–1.04) [12, 22, 35–38]. Substantial divergence between sexes was also seen in two trials that reported results separately for both sexes [38–40]. The most direct evidence supporting the 'treatment of marginal deficiency' explanation is the trial by Baird et al. as they administered only 0.08 g/day vitamin C, yet vitamin C had a significant effect [22, 38]. Modification of the vitamin C supplementation effect by dietary vitamin C was also suggested by the trial of Anderson et al. in Canada [41], as they found greater benefit of vitamin C for those who had low intake of juices (Tab. 1); however, their subgroup analysis was not focused on incidence but on the total number of sickness days during the trial.

Anderson et al. also found other differences between subgroups so that regular vitamin C supplementation appeared more beneficial for people who had contact with children, were often in crowds, or had often colds (Tab. 1).

Table 1: Heterogeneity in the vitamin C effect on the common cold: Anderson et al. trials of 1972 and 1975

Subgroup	Effect on the "total days indoors" per person	
	Regular supplement 1972 study[a]	Therapeutic supplement 1975 study[b]
Daily juice		
0–3 oz	–48%	–33%
≥4 oz	–22%	–22%
Contact with young children		
Yes	–46%	–40%
No	–17%	–13%
Frequently in crowds		
Yes	–34%	–25%
No	–17%	–29%
Usual colds:		
≥2	–43%	
0–1	–13%	

[a]Anderson et al. 1972 [41]: 1 g/day vitamin C was administered regularly and 3 g/day extra was administered during a cold episode for 3 days. For all participants, the effect of vitamin C on "total days indoors" per person was reduced by 30% ($p=0.001$) suggesting that there may be sufficient statistical power to explore subgroup differences, but the authors did not test the significance of the interactions. Based on Anderson's table IV.

[b]Anderson et al. 1975 [42] administered 1.5 g/day vitamin C on the first day of the cold and thereafter 1 g/day for a total of 5 days. For all participants, the effect of vitamin C on "total days indoors" per person was reduced by 25% ($p=0.046$). Based on Anderson's table III.

Duration and severity of the common cold

Regular vitamin C administration reduces the duration of colds that occur during the supplementation period. In 18 trials with 7242 adults, ≥0.2 g/day vitamin C reduced the duration of colds on average by 8% ($p = 0.002$) and in 12 trials with 2434 children by 13% ($p = 0.0008$) [24]. However, these p values underestimate the differences between the study groups, because the calculations are based on the duration of symptoms. For the patient and the society, the days off work or school, or the subjective severity may be much more relevant outcomes than the period the nose is running, and vitamin C might have a different effect on different outcomes.

With 615 Swedish schoolchildren, Ludvigsson et al. [43] found that 1 g/day vitamin C shortened the symptoms of URTI by just 6% ($p = 0.6$), but the 'absence from school' because of URTI by 14% ($p = 0.016$). With 818 Canadian adults, Anderson et al. [41] found that common cold symptoms were shortened by 5% ($p = 0.3$), but days 'confined to house' because of colds were shortened by 21% ($p = 0.015$).

There is evidence suggesting dose dependency in the vitamin C effect [44]. In five trials with adults administered 1 g/day vitamin C, the mean decrease in cold duration was only 7%, whereas in two trials with children administered 2 g/day the mean decrease was four times higher, 26% [14, 44–46]. Children administered 1 g/day and adults administered ≥2 g/day were in the middle [44]. This pattern of results supports dose dependency, given also the lower average weight of children. Nevertheless, the outcomes and study conditions vary between trials hampering the comparison of different trials. The most direct evidence indicating dose dependency was seen in the Karlowski trial with adults, in which 6 g/day caused twice the decrease in common cold duration compared with the dose of 3 g/day [44, 47, 48]. Thus, it seems possible that trials with low doses give an underestimate of the potential benefit of vitamin C.

Therapeutic effect of vitamin C

The great majority of vitamin C trials examined the effect of regular supplementation, meaning that the vitamin was administered each day over the trial. However, if the purpose is to alleviate common cold symptoms, it is much more reasonable to administer vitamin C therapeutically, starting immediately after the first symptoms. Unfortunately, few therapeutic trials have been carried out and their results are heterogeneous. Some of the negative findings may be explained by a low dose or a short treatment of 3 days or less [14, 19, 44, 49].

In a 5-day therapeutic trial, Anderson et al. [42] administered 1.5 g of vitamin C on the first day and 1 g/day on the following days. They found a 25% reduction in 'days confined indoors' and a 29% reduction in 'days felt feverish' ($p < 0.05$ for both). Anderson et al. also found variation between subgroups so that therapeutic vitamin C seemed more beneficial for people who had contact with children or low intake of juices (Tab. 1). Karlowski tested 5-day therapeutic supplementation of 3 g/day vitamin C and found that the duration of colds was decreased by 10% ($p = 0.10$) [47, 48].

In their 1974 trial, Anderson et al. [50] compared 4 g and 8 g when administered only on the first day of the common cold. In the 8-g group, 46% of colds lasted for just 1 day, whereas in the 4-g group, 39% of colds lasted for 1 day only. Thus, about 6% of participants found benefit from the 8 g on the first day of the cold in the form of cold lasting just 1 day instead of longer ($p = 0.046$, [14] p. 42). Thus, this comparison indicates dose dependency in a therapeutic setting.

In the regular supplementation trials, the effect of vitamin C has been greater on children than on adults, but no therapeutic trials with children have been carried out.

Vitamin C is safe in high doses. For example, in a pharmacokinetic study, 100 g vitamin C was administered intravenously over a few hours without reported adverse effects, and this led to plasma concentrations that were 100 times the level reached by oral administration of high doses [51]. High intravenous vitamin C doses, up to 65 g twice per week, have been administered for cancer patients for 10 months [52] also indicating the safety of vitamin C. Several reviewers have concluded that vitamin C is safe in long-term use in doses ranging to several grams per day [53, 54]. Thus, there is no justification to assume that therapeutic high-dose administration of vitamin C for colds for the duration of a week would cause harmful effects.

Finally, although a tablet is practical and the most common form of administering vitamin C, it is worth noting that administering vitamin C powder directly into the nose has also been suggested for treating the common cold [55].

Mechanism of the effect by vitamin C

Proponents of evidence-based medicine emphasize that the evaluation of interventions should be based on controlled trials and not on the biological plausibility. Therefore, this chapter is focused on trials. Nevertheless, dozens of studies have found that vitamin C may affect, for example, phagocytosis and chemotaxis of leukocytes, replication of viruses, and production of interferon [11, 56–60]. Vitamin C is an efficient antioxidant and the effects on the immune system can be explained by the protection against oxidative stress generated during infections [19, 61–65]. Dozens of animal studies found that vitamin C reduces the incidence and severity of bacterial and viral infections, indicating that the vitamin has physiological effects on infections, and not just on laboratory measures of the immune system [66]. Furthermore, heavy physical stress generates oxidative stress [67, 68] and the antioxidant role of vitamin C can thus explain also its effects on respiratory symptoms in physically stressed people.

Problems in influential papers on vitamin C and the common cold

Given the evidence by 1975 indicating that regular ≥2 g/day vitamin C reduces the duration and severity of colds, at the level of $p=0.000002$ [69], it is puzzling that major textbooks have rejected the possibility that vitamin C might be beneficial against colds [14]. The interest in vitamin C and colds disappeared in the middle of the 1970s (Fig. 1). This waning interest was caused by the publication of two negative reviews in wide-circulation journals [70, 71] and a particularly influential trial, carried out at the National Institutes of Health and published in *JAMA*, which concluded that the apparent benefit of vitamin C was explained by the placebo effect [47]. Furthermore, the Karlowski trial [47] and the Dykes and Meier review [71] were published in the same issue of *JAMA*, and Thomas Chalmers, a pioneer of controlled trials, was both the principal investigator of the Karlowski trial [47] and the author of the other review [70]. For such reasons this package of three papers from 1975 still has great impact on discussions on vitamin C and the common cold.

Chalmers' 1975 review [70] contains a large number of serious errors, such as the data being inconsistent with the original published data, errors in calculation, the selection of trials being inconsistent, and in some trials selection of a clinically less meaningful outcome [72, 73]. Dykes and Meier's 1975 review was also biased [69, 74] and Pauling wrote a commentary on their review and submitted his manuscript to *JAMA*. However, Pauling's manuscript was rejected even after he twice made revisions to meet the suggestions of the referees and the manuscript was finally published in a minor journal [75, 76]. The rejection of Pauling's commentary was quite a strange policy by *JAMA*, since the readers were thereby prevented from seeing the other side of an important scientific controversy.

In their 1975 trial, Karlowski et al. [47] carried out a subgroup analysis by participants guessing their treatment and concluded that "The effects demonstrated might be explained equally well by a break in the double blind". However, they excluded 42% of recorded common cold episodes from their subgroup analysis without any explanations and their 'placebo effect' explanation is not even consistent with the data they reported [48, 77–79].

Some other reviews on vitamin C and the common cold [80, 81] are also biased [69, 82, 83]. However, their impact in the medical literature is far lower than that of the three papers from 1975 described above. Nevertheless, the problems in these other reviews also show that there is widespread bias against the potential benefits of vitamin C against the common cold.

On his part, Pauling was too optimistic of the potential benefits of vitamin C [44, 49, 84]. The benefit in the two methodologically best trials that he analyzed [5] can be explained by the low dietary vitamin C intake during the war years in the USA [6] and heavy acute physical stress [7], and, while those findings probably reflect real biological effects, they cannot be extrapolated to the general western communities. Nevertheless, Pauling was correct in his conclusion that the effects of vitamin C are not limited to preventing scurvy.

Vitamin E

Vitamin E has diverse effects on the immune system, which have been assumed to be beneficial [60, 85, 86]. However, in two studies, vitamin E supplementation reduced the bactericidal activity of leukocytes, indicating that it can also cause harm on the immune system [87, 88]. In dozens of animal studies, vitamin E protected against viral and bacterial infections [66]; but increased the severity of infections in a few [89–91].

Two trials examined the effect of 200 mg/day vitamin E on acute respiratory infections in people older than 60 years [92, 93]. Graat et al. [92] carried out a 15-month trial with 652 noninstitutionalized Dutch people. Vitamin E had no effect on the number of respiratory infections, but, paradoxically, it made the episodes more severe. In the vitamin E group, there were more participants with fever ($p=0.009$) and restriction of activity ($p=0.02$), and the median number of symptoms was higher ($p=0.03$) and the total duration of illness was longer ($p=0.02$). Thus, vitamin E was harmful for this population and the trial should not be dismissed when considering the potential harms of vitamin E supplementation [94].

Meydani et al. [93] carried out a 1-year trial with 617 nursing home residents in the USA. They reported the intention-to-treat results, favored by biostatisticians, in their table 3 calculating 13 separate comparisons between the vitamin E and placebo groups. Thus, the table is an example of the multiple comparisons problem. If we calculate 20 statistical tests, when no real difference exists, random variation generates on average one false positive finding, $p<0.05$. The 13 calculations found only one significant difference and very marginally so: $p=0.048$ [93]. Therefore the variations in their table 3 are explained by chance, yet the authors made an unjustified extrapolation that vitamin E supplementation would lead to “more than 5 million fewer elderly nursing home residents contracting upper respiratory infections in a year” in the USA [95].

The large scale ATBC Study with 29 133 Finnish male smokers examined the effects of 6-year vitamin E supplementation [96]. Vitamin E, 50 mg/day, had no overall effect on common cold incidence: RR=0.99 [97]. However, there was heterogeneity so that age and smoking modified the effect of vitamin E (Fig. 2, Tab. 2).

In the young and less smoking males vitamin E increased the incidence of colds. In the old males, the effect diverged so that vitamin E increased

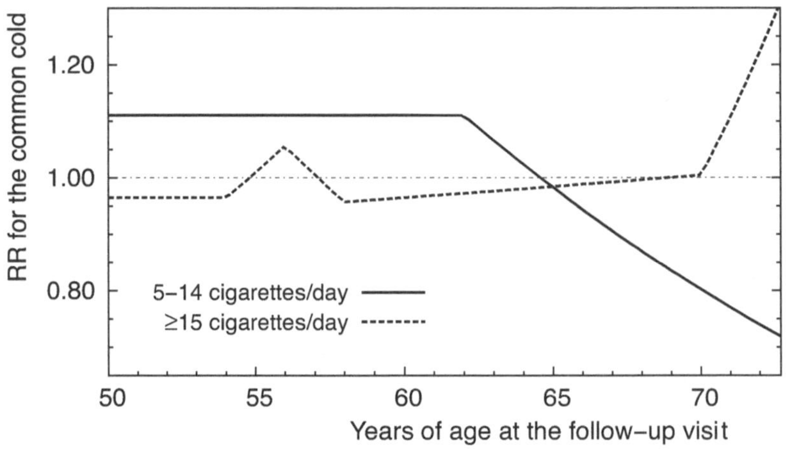

Figure 2. Risk ratio (RR) of the common cold incidence in the vitamin E arm compared with the placebo arm; the ATBC Study, 1985–1993.
Participants are divided to those who smoked 5–14 cigarettes per day at baseline and those who smoked 15 cigarettes or more. The placebo group level is marked by a thin line at the RR=1.00. Adding four knots to the spline curve of the heavy smokers improves the statistical model by $\chi^2(4\ \text{df}) = 25.4$, corresponding to $p = 0.00005$. Adding one knot to the less smoking participants improves the spline model by $\chi^2(1\ \text{df}) = 41.4$, corresponding to $p = 10^{-10}$. Vitamin E dose was 50 mg/day. These curves are based on 55 770 common cold episodes recorded for 14 573 participants. For the construction of these spline models, see [98], except that the first knot was added at 54 years in these curves.

the incidence of colds in heavy smokers but reduced it in those who smoked less. Smoking also modified the effect of vitamin E on pneumonia risk, reducing the risk in those who were least exposed to smoking [99].

Heavy exercise causes oxidative stress and, as an antioxidant, vitamin E might protect against it [67, 68]. In the ATBC Study, vitamin E had no effect on the incidence of colds in those who exercised during their leisure time [100] but halved the incidence of pneumonia [101].

Thus, in the ATBC Study vitamin E supplementation increased, decreased or had no effect on the incidence of the common cold, depending on age and the level of smoking. The numerical estimates of Table 2 are less essential than the evidence of heterogeneity. When the effect of vitamin E depends on the characteristics of people, the estimates of intervention effect obtained in a trial or a subgroup cannot be confidently generalized to other population groups.

The firm evidence of heterogeneity in the effect of vitamin E on respiratory infections refutes the notion that it is noneffective for all people. Nevertheless, the effect of vitamin E on the common cold is modest even in the old and less smoking males (Tab. 2). Considering the cost of taking supplements over a year, and the mild character of the disease occurring less frequently than once per year, it does not seem justified to propose that people take vitamin E to prevent respiratory infections. Furthermore,

Table 2. Vitamin E and common cold incidence: Modification of the effect by age and the level of smoking: the ATBC Study 1985–1993

Age group Cigarettes per day	Visits	Colds per visit vitamin E/placebo	RR (95% CI)	Test of interaction p value
50–54 years				
5–14	4972	0.340/0.289	1.18 (1.06–1.30)	0.001
≥15	28742	0.323/0.330	0.98 (0.94–1.02)	
63–66 years				
5–14	8819	0.255/0.259	0.98 (0.90–1.07)	0.7
≥15	28467	0.241/0.241	1.00 (0.95–1.05)	
≥69 years				
5–14	4755	0.193/0.260	0.74 (0.65–0.84)	0.00000001
≥15	10286	0.236/0.206	1.14 (1.05–1.24)	

Abbreviations: RR, risk ratio; CI, confidence interval.
In the ATBC Study, there were three follow-up visits per year so that the annual common cold incidence is three times the average per visit. For methods, see [98].

vitamin E has increased the incidence and severity of respiratory infections in some population groups (Tab. 2 and [92]). Nevertheless, further studies with old people are warranted.

β-Carotene

The carotenoids are a group of hundreds of pigments that are widespread in plants, of which only about a dozen occur in human food. β-Carotene is important as a precursor of vitamin A, but there is also interest in the effect of β-carotene per se on health. β-Carotene has effects on the immune system and it has been considered potentially beneficial for improving the immune system in aged people [60, 85, 102, 103]. However, few controlled trials have examined the effect of β-carotene on infections.

In the ATBC Study, 20 mg/day β-carotene had no overall effect on the incidence of the common cold: RR=1.00 [97]. Nevertheless, there was significant age- and smoking-dependent variation in the β-carotene effect. In the young and less smoking participants and in the old heavily smoking participants, β-carotene increased the incidence of colds, but had no effect in other subgroups (Fig. 3, Tab. 3). Smoking also modified the effect of β-carotene on pneumonia risk [99].

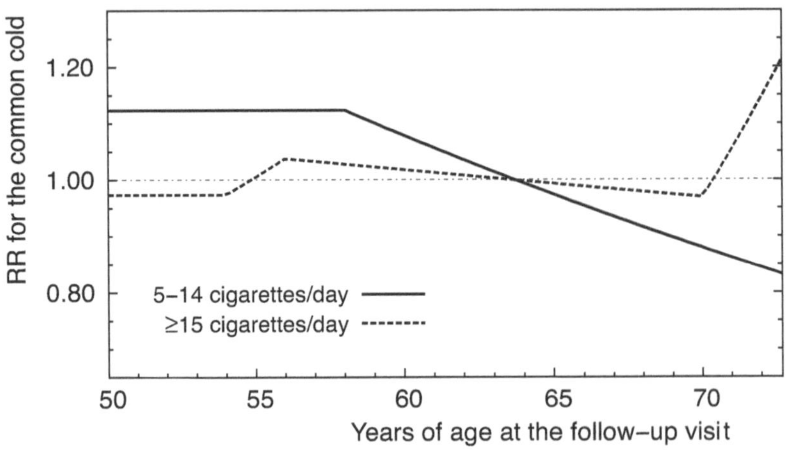

Figure 3. Risk ratio (RR) of the common cold incidence in the β-carotene arm compared with the placebo arm; the ATBC Study, 1985–1993.
Participants are divided to those who smoked 5–14 cigarettes per day at baseline and those who smoked 15 cigarettes or more. The placebo group level is marked by a thin line at the RR = 1.00. Adding three knots to the spline curve of the heavy smokers improves the statistical model by $\chi^2(3\ \text{df}) = 12.8$, corresponding to $p = 0.005$. Adding one knot to the less smoking participants improves the spline model by $\chi^2(1\ \text{df}) = 22.6$, corresponding to $p = 0.000002$. β-Carotene dose was 20 mg/day. These curves are based on 55905 common cold episodes recorded for 14569 participants. For the construction of these spline models, see [98], except that the first knot was added at 54 years in these curves.

In several multivitamin-multimineral trials with old people, β-carotene was one constituent of the supplements in the range of 1.2–6 mg/day (next section). These trials did not find benefit of supplementation, which refutes the notion that increasing β-carotene intake might effectively reduce respiratory infections in old people.

β-Carotene is an antioxidant and potential benefits might be emphasized in physically stressed people. In the ATBC Study, β-carotene increased the incidence of colds in males who exercised heavily during leisure time: RR = 1.25 (95% CI: 1.09–1.44) [100]. In physically active ATBC Study participants, β-carotene nonsignificantly increased pneumonia risk [101].

Two large trials found that β-carotene supplementation increased mortality of people who had been smoking cigarettes or exposed to asbestos [96, 104]. Given the harmful effects of β-carotene, as seen by the increase in respiratory infections and mortality, self-supplementation should be discouraged. There should be firm justification for further trials exposing people to it.

Table 3. β-Carotene and common cold incidence: Modification of the effect by age and the level of smoking: the ATBC Study 1985–1993

Age group Cigarettes per day	Visits in group	Colds per visit β-carotene/placebo	RR (95% CI)	Test of interaction *p* value
50–53 years				
5–14	3038	0.354/0.301	1.17 (1.04–1.33)	0.002
≥15	18528	0.324/0.344	0.94 (0.90–0.99)	
58–67 years				
5–14	23941	0.255/0.253	1.01 (0.96–1.06)	0.9
≥15	85820	0.260/0.259	1.00 (0.98–1.03)	
≥70 years				
5–14	3475	0.223/0.251	0.89 (0.77–1.02)	0.008
≥15	6993	0.217/0.193	1.12 (1.01–1.25)	

Abbreviations: RR, risk ratio; CI, confidence interval.
In the ATBC Study, there were three follow-up visits per year so that the annual common cold incidence is three times the average per visit. For methods, see [98].

Multivitamin and multimineral supplements

If a multivitamin-multimineral supplement has no effect on infections, it seems justified to argue that there is a lack of effect for each constituent of the supplement. Another way to interpret a negative finding is to assume that some constituent is beneficial, whereas some other constituent(s) annuls that benefit, but such reasoning requires explicit supportive evidence. In contrast, if a multivitamin-multimineral group does differ from the placebo group, we cannot draw specific conclusions because the effect can be caused by any single substance or the combination of several of them together. In this respect the implications are quite different when the result of a multivitamin and multimineral trial is positive or negative.

The multivitamin-multimineral trials have examined old people with the rationale that nutritional supplements, and antioxidants in particular, might prevent the decline in immune functions of the aged [85]. The frequently cited multivitamin-multimineral trial by Chandra [105] is excluded because a later paper based on the same data was shown to be fabricated and severe suspicions of the original 1992 paper were also expressed [106–108].

The definition of infection outcome has been variable in the trials of Table 4. Whereas Liu et al. [114] separated URTI and LRTI, the majority

Table 4. Multivitamins and multiminerals for respiratory infections

Study [ref.] Age, duration of study[a]	No. of episodes/ no. of participants[b]		RR (95% CI)[b]	Outcome/ subgroup
	Treatment	Placebo		
Chavance 1993 [109] ≥60 years, 4 months				
vitamin C 90 mg vitamin E 30 mg Zn 22 mg +18 others	61/103	42/101	1.42 (0.96–2.11)	Infections[c]
Girodon 1997 [110] ≥65 years, 2 years				
vitamin C 120 mg vitamin E 15 mg β-carotene 6 mg	47/41	47/40	0.98 (0.65–1.46)	Infections[d]
Zn 20 mg Se 0.1 mg	35/41	59/40	0.58 (0.30–0.88)	Infections[d]
Girodon 1999 [111] ≥65 years, 2 years				
vitamin C 120 mg vitamin E 15 mg β-carotene 6 mg	229/361	239/364	0.97 (0.80–1.16)	Respiratory infections[e]
Zn 20 mg Se 0.1 mg	223/363	245/362	0.92 (0.76–1.10)	Respiratory infections[e]
Graat 2002 [92] ≥60 years, 1.25 years				
vitamin C 60 mg vitamin E 10 mg β-carotene 1.2 mg Zn 10 mg Se 0.025 mg +21 others	514/335	510/317	0.95 (0.84–1.07)	Acute respiratory infections[f]
Barringer 2003 [112] ≥45 years, 1 year				
vitamin C 120 mg vitamin E 60 mg	23/39	24/40	0.98 (0.68–1.41)	Participants with infections[g] / Not diabetic
β-carotene 6 mg Zn 22 mg Se 0.1 mg +18 others	4/24	25/27	0.18 (0.07–0.44)	Participants with infections[g] / DM type II
Avenell 2005 [113] ≥65 years, 1 year				
vitamin C 60 mg vitamin E 10 mg Zn 15 mg +13 others	879/456	930/454	0.94 (0.86–1.03)	Contact with primary care for infections[h]
Liu 2007 [114] ≥65 years, 1.5 years				
vitamin C 80 mg vitamin E 44 mg β-carotene 16 mg	187/375	212/373	0.88 (0.72–1.07)	URTI
Zn 14 mg Se 0.02 mg +13 others	212/375	243/373	0.87 (0.72–1.04)	LRTI

of the trials combined all respiratory infections or all infections together. However, the majority of infections in the general community consist of URTI, and therefore the group of all infections largely reflects the incidence of the URTI.

There is a nearly uniform lack of benefit from multivitamin and multimineral supplementation against respiratory infections (Tab. 4). Girodon et al. [110] found reduction in infections by the combination of zinc and selenium. However, no effect of zinc and selenium was found in the larger trial by the same authors [111], or in trials which included zinc or/and selenium in their supplements [92, 109, 113, 114].

Another positive result was reported by Barringer et al. [112] with type 2 diabetics. The effect of vitamin E was divergent between participants who had diabetes and those who did not have (Tab. 4). Still, the results are odd. Among the non-supplemented participants, infections were more common in the diabetic participants: 92% (25/27), compared with the non-diabetics: 60% (24/40), which is reasonable because susceptibility to infections is higher in diabetics. However, the incidence of infections was substantially lower in supplemented diabetics: 17% (4/24), than in supplemented non-diabetics: 59% (23/39). This is illogical because it means that supplementation would make diabetics more resistant to infections than non-diabetics. Thus, Barringer's findings with the small number of diabetics ($n=51$) should be considered as a justification for further trials but not for supplementing diabetics with vitamins.

All studies in this table were placebo-controlled, double-blind randomized trials.

Abbreviations: RR, risk ratio; CI, confidence interval; URTI, upper respiratory tract infection; LRTI, lower respiratory tract infection.

[a]Only the most relevant vitamins and minerals for this review are listed.

[b]Many trials reported only the average number of episodes and the total number of episodes was calculated for this table. All RR estimates were calculated using the STATA poisson program, except the Barringer trial [112], which was calculated using the STATA glm program with the log-link function.

[c]Chavance et al. [109] collected data "dealing with diagnosis or symptoms of respiratory, nose, throat, ear, skin, mouth, urinary and gynecologic infections." However, Chavance et al. do not describe what proportion of infections was respiratory.

[d]Girodon et al. [110]: "Only respiratory and symptomatic urogenital infections were collected." However, Girodon et al. do not describe what proportion of infections were respiratory and urinary.

[e]Girodon et al. [111]: "Respiratory tract infections were based on clinical symptoms (cough, fever, and purulent sputum) and radiological test results." However, Girodon et al. do not describe what proportion of respiratory infections were URTI and LRTI.

[f]Graat et al. [92]: "Main outcomes were incidence and severity of acute respiratory tract infections assessed using a diary in which participants, who received thorough instructions, recorded all acute symptoms." However, Graat et al. do not describe what proportion of respiratory infections were URTI and LRTI.

[g]Barringer et al. [112]: "42% of participants had URTI, 19% had influenza-like syndromes, 7% had LRTI. 20% of persons experienced more than one type of infection over the study year."

[h]Avenell et al. [113] describe that 50% of the number of days of self-reported infections were URTI and 20% were LRTI.

Excluding the two positive findings leaves no evidence that multivitamins and multiminerals would influence the risk of respiratory infections in old people (Tab. 4). Furthermore, following the argument of the first paragraph of this section, these trials also indicate that none of the following substances has a substantial effect on respiratory infections in the old people: vitamin D, folic acid, vitamin A, thiamin, riboflavin, niacin, pyridoxine, panthotenic acid, cyanocobalamin, iodide, iron, calcium, magnesium, manganese and copper, because they were included in the supplement of four or more of the trials in Table 4.

The findings of the trials in Table 4 indicate that there is so far no justification to supplement old people with vitamins for the purpose of reducing respiratory infections. Nevertheless, the heterogeneity seen in the ATBC Study complicates this question (Figs 2 and 3). Vitamin E and β-carotene had no effect in participants who were somewhat over 60 years, whereas both substances had significant effects on those who were over 70 (Tabs 2 and 3). The multivitamin-multimineral trials of Table 4 are small, with a maximum of 1809 infection episodes recorded in Avenell's trial [113]. In contrast, Figure 2 is based on 55 770 common cold episodes providing statistical power to carry out subgroup analyses of age dependency. Thus, there is justification to study the effects of vitamin E in old people, even though the multivitamin supplements containing vitamin E did not find any benefit for old people (Tab. 4).

Zinc

Zinc deficiency affects the immune system and increases the risk of infections. In developing countries zinc supplementation has reduced the risk of childhood pneumonia [115–117] and in Turkey zinc reduced the risk of the common cold in children [118, 119]. Although these studies indicate that the level of zinc intake has clinically important effects on the immune system, the findings cannot be extrapolated to developed countries. For example, multivitamin-mineral supplements containing 10–22 mg/day zinc had no effect on the incidence of respiratory infections in old people (Tab. 4).

In developed countries the interest in zinc for treating the common cold is primarily based on the rationalization that zinc lozenges may cause local effects in the oral cavity. The research on zinc lozenges for treating the common cold started from a serendipitous observation that colds of a young child with leukemia disappeared when she started to dissolve therapeutic zinc tablets in her mouth instead of swallowing them [120].

Zinc has various effects on the immune system [121], inhibits the replication of rhinovirus and respiratory syncytial virus [122–124], and enhances the effect of interferon [125]. Nonimmune mechanisms have also been proposed to explain the effect of zinc lozenges on the common cold [126, 127]. For the interpretation of the controlled trials with zinc lozenges, the most essential hypothesis is that the level of free zinc ions is a crucial determinant of efficacy [128–133].

Effect of zinc lozenges on the duration of common cold symptoms

Table 5 lists the placebo-controlled trials in which the effect of zinc lozenges on natural common cold infections was studied. The trials are ordered by the calculated total daily dose of zinc from the lozenges. The reporting of outcomes is somewhat variable, but most trials reported the average duration of colds. The table shows that a large proportion of the variation in the results can be explained by the zinc dosage. None of the five trials that used less than 70 mg/day zinc found an effect, whereas seven of the eight trials that used over 70 mg/day zinc found significant benefit of the lozenges. Evidently, the 70 mg/day should not be considered as a biological limit, instead it is a pragmatic limit for analyzing the trials by zinc dosage.

In Table 5 the dose-response relation is examined using the total zinc dose as the explanatory variable. However, this is a simplification because several of the lozenges contained substances which bind zinc ions, such as citrate, reducing the free zinc ion levels. This argumentation has been elaborated in detail by several authors [128–133] and the arguments are not repeated here. Martin assumed that chewing a zinc-citric acid lozenge would decrease the pH of saliva to 2.3, and citrate does not form a complex with zinc ion at such a low pH [130]. However, Zarembo et al. [144] studied the saliva of 18 human subjects, and chewing zinc-citrate lozenges resulted in saliva pH ranging between 3.2 and 5.0. Martin [130] calculated that, in the presence of 2% citric acid in a solution at pH 5.1, only 1.5% of zinc is in the form of unbound zinc ions, which underscores the problem of complex formation.

The solution chemistry of zinc complexes gives further explanations for the variations between the zinc trials. Godfrey et al. [135] administered a particularly high dose of zinc, but glycinate in the lozenge bound 80–90% of the zinc ion to complexes [131–133], which can explain the rather small benefit compared with the other trials using high zinc doses (Tab. 5). The lozenge of Douglas et al. [141] contained tartaric acid, which effectively binds zinc [131, 133].

Two controlled trials examined the effect of 23 mg zinc lozenges on experimental rhinovirus colds. Whereas Al-Nakib et al. [145] found significant benefit of the zinc lozenges, Farr et al. [146] found no benefit. The lozenge of Farr contained 2% citric acid which bound essentially all zinc ions, whereas the lozenge of Al-Nakib did not form complexes of zinc ions, and this difference in the composition of lozenges can explain the divergence in the results [130–133]. Although the solution chemistry calculations of free zinc ion concentrations give further explanations to the variations between trials, the power of dose-response analysis can be seen even by counting the total dosage of zinc (Tab. 5).

Table 5. Zinc lozenges for treating the common cold

Study [ref.]	No. of participants	Zn dose (mg/day)[a]	Days of symptoms[b] Zn/Placebo	Effect of Zn	p[b]
Eby 1984 [120]	65	207	3.9/10.8	–64%[c]	<0.001
Smith 1989 [134]	110	207	5.5/7.0	–22%[d]	0.02
Godfrey 1992 [135]	73	192	4.9/6.1	–21%	0.048
Prasad 2008 [136]	50	92	4.0/7.1	–44%	<0.001
Petrus 1998 [137]	101	89	3.8/5.1	–25%	0.008
Turner 2000 [138]	139	80	6.0/5.5		
Mossad 1996 [139]	99	80	4.4/7.6	–42%	<0.001
Prasad 2000 [140]	48	79	4.5/8.1	–44%	<0.001
Turner 2000 [138]	139	69	5.5/5.5		
Douglas 1987 [141]	58[e]	64	12.1/7.7		0.08
Macknin 1996 [142]	249	55	9.0/9.0		
Weissman 1990 [143]	130	45	7/6		
Turner 2000 [138]	143	30	6.0/5.5		

All studies in this table were placebo-controlled double-blind trials. Weissman et al. [143] did not report the method of allocation, but all the other trials were randomized. All studies examined young and middle-aged adults, except the Macknin et al. [142] trial which examined school children.

[a]The daily dose of zinc is calculated as the product of elemental zinc dose in the lozenge and the planned or counted number of lozenges per day. The lowest zinc doses in the lozenges were in the Weissman et al. [143] trial and in one arm of the Turner et al. trial [138]: 4.5 and 5 mg/lozenge, respectively, and the highest were in Eby et al. [120] and Godfrey et al. [135] trials: 23 and 23.7 mg/lozenge, respectively. In some trials, the used lozenges were counted [135–137, 139–141] and the mean usage was used to calculate the total zinc per day. In other trials, the planned usage was the basis for the calculation so that dosage "every 2 h awake" was interpreted as nine lozenges per day.

[b]The outcome is the average days of symptoms (mean or median) except when otherwise stated. The p value was recalculated when appropriate data was reported in the paper.

[c]Eby et al. [120] did not report the mean or median duration, but estimated the time half of the participants were cured from an exponential fit of the results.

[d]Smith et al. [134] reported that "subjects taking zinc gluconate had lower severity scores than those in the corresponding placebo group on days 4–7 of treatment. This difference is statistically significant ($p = 0.02$)." From Smith's figure 2, I measured the days needed for 80% reduction in severity score, which occurred in the 4–7 days time range, and thereby the effect was transformed to time scale for this table. Smith et al. did not observe difference between the study groups in the median duration of colds.

[e]The number of treatment courses was 63; some of the 55 participants had more than one cold episode.

Concluding from Table 5, the benefit of zinc lozenges can be obtained with substantially lower doses than Eby used in the first trial with zinc gluconate lozenges [120]. Four trials used zinc doses in the range of 80–90 mg/day and observed significant benefit from the lozenges. Three of these trials used lozenges containing zinc acetate [136, 137, 140], which does not involve the problem of forming zinc complexes [133].

New trials should confirm the benefit of zinc lozenges in the dose range of 80–90 mg/day and examine whether benefit could be obtained with even lower doses with lozenges that do not contain substances that bind zinc ions. With the available evidence, a patient suffering from the common cold can test the effects of zinc lozenges as a personal experimentation.

Safety of zinc

In the controlled trials zinc lozenges have caused acute adverse effects, such as bad taste. However, none of the common cold trials reported long-term harm caused by the zinc lozenges. High-dose zinc supplementation, 150 mg/day, has been administered for therapeutic purposes over months and years [147–149]. Copper deficiency has been reported as a consequence in some patients because of several years of high-dose zinc supplementation [148, 149]. However, a 6-week study did not find any detrimental effects of 150 mg/day zinc on plasma copper levels [150]. Consequently, there does not seem to be any reason to assume that treating the common cold for a week with doses that have been used in the zinc lozenge trials would cause unanticipated long-term harm. As regards the bad taste and other acute effects, the patient can simply stop taking the lozenge if such discomforts are annoying.

Nasal sprays or gels of zinc have also been studied for treating the common cold and some studies reported benefit. However, several cases of long-lasting or permanent anosmia have been reported as a consequence of intranasal zinc administration [151, 152]. Given the benign character of the common cold, anosmia is an unacceptable adverse effect. Nasal application of zinc should be discouraged, unless application methods are developed that do not involve the risk of anosmia.

Reviews on zinc and the common cold

Given the number of placebo-controlled trials reporting highly significant benefit of zinc lozenges for treating the common cold (Tab. 5), it is puzzling that some reviews have concluded that there is no evidence that zinc would be beneficial against colds.

Jackson et al. [153, 154] searched the literature on zinc and the common cold and found statistically significant heterogeneity between the trials. They calculated a pooled estimate of effect, although firm evidence of heterogeneity introduces serious doubt about the relevance of any one overall estimate. Instead, the main focus should be on trying to understand the sources of heterogeneity [155]. Although Jackson noted that some of the negative results might have been caused by low zinc availability, they did not carry out subgroup analysis by zinc doses. Jackson et al. [154] concluded that their "meta-analysis suggests that the evidence of zinc effectiveness is still lacking", which is based on their inappropriate pooling of the low and high dose trials together.

In their systematic review, Caruso et al. [156] identified 14 zinc trials. They used the quality scoring approach so that for the identified trials they gave one point for each of 11 quality items if it was satisfied. Four of the identified trials reached the maximum of 11 points, two reached 10 points, and eight trials reached 8 points or less. In two tables and one figure, Caruso et al. described the distribution of quality scores and the individual quality features of the trials. They proposed that the positive findings with zinc could be explained by methodological faults.

The approach to evaluate trial quality by a set of explicit criteria was initiated by Chalmers et al. [157] in the early 1980s and thereafter dozens of quality scales have been developed. However, the approach was not successful and it is discouraged, for example in the Cochrane Handbook, which states that "the use of scales for assessing quality or risk of bias is explicitly discouraged in Cochrane reviews. While the approach offers appealing simplicity, it is not supported by empirical evidence" [158].

One major problem of quality scoring is the focus on reporting in contrast to the scientific quality of the trial. For example, Caruso et al. give one point if there was "measurement of dropout rate" in the trial. This means that a trial can report high dropout rate, which means low scientific quality, yet the trial gets one point from Caruso et al., because the high dropout rate was reported explicitly. Caruso et al. give one point for "sample size calculation", which is important when a trial is planned, because it can show that the planned trial is too small, whereas it is irrelevant after the trial is published, because then the confidence interval reveals the accuracy of the result. Most of Caruso et al.'s remaining nine quality items have similar problems.

Although it is important to consider the methods of a trial, there are no simple criteria that describe whether a trial is reliable or not. In a meta-analysis of 276 randomized controlled trials, Balk et al. [159] concluded that "double blinding and allocation concealment, two quality measures that are frequently used in meta-analyses, were not associated with treatment effect" meaning that valid estimates of treatment effect can be reached without them. Furthermore, Glasziou et al. [160] pointed out that firm conclusions of treatment benefit can be drawn even without any control groups.

Finally, Caruso et al. did not discuss the possibility that the dose of zinc might have an effect on trial results, nor did they refer to any of the numerous papers that discussed the possibility that the level of free zinc ion might be important [128–133, 161].

Thus, the conclusions from Table 5 diverge from the conclusions of two groups of earlier reviewers, but there are reasonable explanations for the divergence in the conclusions.

Bias against vitamins and minerals

In the early 1970s, there was academic interest in the effect of vitamin C on the common cold, but then the interest vanished (Fig. 1). The evaporation of interest can be traced to three influential papers published in 1975 [47, 70, 71]. Although the three papers are severely biased, they have been used singly or as a doublet, for example, as references in nutritional recommendations, in textbooks of medicine, infectious diseases, and nutrition when authors argued that vitamin C has been shown to be useless for colds [48, 69, 72–79]. For example, the American Medical Association based its official statement that "One of the most widely misused vitamins is ascorbic acid. There is no reliable evidence that large doses of ascorbic acid prevent colds or shorten their duration" wholly on Chalmers' 1975 review ([162] p. 1934).

Bias against zinc lozenges is seen, for example, in Caruso et al.'s recent review [156], which focused on methodological features mostly irrelevant to trial validity, without even presenting the study results. Furthermore, they stated that a "common deficiency [in the zinc trials] was proof of blinding which was lacking in seven studies. The placebo effect in the treatment of colds was first shown >70 years ago and has since been demonstrated in subsequent studies". As a justification for this statement, Caruso et al. referred to the doublet of the Karlowski trial [47] and the Chalmers review [70], although they knew that the two papers were erroneous, because I pointed that out in a criticism of their earlier biased review on *Echinacea* and the common cold [163, 164].

Prejudice against nonconventional treatments is not limited to the common cold. Bias against vitamin C was documented by Richards who compared the attitudes and arguments of physicians to three putative cancer medicines: 5-fluorouracil, interferon, and vitamin C [165–169].

Goodwin and Tangum [170] provided several examples to support the conclusion that there has been systematic bias against the concept that vitamins might be beneficial in levels higher than the minimum required to avoid classic deficiency diseases: "Throughout much of the 20th century, American academic medicine was resistant to the concept that micronutrient supplementation might prove beneficial. This resistance is evident in several ways: (1) by uncritical acceptance of bad news about micronutrient supplements; reports of toxic effects were rarely questioned and widely quoted; (2) by the scornful, dismissive tone of the discussions about micronutrient supplementation in textbooks of medicine, a tone avoided in most medical controversies; and (3) by the sceptical reaction greeting any claim of efficacy of a micronutrient, relative to other therapies; indeed, most claims were simply ignored."

Although the proponents of evidence-based medicine emphasize the primary importance of controlled trials as the source of reliable knowledge of treatment effects, the possibility of biologically rationalizing the method usually has a great importance [171]. Goodwin and Goodwin [172, 173] reviewed several cases in which an effective method of treatment was erroneously rejected due to a lack of understanding of the physiological mechanism of the effect. They designated this problem 'the tomato effect', since the tomato was considered poisonous in the USA in the 1700s because several other plants in the same family were poisonous: "The tomato effect in medicine occurs when an efficacious treatment for a certain disease is ignored or rejected because it does not 'make sense' in the light of accepted theories of disease mechanism and drug action."

Finally, in a paper discussing great scientific discoveries, Barber [174] noted "Medical experts have a long history of resisting scientific innovations from what they define as 'the outside'." Thus, it is possible that this mechanism is a further reason for prejudices against vitamin C and zinc in the medical community, as the most active proponents, Pauling and Eby, are not physicians.

Goodwin and Tangum [170] conclude their paper on micronutrient supplements in academic medicine as follows: "There are only three important questions when evaluating a potential treatment. Does it work? What are the adverse effects? How much does it cost? Ideally, issues such as the theory underlying the treatment or the guild to which the proponents of the treatment belong should be irrelevant to the fundamental questions of efficacy, toxicity, and cost. The history of the response of academic medicine to micronutrient supplementation suggests that we have not attained that ideal."

Conclusions

Regular vitamin C supplementation reduces common cold symptoms and probably vitamin C is beneficial when administered therapeutically, starting immediately after the onset of symptoms. However, few therapeutic vitamin C trials have been published, and none with children, although regular vitamin C has greater effect on children than on adults. In the controlled trials, the largest doses were 6 g/day for adults and 2 g/day for children and such doses may be safely tested as a treatment option by common cold patients.

The results of zinc lozenge trials have diverged, but the divergence is explained largely by the variation in dosage, so that doses over 70 mg/day have quite consistently reduced the duration of colds. Zinc lozenges have caused high frequency of adverse effects, such as bad taste, but there is no evidence that zinc lozenges would cause actual long-term harm. A large proportion of trial participants remained without adverse effects and consequently zinc lozenges might be useable by them.

Thus, both vitamin C and zinc supplementation have a potential for becoming options for treating the common cold. Both of them are safe in the doses that have been tested, there is strong evidence that they differ from placebo, they are inexpensive and, unlike the antibiotics [175], they do not cause harm to microbial ecology.

In the case of vitamin C and zinc, the most reasonable approach would seem to be to test them at the individual level so that the patient decides whether the benefits are worth the cost, the side effects and the involved effort. This kind of approach is not different from ordinary treatments for acute medical problems in the community. Although a controlled trial can show that an analgesic differs on average from a placebo, it is the patient who decides whether a particular drug is effective for him or her. Thus, experimentation at the individual level may be encouraged, yet simultaneously more research is needed on vitamin C tablets and zinc lozenges to determine optimal doses and treatment strategies.

Vitamin C has no prophylactic effect in the general community, but it may reduce the incidence of respiratory symptoms in restricted population groups such as people under heavy acute physical stress and people who have particularly low dietary vitamin C intake. The effect of vitamin E on the common cold incidence is heterogeneous which means that it is not ineffective over all the population. Nevertheless, further studies are needed to specify the population groups that might possibly benefit from vitamin E supplementation.

Vitamin D and folic acid have been constituents in five multivitamin supplements that have been tested for old people. Those supplements did not prevent respiratory infections implying that vitamin D and folic acid do not have substantial preventive effects against respiratory infections. There is no evidence suggesting that β-carotene would be beneficial against the common cold, whereas it increased mortality in two large-scale trials, and therefore self-supplementation should be discouraged.

References

Links to the full texts or abstracts of the following reference list that are available *via* the internet can be found at: http://www.ltdk.helsinki.fi/users/hemila/birkhauser. Some of the publications are located at the publisher's pages and require permissions to be reached, but several are freely available. The file will be updated so that new controlled trials on the substances discussed in this chapter will be appended at the end of the file.

1 Mäkelä MJ, Puhakka T, Ruuskanen O, Leinonen M, Saikku P, Kimpimäki M, Blomqvist S, Hyypiä T, Arstila P (1998) Viruses and bacteria in the etiology of the common cold. *J Clin Microbiol* 36: 539–542

2 Syrjälä H, Broas M, Suramo I, Ojala A, Lähde S (1998) High resolution computed tomography for the diagnosis of community-acquired pneumonia. *Clin Infect Dis* 27: 358–363

3 Millen AE, Dodd KW, Subar AF (2004) Use of vitamin, mineral, nonvitamin, and nonmineral supplements in the United States: The 1987, 1992, and 2000 National Health Interview Survey results. *J Am Diet Assoc* 104: 942–950

4 Pauling L (1971) The significance of the evidence about ascorbic acid and the common cold. *Proc Natl Acad Sci USA* 68: 2678–2681
5 Pauling L (1971) Ascorbic acid and the common cold. *Am J Clin Nutr* 24: 1294–1299
6 Cowan DW, Diehl HS, Baker AB (1942) Vitamins for the prevention of colds. *JAMA* 120: 1268–1271
7 Ritzel G (1961) Kritische Beurteilung des Vitamins C als Prophylacticum und Therapeuticum der Erkältungskrankheiten [Critical analysis of the role of vitamin C in the treatment of the common cold]. *Helv Med Acta* 28: 63–68. Translation at: http://www.ltdk.helsinki.fi/users/hemila/T3.pdf (accessed 29 December 2008)
8 Hess AF (1920) *Scurvy: Past and Present.* Lippincott, Philadelphia. A digitalized version is available at the Cornell University Library: http://chla.library.cornell.edu/ (accessed 29 December 2008)
9 Robertson EC (1934) The vitamins and resistance to infection: Vitamin C. *Medicine* 13: 190–206
10 Perla D, Marmorston J (1937) Role of vitamin C in resistance. Parts I and II. *Arch Pathol* 23: 543–575, 683–712
11 Bourne GH (1949) Vitamin C and immunity. *Br J Nutr* 2: 341–347
12 Glazebrook AJ, Thomson S (1942) The administration of vitamin C in a large institution and its effect on general health and resistance to infection. *J Hygiene* 42: 1–19
13 Hemilä H, Louhiala P (2007) Vitamin C may affect lung infections. *J R Soc Med* 100: 495–498
14 Hemilä H (2006) *Do vitamins C and E affect respiratory infections?* [PhD Thesis]. University of Helsinki, Helsinki, Finland, pp. 11–16, 35–51. Available at: http://ethesis.helsinki.fi/julkaisut/laa/kansa/vk/hemila/ (accessed 29 December 2008)
15 Bartley W, Krebs HA, O'Brien JRP (1953) *Vitamin C Requirement of Human Adults. A Report by the Vitamin C Subcommittee of the Accessory Food Factors Committee.* Spec Rep Ser Med Res Counc (GB) No. 280. HMSO, London, p. 43
16 Mason SF (1997) The science and humanism of Linus Pauling (1901–1994). *Chem Soc Rev* 26: 29–39
17 Pauling L (1970) *Vitamin C and the Common Cold.* Freeman, San Francisco
18 Pauling L (1976) *Vitamin C, the Common Cold, and the Flu.* Freeman, San Francisco
19 Hemilä H (1992) Vitamin C and the common cold. *Br J Nutr* 67: 3–16
20 Himmelstein SA, Robergs RA, Koehler KM, Lewis SL, Qualls CR (1998) Vitamin C supplementation and upper respiratory tract infections in marathon runners. *J Exercise Physiology online* 1(2; July). Available at: http://faculty.css.edu/tboone2/asep/jan9.htm (accessed 29 December 2008)
21 van Straten M, Josling P (2002) Preventing the common cold with a vitamin C supplement: A double-blind, placebo-controlled survey. *Adv Ther* 19: 151–159
22 Hemilä H (1997) Vitamin C intake and susceptibility to the common cold. *Br J Nutr* 77: 59–72; discussion: 1997;78: 857–866
23 Briggs M (1984) Vitamin C and infectious disease: A review of the literature

and the results of a randomized, double-blind, prospective study over 8 years. In: MH Briggs (ed) *Recent Vitamin Research.* CRC Press, Boca Raton, pp 39–82
24 Hemilä H, Chalker EB, Treacy B, Douglas RM (2007) Vitamin C for preventing and treating the common cold. *Cochrane Database Syst Rev* CD000980
25 Hemilä H (1996) Vitamin C and common cold incidence: A review of studies with subjects under heavy physical stress. *Int J Sports Med* 17: 379–383
26 Hemilä H (2004) Vitamin C supplementation and respiratory infections: A systematic review. *Mil Med* 169: 920–925
27 Peters EM, Goetzsche JM, Grobbelaar B, Noakes TD (1993) Vitamin C supplementation reduces the incidence of postrace symptoms of upper-respiratory-tract infection in ultramarathon runners. *Am J Clin Nutr* 57: 170–174
28 Peters EM, Goetzsche JM, Joseph LE, Noakes TD (1996) Vitamin C as effective as combinations of anti-oxidant nutrients in reducing symptoms of upper respiratory tract infection in ultramarathon runners. *S Afr J Sports Med* 11 (March): 23–27
29 Moolla ME (1996) *The effect of supplemental anti-oxidants on the incidence and severity of upper respiratory tract infections in ultra-marathon runners* [MSc Thesis]. University of Cape Town, South Africa
30 Sabiston BH, Radomski MW (1974) *Health Problems and Vitamin C in Canadian Northern Military Operations.* DCIEM Report no. 74-R–1012. Defence and Civil Institute of Environmental Medicine; Downsview, Ontario, Canada. 10 pp. Available at: http://www.ltdk.helsinki.fi/users/hemila/CC/Sabiston_1974_ch.pdf (accessed 29 December 2008)
31 Anderson SD, Kippelen P (2008) Airway injury as a mechanism for exercise-induced bronchoconstriction in elite athletes. *J Allergy Clin Immunol* 122: 225–235; discussion: 2009; 123: 274–275
32 Schachter EN, Schlesinger A (1982) The attenuation of exercise-induced bronchospasm by ascorbic acid. *Ann Allergy* 49: 146–151
33 Cohen HA, Neuman I, Nahum H (1997) Blocking effect of vitamin C in exercise-induced asthma. *Arch Pediatr Adolesc Med* 151: 367–370
34 Tecklenburg SL, Mickleborough TD, Fly AD, Bai Y, Stager JM (2007) Ascorbic acid supplementation attenuates exercise-induced bronchoconstriction in patients with asthma. *Respir Med* 101: 1770–1778
35 Charleston SS, Clegg KM (1972) Ascorbic acid and the common cold. *Lancet* 299: 1401–1402
36 Clegg KM, Macdonald JM (1975) L-ascorbic acid and D-isoascorbic acid in a common cold survey. *Am J Clin Nutr* 28: 973–976
37 Elwood PC, Lee HP, Leger AS, Baird IM, Howard AN (1976) A randomized controlled trial of vitamin C in the prevention and amelioration of the common cold. *Br J Prev Soc Med* 30: 193–196
38 Baird IM, Hughes RE, Wilson HK, Davies JE, Howard AN (1979) The effects of ascorbic acid and flavonoids on the occurrence of symptoms normally associated with the common cold. *Am J Clin Nutr* 32: 1686–1690
39 Tyrrell DAJ, Craig JW, Meade TW, White T (1977) A trial of ascorbic acid in the treatment of the common cold. *Br J Prev Soc Med* 31: 189–191

40 Hemilä H (2008) Vitamin C and sex differences in respiratory tract infections. *Respir Med* 102: 625–626
41 Anderson TW, Reid DBW, Beaton GH (1972) Vitamin C and the common cold: A double-blind trial. *Can Med Assoc J* 107: 503–508; corrections: 1973;108: 133 and 1973;108: 492
42 Anderson TW, Beaton GH, Corey PN, Spero L (1975) Winter illness and vitamin C: The effect of relatively low doses. *Can Med Assoc J* 112: 823–826
43 Ludvigsson J, Hansson LO, Tibbling G (1977) Vitamin C as a preventive medicine against common colds in children. *Scand J Infect Dis* 9: 91–98
44 Hemilä H (1999) Vitamin C supplementation and common cold symptoms: Factors affecting the magnitude of the benefit. *Med Hypotheses* 52: 171–178
45 Coulehan JL, Reisinger KS, Rogers KD, Bradley DW (1974) Vitamin C prophylaxis in a boarding school. *N Engl J Med* 290: 6–10
46 Bancalari A, Seguel C, Neira F, Ruiz I, Calvo C (1984) Valor profilactico de la vitamina C en infecciones respiratorias agudas del escolar [Prophylactic value of vitamin C in acute respiratory infections of schoolchildren]. *Rev Med Chil* 112: 871–876. Translation at: http://www.ltdk.helsinki.fi/users/hemila/T6.pdf (accessed 29 December 2008)
47 Karlowski TR, Chalmers TC, Frenkel LD, Kapikian AZ, Lewis TL, Lynch JM (1975) Ascorbic acid for the common cold. *JAMA* 231: 1038–1042
48 Hemilä H (1996) Vitamin C, the placebo effect, and the common cold: A case study of how preconceptions influence the analysis of results. *J Clin Epidemiol* 49: 1079–1084
49 Hemilä H (1997) Vitamin C supplementation and the common cold: Was Linus Pauling right or wrong? *Int J Vitam Nutr Res* 67: 329–335
50 Anderson TW, Suranyi G, Beaton GH (1974) The effect on winter illness of large doses of vitamin C. *Can Med Assoc J* 111: 31–36
51 Padayatty SJ, Sun H, Wang Y, Riordan HD, Hewitt SM, Katz A, Wesley RA, Levine M (2004) Vitamin C pharmacokinetics: Implications for oral and intravenous use. *Ann Intern Med* 140: 533–537
52 Padayatty SJ, Riordan HD, Hewitt SM, Katz A, Hoffer LJ, Levine M (2006) Intravenously administered vitamin C as cancer therapy: Three cases. *CMAJ* 174: 937–942
53 Rivers JM (1987) Safety of high-level vitamin C ingestion. *Ann NY Acad Sci* 498: 445–454
54 Hathcock JN, Azzi A, Blumberg J, Bray T, Dickinson A, Frei B, Jialal I, Johnston CS, Kelly FJ, Kraemer K et al. (2005) Vitamins E and C are safe across a broad range of intakes. *Am J Clin Nutr* 81: 736–745
55 Gotzsche AL (1989). Pernasal vitamin C and the common cold. *Lancet* 2: 1039
56 Thomas WR, Holt PG (1978) Vitamin C and immunity: An assessment of the evidence. *Clin Exp Immunol* 32: 370–379
57 Beisel WR (1982) Single nutrients and immunity: Vitamin C. *Am J Clin Nutr* 35(Feb suppl): 423–428, 460–461
58 Gross RL, Newberne PM (1980) Role of nutrition in immunologic function: Vitamin C. *Physiol Rev* 60: 255–260, 290–302
59 Jariwalla RJ, Harakeh S (1996) Antiviral and immunomodulatory activities of ascorbic acid. *Subcell Biochem* 25: 215–231

60 Webb AL, Villamor E (2007) Effects of antioxidant and non-antioxidant vitamin supplementation on immune function. *Nutr Rev* 65: 181–217
61 Akaike T, Noguchi Y, Ijiri S, Setoguchi K, Suga M, Zheng YM, Dietzschold B, Maeda H (1996) Pathogenesis of influenza virus-induced pneumonia: Involvement of both nitric oxide and oxygen radicals. *Proc Natl Acad Sci USA* 93: 2448–2453
62 Peterhans E (1997) Oxidants and antioxidants in viral diseases. *J Nutr* 127: 962S–965S
63 Akaike T (2001) Role of free radicals in viral pathogenesis and mutation. *Rev Med Virol* 11: 87–101
64 Snelgrove RJ, Edwards L, Rae AJ, Hussell T (2006) An absence of reactive oxygen species improves the resolution of lung influenza infection. *Eur J Immunol* 36: 1364–1273
65 Castro SM, Guerrero-Plata A, Suarez-Real G, Adegboyega PA, Colasurdo GN, Khan AM, Garofalo RP, Casola A (2006) Antioxidant treatment ameliorates respiratory syncytial virus-induced disease and lung inflammation. *Am J Respir Crit Care Med* 174: 1361–1369
66 Hemilä H (2006) *Do vitamins C and E affect respiratory infections?* [PhD Thesis]. Helsinki, Finland: University of Helsinki; pp. 5–10, 105–131. Available at: http://ethesis.helsinki.fi/julkaisut/laa/kansa/vk/hemila/ (accessed 29 December 2008)
67 Witt EH, Reznick AZ, Viguie CA, Starke-Reed P, Packer L (1992) Exercise, oxidative damage and effects of antioxidant manipulation. *J Nutr* 122: 766–773
68 Packer L (1997) Oxidants, antioxidant nutrients and the athlete. *J Sports Sci* 15: 353–363
69 Hemilä H (1996) Vitamin C supplementation and common cold symptoms: Problems with inaccurate reviews. *Nutrition* 12: 804–809
70 Chalmers TC (1975) Effects of ascorbic acid on the common cold: An evaluation of the evidence. *Am J Med* 58: 532–536
71 Dykes MHM, Meier P (1975) Ascorbic acid and the common cold: Evaluation of its efficacy and toxicity. *JAMA* 231: 1073–1079
72 Hemilä H, Herman ZS (1995) Vitamin C and the common cold: A retrospective analysis of Chalmers' review. *J Am Coll Nutr* 14: 116–123
73 Hemilä H (2008) Chalmers' meta-analysis 1975. Available at: http://www.ltdk.helsinki.fi/users/hemila/reviews/chalmers (accessed 29 December 2008)
74 Hemilä H (2008) The Dykes and Meier review 1975. Available at: http://www.ltdk.helsinki.fi/users/hemila/reviews/dykes (accessed 29 December 2008)
75 Pauling L (1976) Ascorbic acid and the common cold: Evaluation of its efficacy and toxicity. Part I. *Med Tribune* 17(12): 18–19
76 Pauling L (1976) Ascorbic acid and the common cold. Part II. *Med Tribune* 17(13): 37–38
77 Chalmers TC (1996) Dissent to the preceding article by H. Hemilä. *J Clin Epidemiol* 49: 1085
78 Hemilä H (1996) To the dissent by Thomas Chalmers. *J Clin Epidemiol* 49: 1087
79 Hemilä H (2008) The most influential trial on vitamin C and the common cold: Karlowski et al. 1975. Available at: http://www.ltdk.helsinki.fi/users/hemila/karlowski (accessed 29 December 2008)

80 Truswell AS (1986) Ascorbic acid. *N Engl J Med* 315: 709
81 Kleijnen J, Riet G, Knipschild PG (1989) Vitamine C en verkoudheid; overzicht van een megadosis literatuur [in Dutch; Vitamin C and the common cold; a review of the megadose literature]. *Ned Tijdschr Geneeskd* 133: 1532–1535
82 Hemilä H (2008) Truswell's mini-review 1986. Available at: http://www.ltdk.helsinki.fi/users/hemila/reviews/truswell (accessed 29 December 2008)
83 Hemilä H (2008) Kleijnen's meta-analysis 1989. Available at: http://www.ltdk.helsinki.fi/users/hemila/reviews/kleijnen (accessed 29 December 2008)
84 Hemilä H (2008) Pauling's meta-analyses 1971a,b. Available at: http://www.ltdk.helsinki.fi/users/hemila/reviews/pauling (accessed 29 December 2008)
85 Meydani SN, Wu D, Santos MS, Hayek MG (1995) Antioxidants and immune response in aged persons: Overview of present evidence. *Am J Clin Nutr* 62: 1462S–1476S
86 Moriguchi S, Muraga M (2000) Vitamin E and immunity. *Vitam Horm* 59: 305–336
87 Baehner RL, Boxer LA, Allen JM, Davis J (1977) Autoxidation as a basis for altered function by polymorphonuclear leukocytes. *Blood* 50: 327–335
88 Prasad JS (1980) Effect of vitamin E supplementation on leukocyte function. *Am J Clin Nutr* 33: 606–608
89 Eckman JR, Eaton JW, Berger E, Jacob HS (1976) Role of vitamin E in regulating malaria expression. *Transact Assoc Am Physicians* 89: 105–115
90 Taylor DW, Levander OA, Krishna VR, Evans CB, Morris VC, Barta JR (1997) Vitamin E-deficient diets enriched with fish oil suppress lethal Plasmodium yoelii infections in athymic and scid/bg mice. *Infect Immun* 65: 197–202
91 Garg R, Singh N, Dube A (2004) Intake of nutrient supplements affects multiplication of Leishmania donovani in hamsters. *Parasitology* 129: 685–691
92 Graat JM, Schouten EG, Kok FJ (2002) Effects of daily vitamin E and multivitamin-mineral supplementation on acute respiratory tract infections in elderly persons: A randomized controlled trial. *JAMA* 288: 715–721
93 Meydani SN, Leka LS, Fine BC, Dallal GE, Keusch GT, Singh MF, Hamer DH (2004) Vitamin E and respiratory tract infections in elderly nursing home residents: A randomized controlled trial. *JAMA* 292: 828–836; corrections: 2004;292: 1305 and 2007;297: 1882; discussion: 2004;292: 2834
94 Hemilä H (2005) Potential harm of vitamin E supplementation. *Am J Clin Nutr* 82: 1141–1142
95 Hamer DH, Meydani SN (2004) Vitamin E and respiratory tract infections in elderly people. *JAMA* 292: 2834
96 The Alpha-Tocopherol, Beta-Carotene Cancer Prevention Study Group (1994) The effect of vitamin E and beta-carotene on the incidence of lung cancer and other cancers in male smokers. *N Engl J Med* 330: 1029–1035
97 Hemilä H, Kaprio J, Albanes D, Heinonen OP, Virtamo J (2002) Vitamin C, vitamin E, and beta-carotene in relation to common cold incidence in male smokers. *Epidemiology* 13: 32–37
98 Hemilä H, Virtamo J, Albanes D, Kaprio J (2006) The effect of vitamin E on common cold incidence is modified by age, smoking and residential neighborhood. *J Am Coll Nutr* 25: 332–339
99 Hemilä H, Virtamo J, Albanes D, Kaprio J (2004) Vitamin E and beta-carotene

supplementation and hospital-treated pneumonia incidence in male smokers. *Chest* 125: 557–565
100 Hemilä H, Virtamo J, Albanes D, Kaprio J (2003) Physical activity and the common cold in men administered vitamin E and β-carotene. *Med Sci Sports Exerc* 35: 1815–1820
101 Hemilä H, Kaprio J, Albanes D, Virtamo J (2006) Physical activity and the risk of pneumonia in men administered vitamin E and β-carotene. *Int J Sports Med* 27: 336–341
102 Bendich A (1989) Carotenoids and the immune response. *J Nutr* 119: 112–115
103 Hughes DA (1999) Effects of carotenoids on human immune function. *Proc Nutr Soc* 58: 713–718
104 Omenn GS (1998) Chemoprevention of lung cancer: The rise and demise of beta-carotene. *Annu Rev Public Health* 19: 73–99
105 Chandra RK (1992) Effect of vitamin and trace-element supplementation on immune responses and infection in elderly subjects. *Lancet* 340: 1124–1127
106 Carpenter KJ, Roberts S, Sternberg S (2003) Nutrition and immune function: A 1992 report. *Lancet* 361: 2247–2248
107 White C (2004) Three journals raise doubts on validity of Canadian studies. *BMJ* 328: 67; correction: 2004;328: 257
108 Smith R (2005) Investigating the previous studies of a fraudulent author. *BMJ* 331: 288–291
109 Chavance M, Herbeth B, Lemoine A, Zhu BP (1993) Does multivitamin supplementation prevent infections in healthy elderly subjects? A controlled trial. *Int J Vitam Nutr Res* 63: 11–16
110 Girodon F, Lombard M, Galan P, Brunet-Lecomte P, Monget AL, Arnaud J, Preziosi P, Hercberg S (1997) Effect of micronutrient supplementation on infection in institutionalized elderly subjects. *Ann Nutr Metab* 41: 98–107
111 Girodon F, Galan P, Monget AL, Boutron-Ruault MC, Brunet-Lecomte P, Preziosi P, Arnaud J, Manuguerra JC, Hercberg S (1999) Impact of trace elements and vitamin supplementation on immunity and infections in institutionalized elderly patients. *Arch Intern Med* 159: 748–754
112 Barringer TA, Kirk JK, Santaniello AC, Foley KL, Michielutte R (2003) Effect of multivitamin and mineral supplement on infection and quality of life. *Ann Intern Med* 138: 365–371
113 Avenell A, Campbell MK, Cook JA, Hannaford PC, Kilonzo MM, McNeill G, Milne AC, Ramsay CR, Seymour DG, Stephen AI et al. (2005) Effect of multivitamin and multimineral supplements on morbidity from infections in older people (MAVIS trial): Pragmatic, randomised, double blind, placebo controlled trial. *BMJ* 331: 324–329
114 Liu BA, McGeer A, McArthur MA, Simor AE, Aghdassi E, Davis L, Allard JP (2007) Effect of multivitamin and mineral supplementation on episodes of infection in nursing home residents: A randomized, placebo-controlled study. *J Am Geriatr Soc* 55: 35–42; correction: 2007; 55: 478; discussion: 2007; 55: 1311–1314
115 Fischer Walker C, Black RE (2004) Zinc and the risk for infectious disease. *Annu Rev Nutr* 24: 255–275
116 Aggarwal R, Sentz J, Miller MA (2007) Role of zinc administration in preven-

tion of childhood diarrhea and respiratory illnesses: A meta-analysis. *Pediatrics* 119: 1120–1130
117 Coles CL, Bose A, Moses PD, Mathew L, Agarwal I, Mammen T, Santosham M (2007) Infectious etiology modifies the treatment effect of zinc in severe pneumonia. *Am J Clin Nutr* 86: 397–403
118 Kurugöl Z, Akilli M, Bayram N, Koturoglu G (2006) The prophylactic and therapeutic effectiveness of zinc sulphate on common cold in children. *Acta Paediatr* 95: 1175–1181
119 Kurugöl Z, Bayram N, Atik T (2007) Effect of zinc sulfate on common cold in children: Randomized, double blind study. *Pediatr Int* 49: 842–847
120 Eby GA, Davis DR, Halcomb WW (1984) Reduction in duration of common cold by zinc gluconate lozenges in a double-blind study. *Antimicrob Agents Chemother* 25: 20–24
121 Prasad AS (2008) Zinc in human health: Effect of zinc on immune cells. *Mol Med* 14: 353–357
122 Korant BD, Butterworth BE (1976) Inhibition by zinc of rhinovirus protein cleavage: Interaction of zinc with capsid polypeptides. *J Virol* 18: 298–306
123 Geist FC, Bateman JA, Hayden FG (1987) *In vitro* activity of zinc salts against human rhinoviruses. *Antimicrob Agents Chemother* 31: 622–624
124 Suara RO, Crowe JE (2004) Effect of zinc salts on respiratory syncytial virus replication. *Antimicrob Agents Chemother* 48: 783–790
125 Berg K, Bolt G, Andersen H, Owen TC (2001) Zinc potentiates the antiviral action of human IFN-alpha tenfold. *J Interferon Cytokine Res* 21: 471–474
126 Novick SG, Godfrey JC, Godfrey NJ, Wilder HR (1996) How does zinc modify the common cold? Clinical observations and implications regarding mechanisms of action. *Med Hypotheses* 46: 295–302
127 Novick SG, Godfrey JC, Pollack RL, Wilder HR (1997) Zinc-induced suppression of inflammation in the respiratory tract, caused by infection with human rhinovirus and other irritants. *Med Hypotheses* 49: 347–357
128 Godfrey JC (1988) Zinc for the common cold. *Antimicrob Agents Chemother* 32: 605–606
129 Eby GA (1988) Stability constants of zinc complexes affect common cold treatment results. *Antimicrob Agents Chemother* 32: 606–607
130 Martin RB (1988) pH as a variable in free zinc ion concentration from zinc-containing lozenges. *Antimicrob Agents Chemother* 32: 608–609
131 Eby GA (1997) Zinc ion availability – The determinant of efficacy in zinc lozenge treatment of common colds. *J Antimicrob Chemother* 40: 483–493
132 Bakar NKA, Taylor DM, Williams DR (1999) The chemical speciation of zinc in human saliva: Possible correlation with reduction of the symptoms of the common cold produced by zinc gluconate-containing lozenges. *Chem Speciat Bioavail* 11: 95–101
133 Eby GA (2004) Zinc lozenges: Cold cure or candy? Solution chemistry determinations. *Biosci Rep* 24: 23–39
134 Smith DS, Helzner EC, Nuttall CE, Collins M, Rofman BA, Ginsberg D, Goswick CB, Magner A (1989) Failure of zinc gluconate in treatment of acute upper respiratory tract infections. *Antimicrob Agents Chemother* 33: 646–648
135 Godfrey JC, Conant-Sloane B, Smith DS, Turco JH, Mercer N, Godfrey NJ

(1992) Zinc gluconate and the common cold: A controlled clinical study. *J Int Med Res* 20: 234–246
136 Prasad AS, Fitzgerald JT, Bao B, Beck FW, Chandrasekar PH (2008) Duration and severity of symptoms and levels of plasma interleukin–1 receptor antagonist, soluble tumor necrosis factor receptor, and adhesion molecules in patients with common cold treated with zinc acetate. *J Infect Dis* 197: 795–802
137 Petrus EJ, Lawson KA, Bucci LR, Blum K (1998) Randomized, double-masked, placebo-controlled clinical study of the effectiveness of zinc acetate lozenges on common cold symptoms in allergy-tested subjects. *Curr Ther Res* 59: 595–607
138 Turner RB, Cetnarowski WE (2000) Effect of treatment with zinc gluconate or zinc acetate on experimental and natural colds. *Clin Infect Dis* 31: 1202–1208; discussion in: 2001;32: 1520
139 Mossad SB, Macknin ML, Medendorp SV, Mason P (1996) Zinc gluconate lozenges for treating the common cold: A randomized, double-blind, placebo-controlled study. *Ann Intern Med* 125: 81–88
140 Prasad AS, Fitzgerald JT, Bao B, Beck FW, Chandrasekar PH (2000) Duration of symptoms and plasma cytokine levels in patients with the common cold treated with zinc acetate; a randomized, double-blind, placebo-controlled trial. *Ann Intern Med* 133: 245–252
141 Douglas RM, Miles HB, Moore BW, Ryan P, Pinnock CB (1987) Failure of effervescent zinc acetate lozenges to alter the course of upper respiratory infection in Australian adults. *Antimicrob Agents Chemother* 31: 1263–1265
142 Macknin ML, Piedmonte M, Calendine C, Janosky J, Wald E (1998) Zinc gluconate lozenges for treating the common cold in children: A randomized controlled trial. *JAMA* 279: 1962–1967
143 Weismann K, Jakobsen JP, Weismann JE, Hammer UM, Nyholm SM, Hansen B, Lomholt KE, Schmidt K (1990) Zinc gluconate lozenges for common cold: A double-blind clinical trial. *Dan Med Bull* 37: 279–281
144 Zarembo JE, Godfrey JC, Godfrey NJ (1992) Zinc(II) in saliva: Determination of concentrations produced by different formulations of zinc gluconate lozenges containing common excipients. *J Pharm Sci* 81: 128–130
145 Al-Nakib W, Higgins PG, Barrow I, Batstone G, Tyrrell DA (1987) Prophylaxis and treatment of rhinovirus colds with zinc gluconate lozenges. *J Antimicrob Chemother* 20: 893–901
146 Farr BM, Conner EM, Betts RF, Oleske J, Minnefor A, Gwaltney JM (1987) Two randomized controlled trials of zinc gluconate lozenge therapy of experimentally induced rhinovirus colds. *Antimicrob Agents Chemother* 31: 1183–1187
147 Simkin PA (1976) Oral zinc sulphate in rheumatoid arthritis. *Lancet* 2: 539–542
148 Prasad AS, Brewer GJ, Schoomaker EB, Rabbani P (1978) Hypocupremia induced by zinc therapy in adults. *JAMA* 240: 2166–2168
149 Hoffman HN, Phyliky RL, Fleming CR (1988) Zinc-induced copper deficiency. *Gastroenterology* 94: 508–512
150 Samman S, Roberts DC (1987) The effect of zinc supplements on plasma zinc

and copper levels and the reported symptoms in healthy volunteers. *Med J Aust* 146: 246–249
151 Jafek BW, Linschoten MR, Murrow BW (2004) Anosmia after intranasal zinc gluconate use. *Am J Rhinol* 18: 137–141
152 Alexander TH, Davidson TM (2006) Intranasal zinc and anosmia: The zinc-induced anosmia syndrome. *Laryngoscope* 116: 217–220; discussion: 2006;116: 1720–1723
153 Jackson JL, Peterson C, Lesho E (1997) A meta-analysis of zinc salts lozenges and the common cold. *Arch Intern Med* 157: 2373–2376
154 Jackson JL, Lesho E, Peterson C (2000) Zinc and the common cold: A meta-analysis revisited. *J Nutr* 130 (5S Suppl): 1512S–1515S
155 Thompson SG (1994) Why sources of heterogeneity in meta-analysis should be investigated. *BMJ* 309: 1351–1355
156 Caruso TJ, Prober CG, Gwaltney JM (2007) Treatment of naturally acquired common colds with zinc: A structured review. *Clin Infect Dis* 45: 569–574
157 Chalmers TC, Smith H, Blackburn B, Silverman B, Schroeder B, Reitman D, Ambroz A (1981) A method for assessing the quality of a randomized control trial. *Control Clin Trials* 2: 31–49
158 Higgins JPT, Green S (eds) (2008) Cochrane Handbook for Systematic Reviews of Interventions Version 5.0.1 [updated September 2008]. Section 8.3.3. The Cochrane Collaboration. Available at: www.cochrane-handbook.org (accessed 29 December 2008)
159 Balk EM, Bonis PA, Moskowitz H, Schmid CH, Ioannidis JP, Wang C, Lau J (2002) Correlation of quality measures with estimates of treatment effect in meta-analyses of randomized controlled trials. *JAMA* 287: 2973–2982
160 Glasziou P, Chalmers I, Rawlins M, McCulloch P (2007) When are randomised trials unnecessary? Picking signal from noise. *BMJ* 334: 349–351
161 Eby GA (2008) Therapeutic effectiveness of ionic zinc for common colds. *Clin Infect Dis* 46: 483–484
162 Council of Scientific Affairs, American Medical Association (1987) Vitamin preparations as dietary supplements and as therapeutic agents. *JAMA* 257: 1929–1936
163 Caruso TJ, Gwaltney JM (2005) Treatment of the common cold with *Echinacea*: A structured review. *Clin Infect Dis* 40: 807–810
164 Hemilä H (2005) *Echinacea*, vitamin C, the common cold, and blinding. *Clin Infect Dis* 41: 762–763
165 Richards E (1988) The politics of therapeutic evaluation: The vitamin C and cancer controversy. *Soc Stud Sci* 18: 653–701
166 Richards E (1991) *Vitamin C and Cancer: Medicine or Politics?* St Martins Press, New York
167 Galloway J (1991) Crusades and rackets. *Nature* 353: 125
168 Segerstråle U (1992) Vitamin C and cancer – Medicine or politics. *Science* 255: 613–615
169 Huxtable RJ (1992) C for controversy. *Trends Pharmacol Sci* 13: 82–83
170 Goodwin JS, Tangum MR (1998) Battling quackery: Attitudes about micronutrient supplements in American Academic medicine. *Arch Intern Med* 158: 2187–2191

171 Vandenbroucke JP, de Craen AJM (2001) Alternative medicine: A mirror image for scientific reasoning in conventional medicine. *Ann Intern Med* 135: 507–513
172 Goodwin JS, Goodwin JM (1981) Failure to recognize efficacious treatments: A history of salicylate therapy in rheumatoid arthritis. *Perspect Biol Med* 31: 78–92
173 Goodwin JS, Goodwin JM (1984) The tomato effect: Rejection of highly efficacious therapies. *JAMA* 251: 2387–2390
174 Barber B (1961) Resistance by scientists to scientific discovery. *Science* 134: 596–602
175 Gonzales R, Sande M (1995) What will it take to stop physicians from prescribing antibiotics in acute bronchitis? *Lancet* 345: 665–666

Common Cold
ed. by R. Eccles and O. Weber

Herbal, traditional and alternative remedies

Florin Mihail

Am Ringofen 7, 42327 Wuppertal, Germany

Introduction

This chapter is composed of sections dealing with some of the well known but, with respect to clinical studies, not always well investigated traditional and alternative treatments against common cold. It includes data on phytotherapy, apitherapy, ayurvedic remedies, homeopathic remedies, Schuessler's biochemistry, acupuncture and acupressure, nasal irrigation and inhalation.

Efforts to relieve annoyances produced by the common cold started probably already in the prehistoric times. What we call today "traditional methods" originated from the use of simple means and preparations such as autochthon herbs, fruits, vegetables and spices used for daily nutrition, partial or total fasting, exposure to a heat/fire source, smoke, water etc.

Some of the traditional methods are really ubiquitous, e.g., use of garlic, honey products, inhalation of water vapors with some drops of etherical oil. Others were for a long time restricted to a certain geographic region. Traditional Chinese Medicine as well the tradition of Ayurveda are briefly reviewed in this section.

In order to provide a comprehensive review of herbal, alternative and traditional remedies, homeopathy is also briefly reviewed in this chapter. Although discussed controversially in the modern scientific literature, homeopathic methods are in practice frequently used to intervene with common cold.

An updated view about existing methods of phytotherapy and beyond is provided within this chapter. The limited space, however, required opting for a certain selection of remedies and it should be noticed that not all existing products and methods could be reviewed here for this reason.

Phytotherapy

Andrographis paniculata

Andrographis (the king of Bitters, Acanthaceae) is a shrub found in most Asian countries with a long tradition of use in Chinese and Ayuverdic medicine for the treatment of infection, inflammation, common cold, fever, malaria and diarrhea. The plant contains potentially anti-inflammatory and immunomodulatory bicyclic diterpenoid lactones (as andrographolide, neoandrographolide, etc.).

Clinical studies with *Andrographis paniculata*

Three recent reviews assessed the effectivity of *A. paniculata* in the symptomatic treatment of uncomplicated upper respiratory tract infections (URTIs). One article reported the statistical evaluation of results of three studies with 433 patients that received *A. paniculata* in the fixed-dose combination with *Eleutherococcus* (*Acanthopanax*) *senticosus*. The authors conclude that the combination was more effective than placebo in the reduction in symptom severity score ($p = 0.0002$). Hence, *A. paniculata* extract alone or in combination with *A. senticosus* was regarded by the authors as an appropriate alternative treatment of uncomplicated URTIs [1]. The second review, using seven double-blind, controlled trials ($n = 896$) confirmed this conclusion and pointed to some evidence of a preventive effect. Short-term treatment, at recommended dose, is associated with only few reports on adverse effects [2].

These conclusions are again endorsed by the third review [3], which incorporated the results of the first two cited above.

Several individual studies present the results obtained in the treatment of URTIs with Kan Jang [a standardized fixed combination of *A. paniculata* (SHA-10 extract) with *E. senticosus*]. Throat and nasal symptoms as well as general malaise and headache were the symptoms showing most significant improvement under the treatment [4, 5]. In a three-arm study with a total of 130 children, Kan Jang tablets had the most pronounced effect on the amount of nasal secretion and nasal congestion [6]. Children who received 200 mg of a standardized *A. paniculata* extract daily over 3 months showed a significant decreased number of common cold cases (30% *versus* 62% in the placebo group) [7, 8].

Adverse and side effects

No significant adverse effects have been reported in human studies of *A. paniculata*; however, there were some concerns from animal studies that *Andrographis* may impair fertility. In a newer Phase I clinical study, Kan

Jang did not reveal negative effects on male semen quality and spermatogenesis [9].

Natural product-drug interactions

No significant interactions have been reported.

Echinacea (E. purpurea, E. angustifolia, E. pallida)

Echinacea is the name of a genus of plants native to midwestern North America. *Echinacea* preparations are derived from three of the nine species: *E. purpurea* (purple coneflower), *E. angustifolia* (narrow-leaf coneflower), and *E. pallida* (pale purple coneflower). Medicinal use of this herb began with Native Americans, who used *E. angustifolia* rhizome to treat a wide variety of health problems including respiratory infections, relief of pain and snakebites. During the 19th century, *Echinacea* was used as a blood purifier, a basic antimicrobial herb and a treatment for dizziness. In the early 20th century, it was used as a cold and flu remedy, and as an anti-infective until the advent of modern antibiotics [10].

Preparations of *Echinacea* are intended for oral [capsules/tablets, dried root or herb for tea, expressed juice, extract (mostly alcoholic) or tincture] or topical application. The use of *Echinacea* in injectable form is questionable. The most commonly used preparations at present are root or whole-plant extracts of *E. purpurea*.

Present uses include URTIs (preventing, "aborting" or treating a cold), chronic bronchitis, otitis, urinary tract infections, recurrent vaginal yeast infections, skin and oral wound healing. Under investigation are further potential uses, e.g., immune system stimulation in cancer patients receiving radiation or chemotherapy and low-grade uveitis.

Dosage in adults

For treatment of URTIs, the most often recommended dose is 500–1000 mg in capsules, three times per day. In case of expressed juice, the daily dose should be 6–9 ml. Tinctures (1:5) are suggested in a dose range of 0.75-1.5 ml; they should be gargled and swallowed two to five times per day. Independent of the formulation type, 5–7 days is considered as the standard treatment time [11, 12].

Pediatric dosing (younger than 18 years)

In the case of expressed juice, Schapowal recommends 3 ml for children 1–4 years old, 3–5 ml for children 4–10 years old and 6–9 ml for older children and adolescents [13].

Echinacea has been studied alone or in combination preparations in numerous *in vitro* and *in vivo* studies (including human studies). The test samples expressed a large variation as they may differ with respect to the chosen species, part of the plant selected (above ground, root or whole plant), differences in the manufacturing process or kind of formulation. Active constituents include alkylamides, alkaloids, arabinolactan, cichoric acid, flavonoids, isobutylamides, polyenes and polysaccharides [14, 15].

Mode of action

Preparations of *Echinacea* sp. are touted as stimulants or modulators of the immune system.

Herbal extracts of the leaves and root of *E. purpurea* increase counts of natural killer (NK) cells and monocytes (both mediators of nonspecific immunity) in the spleen and bone marrow of rats [16], and also the number of leukocytes and lymphocytes, especially T lymphocytes, in peripheral blood of rabbits as compared with the control group. Activation of phagocytosis of neutrophils *in vitro* and *in vivo* was demonstrated in humans [17].

Further (nonspecific) effects include secretion of interferon (IFN), tumor necrosis factor (TNF) and interleukin (IL)-1 and IL-10 [18, 19].

Echinacea enhances besides NK cell activity also the cellular immune function of human peripheral blood mononuclear cells against human herpesvirus 6-infected H9 cells [20]. *E. purpurea* activates macrophages to stimulate IFN-γ production in association with the secondary activation of T lymphocytes [21]. New *in vitro* studies confirm the macrophage activation, which results in stimulating production of IL-6, TNF, IL-12, and NO [22].

In spite of the promising results regarding the mechanism of action, it should be mentioned that newer human studies that included a battery of parameters to assess the reaction of the immune system deliver contradictory facts. Schwarz et al. [23] could not find an influence on phagocytic activity of polymorphonuclear leukocytes or monocytes or an influence on the production TNF-α and IL-1β by LPS-stimulated monocytes. In a subsequent investigation on lymphocyte subpopulations only minor effects (of questionable physiological relevance) on 2 of the 12 subtypes of lymphocytes were detected [24].

In contrast, Goel et al. [25] reported a significant and sustained increase in the number of circulating total white blood cells, monocytes, neutrophils and NK cells as a result of administration of *Echinacea* preparation to volunteers.

Clinical studies with *Echinacea*

A discussion of every one of the 400 plus studies and observations in humans would surely be beyond the capacity of this chapter. Therefore, we opted to present and discuss reviews, collections and meta-analyses of clinical studies, which have already passed a preselection in terms of test design, quality and meaningfulness. Whenever necessary individual studies are mentioned and discussed.

A comprehensive review of controlled clinical trials was published in 1994 by Melchart et al. [26]. The paper encompassed six studies on treatment and six studies on prevention of URTIs published between 1961 and 1992. Although the original authors of the most studies concluded that *Echinacea* was superior to placebo, the analysis of the reviewers pointed to a variety of flaws and deficiencies in 11 out of 12 trials. Only 1 study [27] using 900 mg/day of *E. purpurea* root extract was thought to have verified efficacy for URTIs symptoms.

In total, the results of the 12 studies were regarded as not sufficient to allow safe recommendations with respect to dosage or formulation, although some evidence existed to support the use of *Echinacea* for preventing and treating URTIs.

A second review by Barrett et al. in 1999 [28] analyzed 9 clinical trials on treatment and 4 on prevention of URTIs. All 13 studies were designed as randomized, double-blind, placebo-controlled trials. The original authors concluded that *Echinacea* had a positive effect against URTI symptoms in 8 of the 9 treatment trials. On the other hand, the prevention trials did not deliver evidence on a prophylactic efficacy. Barrett et al. concluded that despite methodological deficiencies there is evidence for a role of *Echinacea* in the treatment of URTIs.

Five studies on prevention and treatment of common cold published between 1997 and 1999 were reviewed by Giles et al. [29] in 2000. The evaluation is positive with regard to the treatment potential of URTIs, although the effects are not dramatic. The improvements comprise a decreased time to resolution of signs and somewhat milder symptoms. Again, no prophylactic effect was seen.

An evidence-based systematic review of studies performed with the three *Echinacea* species was prepared by Basch et al. in 2005 [12]. The authors used studies of the three aforementioned reviews and the 2000 edition of the Cochrane monograph published by Melchart and coauthors [30]. The results are summarized here under three categories:

- URTIs – Treatment (adults): The sum of existing positive evidence is regarded as highly suggestive, albeit not definitive. Variations in frequency of administration, dosage, choice of *Echinacea* species and of the suitable part of plant used as raw material prevent a more distinct statement.
- URTIs – Prevention (adults and children): The evidence is equivocal. The available randomized studies have moderate sample size and brief follow-up periods. Even if there is a preventive effect of *Echinacea* (see study of Cohen et al. [31]), it is likely small at best.

- URTIs – Treatment (children): Initial research suggests that *Echinacea* may not be helpful in children for alleviation of cold symptoms. Additional research is recommended. Furthermore, adverse effects (skin rash) may outweigh the potential benefits.

Caruso and Gwaltney [32] published also in 2005 a structured review on the treatment of common cold with *Echinacea.* From a total of 322 retrieved articles, 9 placebo-controlled trials were selected. The quality of experimental design and methods of statistical analysis were in the focus of this report, which used no less than 11 criteria to judge the validity of the studies. Only 2 studies [33, 34] both negative to the therapeutic benefit) met all quality criteria imposed by the authors. From the 9 selected clinical studies, 6 yielded positive and 3 negative results. Caruso and Gwaltney concluded their report stating that on the basis of the limited information the possible value of *Echinacea* in treating the common cold cannot be established.

A meta-analysis on the effectiveness of *Echinacea* to prevent induced rhinovirus colds was provided in 2006 by Schoop et al. [35]. Three inoculation studies fulfilled the quality criteria on study design. The results were pooled and underwent statistical evaluation. The pooled estimate included 223 subjects who received *Echinacea* and 167 who received placebo. *Echinacea* did not influence the number of infections but the likelihood of developing a clinical cold with its typical symptoms was 55 % higher in the placebo group than in the *Echinacea* group ($p<0.043$). It has to be remarked that the results of the meta-analysis do not fully concur with those of the individual studies, a fact that may be explained by the different size of samples on which statistics was performed.

A newer meta-analysis with outcome incidence and duration of common cold was done by Shah et al. in 2007 [36]. Fourteen randomized, placebo-controlled trials with endpoints of cold incidence or cold duration were selected. Seven out of 14 studies evaluated monotherapy with *E. purpurea* and 2 out of 14 were performed in children. *Echinacea*'s efficacy was assessed both in the presence and absence of other active ingredients in the test sample. Studies included in the meta-analysis examined patients who either contracted a cold naturally or as a result of experimental inoculation.

The statistical calculation showed that *Echinacea* lowered the odds of a patient contracting a cold by 58% and also decreased the duration of a cold by 1.4 days. A subgroup analysis could not discover differences in the incidence of common cold between groups receiving *Echinacea* alone or in the presence of other supplements or nutraceuticals. On the other hand, the subgroup of those patients receiving *Echinacea* with a supplement showed a significant effect on shortening the duration of cold in its own right, compared with only a trend towards benefit in the *Echinacea*-only group.

A first version of the Cochrane review of *Echinacea* for preventing and treating the common cold was completed in 1998 [30]. A new version, subjected to regular updates, was provided in 2006. The version used in this chapter described and assessed the results of a literature search up to September 2007 [37]. The authors selected randomized, controlled trials for prevention or treatment of common colds in which only *Echinacea* mono-preparations were used. Special care was also taken to include only studies with patients clearly diagnosed with URTI. Sixteen studies including a total of 22 comparisons of *Echinacea* preparations and a control group met the selection criteria. Two studies were in children, the remaining 14 in adults. Three comparisons investigated prevention, while the other 19 investigated treatment of colds.

Comparing an *Echinacea* preparation with placebo as treatment, a significant effect was reported in 9 comparisons, a trend in 1, and no difference in 6. Evidence for more than 1 trial was available from the preparations based on the aerial parts of *Echinacea purpurea*, although the results were not fully consistent. Beneficial effects of other *Echinacea* preparations, and of *Echinacea* used for prevention purposes might exist but have not been shown in independently replicated, rigorous randomized studies.

The main results of the outlined eight reviews can be summarized as follows:

- Positive evidence prevails and shows that *Echinacea* has beneficial effects in the treatment of common cold. More positive data were reported for *E. purpurea*, and here especially for preparations of the above-the-ground parts; however, this can be due in part to the larger number of studies performed with this species.
- A start of treatment with *Echinacea* at the very beginning of the illness may deliver better results. In contrast to this positive experience, preventive studies did not bring evidence of a prophylactic efficacy. Even if a trend for beneficial effects exists more data of modern designed clinical studies are required to substantiate it.
- The available data show that *Echinacea* may not be so helpful in children as it is in the treatment of adults. It is at present not clear, whether more clinical studies may bring clarification on this issue or if the difference is based on particularities of the immune system in children.

In a 2008 evaluation of the existing meta-analyses, Woelkart et al. [38] concluded their paper by underlining that the clinical data for *Echinacea* are still not conclusive and require in the case of *E. purpurea* more studies with precisely standardized products in various clinical settings, also for prevention. Further controlled clinical trials are also needed for *E. angustifolia* and *E. pallida* to provide a better evidence for clinical efficacy.

Adverse and side effects

Data from clinical studies and spontaneous reporting programs suggest that short-term use of *Echinacea* is associated with a relatively good safety profile. Gastrointestinal upsets (nausea, abdominal pain) and rashes (dermatitis, pruritus, erythema nodosum) occur more frequently. However, in rare cases, *Echinacea* can be associated with allergic reactions (anaphylaxis, asthma attacks or exacerbation) that may be severe. Persons with a history of allergy to plants from the *Asteraceae* or *Compositae* family (including ragweed, marigold, daisies and chrysanthemum) may be at greater risk.

Angioedema, leukopenia/potential for immunosuppression (after long-term use), thrombotic thrombocytopenic purpura, arthralgia or myalgia have been reported in isolated cases. The adverse effects tend in general to be infrequent, mild, and transient; however, the increased incidence of rash in children should be considered before such a treatment is initiated [10, 39–41].

The German Commission E monograph10 recommends that *Echinacea* not be used in patients with autoimmune conditions or human immunodeficiency virus (HIV) infection, because of the risk that its immunostimulating effect could lead to exacerbation of autoimmune illness or increase in HIV viral load; however, the risk of *Echinacea* use with these conditions are not clear [40–42].

The use of *Echinacea* products during pregnancy and lactation appears to be rather ill-advised in light of the paucity of data in this area [38].

Natural product-drug interactions

As long-term use of *Echinacea* has been associated with some liver toxicity, its intake should be better avoided by patients under treatment with hepatotoxic drugs such as anabolic steroids, amiodarone, ketokonazole (oral administration), acetaminophen or methotrexate [43, 44].

Studies suggest that *Echinacea* might inhibit activities of the cytochrome P450 family enzymes (as CYP 1A2 and CYP 3A4, respectively) [45, 46, 48]; this inhibition tends to increase levels of drugs metabolized by this system, such as itraconazole, fexofenadine, lovastatin, alprazolam, calcium-channel blockers and protease inhibitors [43]. Nevertheless, there are currently no verifiable reports of drug-herb interactions with any *Echinacea* product, and the weak inhibition is unlikely to be of clinical relevance. Furthermore, additional pharmacokinetic testing is necessary before conclusive statements can be made about *Echinacea* drug-herb interactions [47, 49].

Theoretically, the immune-stimulating properties of *Echinacea* might interfere with the use of immunosuppressive medications in patients with autoimmune disease; however, while such an effect is theoretically possible, it has not been documented in animals or humans.

Echinacea may interact with anesthetics, anti-neoplastics, antioxidants and caffeine. However, these potential interactions are not fully understood [44].

*Elderberry (*Sambucus nigra*)*

Several species of *Sambucus* (Elder or Elderberry) produce elderberries. Most research and publications refer to *S. nigra* or regard the whole group as composed of very similar species.

Flowers and leaves have a long history of use for pain relief, swelling/inflammation, diuresis, diabetes and for facilitating expectoration, while the aged bark serves as diuretic, laxative or emetic.

Flowers and berries are the base of herbal teas or juice. They may improve common cold and flu-like symptoms, such as fever, fatigue, headache, sore throat, cough and aches and shorten the duration of the disease [50]. Children with chronic or "dry" rhinitis and flu accompanied by fever without perspiration show very good results after application of elderberry preparations [51]. *Sambucus* extracts are sometimes combined with zinc in capsules for fighting the common cold and flu, and seem particularly effective in alleviating the pulmonary symptoms.

Elder flowers are often processed to herbal teas to boost transpiration. They are helpful especially in situations in which the feverish person fills chilled and the hot tea accompanied by a hot bath induces a strong sudorific episode.

The usual prescriptions for pediatric use comprise 1–2 g/day for infants and toddlers and up to 10–15 g/day for children between 10 and 16 years [13].

Mode of action

There has been limited research done on mode of action, and much of it involves the flu virus. Apparently, elderberry constituents can effectively neutralize the hemagglutinin spikes found on the surface of several viruses including influenza A and B, disabling the entry of the viral particles into the host cells [52]. Anthocyanins seem (independently of the plant used) to play a major role in this antiviral mode of action [53]. Further constituents of the berries are flavonoids, cyanogenic glycosides, a hemagglutinin protein and vitamins A and C [52].

Clinical studies with elderberry

In a randomized, double-blind, placebo-controlled study, patients suffering from influenza-like symptoms received 15 ml elderberry or placebo syrup (Sambucol, 38% extract) four times a day over 5 days. Symptoms were relieved on average 4 days earlier and use of rescue medication was significantly reduced in the medication group [54]. An earlier placebo-controlled double-blind study on 40 individuals, done also on Sambucol, showed a significant difference ($p<0.001$) for the proportion of patients whose symptoms were resolved within 3 days [55].

Worth mentioning are also the immune modulation *via* cytokine production and the antioxidant properties of elderberry extracts [56].

Adverse and side effects

Only commercially prepared extracts of the berry should be used, because the fresh leaves, bark, young buds, unripe berries and roots contain the cyanogenic glycoside sambunigrin, which is potentially toxic. High doses of elderberry may potentiate insulin release, and thus lower blood sugar levels [56]. Dizziness, headache, convulsions and rapid heart rate have been reported [50]. Elderberry pollen, flowers and berries contain a protein prone to induce the type I allergy in sensitive persons [57].

Natural product-drug interactions

Caution is advised when using diuretics, laxatives or medications that lower blood sugar levels. Patients under theophylline medication should take into account a possible interaction with the elderberry flavonoid quercetin [50].

*Garlic (*Allium sativa*)*

Garlic is a perennial plant native to Central Asia and belonging to the Liliaceae family. It has been used as both food and medicine (e.g., in the Ayurvedic and traditional Chinese medicine) in many cultures for thousands of years. Garlic exhibits some hypolipidemic, anti-platelet and procirculatory effects and can be effective as antibacterial, antifungal and anti-inflammatory agent. In addition, aged garlic possesses hepatoprotective, neuroprotective and antioxidative activities [58, 59].

Garlic has a long and worldwide history of use for relief of cough, colds and rhinitis as well as for preventing respiratory tract infections, possibly through immune enhancement [58]. One may use it in fresh form (chopped or crushed) alone or with honey [60] but is also available as an extract (mostly formulated as a pill). The recommended dose is around 1200 mg/day [59]. The cold-fighting compound in garlic was thought to be allicin; however, on the strength of new findings it is questionable whether allicin plays the major role in the efficacy. Additional effects may be caused by S-allylcysteine, saponins and *N*-α-fructosyl arginine, all compounds found in garlic or aged garlic extract [58].

Clinical studies with garlic

Despite of the very large database on garlic, there are only a limited number of studies in volunteers/patients with a guideline-conform study design. In a randomized study 146 volunteers received one capsule containing either allicin or placebo daily over a 12-week period. In the study performed between November and February a five-point scale was used to assess the symptoms. In the allicin-treatment group, 24 colds were reported compared to 65 in the placebo group. In addition, volunteers of the allicin-treated group appeared to have a significantly shorter duration of symptoms [61].

In a second double-blind placebo-controlled randomized 5-month study, the effects of Allicor (long-releasing garlic tablets) to treat acute respiratory viral infections were compared with those produced by benzimidazole (actually a parasiticide); 42 children aged 10–12 years received 300 mg Allicor/day in comparison to 41 placebo- and 73 benzimidazol-treated children. Allicor reduced acute respiratory viral diseases 1.7-fold compared to placebo and 2.4-fold *versus* benzimidazole. Health index in Allicor-treated group was 1.5-fold higher as compared to placebo children [62, 63].

A third study investigated the possibility to prevent airborne infection by applying an intranasal cellulose powder alone or in combination with powdered garlic extract. The randomized and blinded study was performed in Finland and the United Kingdom over 8 weeks. The volunteers ($n=52$) were instructed to use a five-point scale to assess the health status and to note symptoms.

The group receiving powdered garlic extract recorded significantly fewer infections (20 *versus* 57), and number of days on which an infection was present (126 *versus* 240 days) than the control group [64].

A review of recent randomized, double-blind studies revealed no convincing evidence that garlic may be an effective treatment [65]. As mentioned by the authors more data from rigorous trials on the effectiveness of garlic are needed before a clinical recommendation can be made.

Adverse and side effects

Gastrointestinal disturbances (bloating, nausea), change in body odor through the sweat and breath, headaches, sweating, dizziness (maybe due to low blood pressure) and rarely allergic reactions or hypoglycemia have been reported [66, 67]. When raw garlic is taken in excessive doses, it can cause symptoms, such as stomach upset, heartburn, nausea, vomiting, diarrhea, flatulence, facial flushing, rapid pulse, and insomnia [68]. Sources from open literature mention a possible effect of garlic on thrombocyte aggregation [69]. No effect on thrombocyte function was seen in a more recent study when volunteers ingested 4.2 g raw garlic daily over 1 week [70].

Natural product-drug interactions

Garlic extract decreased the area under the plasma concentration-time curve (AUC) and maximum plasma concentration of saquinavir, but not ritonavir and acetaminophen in volunteers [71]. Although the mechanism of this interaction is not fully understood, garlic supplements should be better avoided by people taking protease inhibitors and non-nucleoside reverse transcriptase inhibitors [69]. It further caused hypoglycemia when taken with chlorpropamide and increased clotting time and international normalized ratio (INR) of warfarin [71]. No agonistic effect on warfarin was noticed, however, when patients received an aged garlic extract in a double-blind, randomized, placebo-controlled pilot study [72]. Even if there is still no clear consensus regarding the blood-coagulation effect of garlic, appropriate caution is necessary when patients are taking anticoagulants or drugs which interfere with platelet function.

*Ginger (*Zingiber officinalis*)*

Ginger is the rhizome of *Z. officinalis* Roscoe (Zingiberaceae family), a perennial herb native to southern Asia. Besides being a common constituent of diets, it has a millennial history of use in the traditional Chinese medicine against nausea, diarrhea, stomachaches, cholera, bleeding or rheumatism, in fighting the early stages of common cold and coughs and also in treating allergic rhinitis. Hot ginger tea is recommended to avert or to ease the infection when taken at the first signs of a fenghan-type of cold. Main modern uses of ginger today include nausea and vomiting during pregnancy, motion and sea sickness and post-surgical nausea.

While direct scientific evidence on the effectiveness of ginger in preventing or fighting common cold is lacking, some studies done on its mode of action might explain the positive experience gathered over centuries.

- Anti-inflammatory and smooth-muscle relaxing effects: In rats, ginger extract attenuates effects of lung inflammation by lipopolysaccharides and trachea hyperreactivity by reducing the serum level of prostaglandin E2 and by inhibiting some inflammation-related enzymes [73]. In a further study using mouse lung slices, it was demonstrated that ginger extract reduces the acetylcholine-induced contraction of smooth muscle cells [74]. An inhibition of inflammation and relieve of airway hyperreactivity was also noticed in an *in vivo* study in sensitized guinea pigs receiving shegan mahuang (a traditional Chinese medicine recipe containing ginger) [75].
- Antiviral effects: Ginger extract showed a clear anti-influenza virus type A (Aichi) effect *in vitro* [76]. Imanishi et al. [77] demonstrated in a series of *in vitro* experiments that ginger extract itself has no inhibitory effects on the replication of influenza virus but was able to exert an antiviral effect *via* macrophage activation of TNF-α. This kind of activation may also play a principal role in the course of an infection with common cold viruses.

Adverse and side effects

In a series of *in vitro* experiments, ginger extract showed the potential to interfere with thrombocytes aggregation [78, 79]; however, on the strength of *in vivo* experiments there is no proof that the dosages of ginger used as a diet component or as a dietary supplement (corresponding to 1–4 g of powdered ginger) would lead to significant side effects [80]. Animal experiments delivered some contradictory results regarding a possible effect of ginger extract on blood glucose levels [80, 82]. No effect on blood sugar was observed when 4 g per day were taken for 3 months in healthy humans and patients with coronary arterial disease [83].

Aqueous ginger extract is only a weak clastogenic agent in mouse bone marrow cells. This can be attributed to the presence of both mutagenic and anti-mutagenic compounds in it. The oral application of ginger oil resulted, on the other hand, in a higher degree of clastogenicity [84]. One report describe a case of occupational asthma and skin sensitization in a production worker exposed to ginger [85], which is somewhat in contrast to its widespread use to treat allergic rhinitis and asthma.

Natural product-drug interactions

One recent paper points to a possible agonistic anticoagulant effect of ginger and phenprocoumon [81]. High doses of ginger might therefore possibly increase the risk of bleeding in patients taking anticoagulants (heparinoids, coumarin derivatives) or drugs that interfere with thrombocytes activity (ASS, clopidogrel); appropriate caution is therefore necessary.

Ginseng

The two most common types of ginseng are *Panax ginseng*, known as Asian or Korean ginseng, and *Panax quinquefolium* (American ginseng). According to traditional Chinese medicine, the American ginseng promotes Yin energy, cleaning excess Yang from the body, which makes it valuable for fever and respiratory tract disorders. East Asian ginseng is strong in Yang energy, which is good for improving circulation.

Both American and Asian ginseng serve as adaptogens (products supposed to increase body's resistance to stress and to build energy and general vitality), as stimulants of the immune system as well as natural drugs in the treatment of type II diabetes and of sexual dysfunctions. Ginseng extracts contain poly- and oligosaccharides, phytoestrogens and antioxidants.

A third kind of ginseng is *Eleutherococcus senticosus* known also as Siberian or Russian ginseng, but this small, woody shrub belongs to the Araliaceae family. For more information please consult the paragraph on *Andrographis*.

Clinical studies with *Panax quinquefolium* and *Panax ginseng*

Asian ginseng had been used for many centuries to prevent and treat respiratory tract infections, and warm ginseng tea is, for example, one of the oldest traditional remedy against common cold in Korea [86]. However, it has been only in the last two decades that science-based studies in humans were performed with ginseng extracts.

Two randomized placebo-controlled trials tested a proprietary extract of *P. quinquefolium*. In the first study 43 adults aged 65 years or older received two capsules per day of either placebo or verum (200 mg/capsule) for a period of 4 months. After the first month of treatment subjects were immunized with influenza vaccine.

During the last two months only 32% of the verum group reported acute respiratory illness compared with 62% in the placebo group. The duration of the symptoms was significantly shorter in the *P. quinquefolium* group (5.6 days) *versus* 12.6 days in the placebo group [87].

The second study used a similar design (start at the onset of the influenza season, 4-month duration) and selected a total of 323 persons between 18 and 65 years. Treatment was started by 130 volunteers in the ginseng group and 149 in the placebo group.

The mean number of colds per person was somewhat lower but still not considered significant (0.68 vs 0.93, $p=0.017$) by the authors and the proportion of subjects with two or more Jackson-verified colds during the 4-month period was significantly lower (10% vs 22.8%, $p=0.004$) in the verum group than in the placebo group. (Please note that Jackson criteria are used to characterize a common cold and to distinguish it from other illnesses of the respiratory tract; see Jackson GG et al, Arch Intern med 101: 267–278; 1958.)

Significant differences between the two groups were also noted with respect to the severity of symptoms and the number of days for which cold symptoms were reported [88]. Two further double-blind, placebo-controlled studies indicated that *P. quinquefolium* may be able to prevent flu-like illness in seniors. For these two studies 89 and 109 subjects with average ages of 81 and 83.5 years, respectively, were selected. Approximately 90% of the volunteers had received influenza vaccine in each of the 2 years of study.

Results showed an overall 89% relative risk reduction of viral acute respiratory illness in the test group. The proprietary ginseng extract (2×200 mg daily) was shown to be both safe and well tolerated [89].

In a multicenter, two-armed, randomized, placebo-controlled double-blind study, 227 volunteers received daily oral doses of placebo or 100 mg of a proprietary *P. ginseng* extract for a period of 12 weeks. An anti-influenza polyvalent vaccination was performed at week 4. The frequency of influenza or common cold was statistically significant lower in the ginseng group. The treatment group showed also significantly higher levels for some immunological markers [90] (see also notes on ginseng mode of action below).

Mode of action

The protective effects of extracts of the two ginseng species against common cold and flu can be explained taking into account their immunomodulating potential. Administration of *P. ginseng* extract to volunteers over 12 weeks almost doubled the influenza virus antibody titers and the NK cell activity levels [90].

P. ginseng enhances the chemotaxis, the phagocytosis index, the phagocytosis fraction and possibly intracellular killing in granulocytes [92]. Furthermore, *P. ginseng* extracts were shown to increase anti-complementary and reticuloendothelial system activities and to induce messenger RNA expression of a multitude of immunity markers [88]. *P. quinquefolium* stimulates *in vitro* the proliferation of murine B lymphocytes and leads to enhanced IL-1, IL-6, TNF-α and NO production. Treated mice showed a stimulation of IgG production [93]. An *ex vivo* study revealed significantly increased Con-A-induced IL-2 and IFN-γ production in splenocytes of mice. The authors concluded that *P. quinquefolium* intake may improve natural immune responses [94].

Adverse and side effects

Nausea, diarrhea, euphoria, insomnia, blood pressure abnormalities, mastalgia, vaginal bleeding have been have been reported [92]. Side effects are rare and most of them the result of intake of high ginseng doses.

Natural product-drug interactions

Both Asian and American ginseng reduce blood glucose and hemoglobin A1c levels in people with type 2 diabetes mellitus. This should be taken into account when ginseng products and anti-diabetic drugs are being taken together [69, 91]. It can also not be ruled out that ginseng has an antagonist effect on anticoagulants like warfarin. Hence, INRs should be supervised more closely in patients taking concomitantly coumarin derivatives and ginseng [69, 95].

Intake of ginseng may also lead to increased digoxin levels [15]. Caution is advised in patients taking ginseng in addition to caffeine or monoamine oxidase inhibitors [92] (although interaction with monoamine oxidases is questionable), and to some antipsychotic drugs.

*Goldenseal (*Hydrastis canadensis*)*

Goldenseal also called Orange-root or Orangeroot belongs to the Ranunculaceae family and is native to southeastern Canada and the northeastern United States. The rhizome and the root are the parts used for medicinal purposes. Goldenseal contains the isoquinoline alkaloids: hydrastine, berberine, berberastine, hydrastinine tetrahydroberberastine, canadine, and canalidine [96].

Goldenseal is an immune-booster and an anti-bacterial agent (containing the natural antibiotic berberine) [97], and has anti-inflammatory, laxative, antiseptic, astringent, emmenagogue and oxytocic properties. Goldenseal extracts and decoctions have also demonstrated some antiviral, antifungal and anti-protozoan activity [98]. It is commonly used to treat several skin, eye, and mucous membrane inflammatory and infectious conditions, and also for sore throats and canker sores. Ready-to-use formulations are mostly tinctures (alcohol extracts), capsules, or herbal teas.

Although no modern controlled clinical studies to demonstrate its efficacy against common cold viruses are available, goldenseal should be mentioned here, as is contained (in combination with *Echinacea*) in some of the most widespread herbal cold treatments. The herb may lessen mucus in the nose and throat; under other conditions, however, it may increase the secretion of the mucous membranes.

In vitro studies addressed the anti-inflammatory effects of goldenseal. Berberine exerts a significant inhibitory effect on transformation of human peripheral lymphocytes, which may be due to inhibition of DNA synthesis in activated lymphocytes [99]. Another study demonstrated the inhibitory effect of berberine on some parameters of the inflammatory process in response to tissue injury [98, 100].

Adverse and side effects

When used at high doses, goldenseal can cause anxiety, depression, paralysis and seizures. Topical use of concentrated solutions can cause ulcerations of mucous membranes (skin, mouth, throat, and vagina). Goldenseal may increase blood pressure and cause an increased sensitivity to sunlight [101–103]. It can also reduce the number of "good" bacteria in the digestive system, which can cause nausea and diarrhea [104].

Berberine in humans can inhibit receptors in smooth muscle, block potassium channels in the heart and reduce ventricular tachycardia, inhibit intestinal ion secretion and toxin formation in the gut and increase bile secretion [105].

Although developmental toxicity studies with goldenseal (in rats), or with berberine (in rats and mice) suggest that the herb extracts at the prescribed human dose are unlikely to produce untoward effects [106, 107], the respective products should be avoided in pregnancy due to their potential to cause uterine contractions [102].

Natural product-drug interactions

One study reported that berberine may decrease the effectiveness of tetracycline antibiotics [101]. Goldenseal inhibits cytochrome P450 3A4 *in vitro*, a fact which might lead to higher levels of drugs that are normally metabolized by this isoenzyme [45]. However, a pharmacokinetic study in volunteers receiving the CYP 3A4 substrate indinavir before and after 14 days of treatment with goldenseal did not reveal any significant interaction [108].

*Ivy leaf (*Hedera helix*)*

Ivy, also called common ivy or English ivy, is a woody, evergreen, climbing or creeping vine ubiquitous in Europe, North America (naturalized), South America, southwest Asia and Australia.

Ivy leaf extracts are used in acute respiratory tract infections and in cases of irritating cough in consequence of common cold. The therapeutical range also covers management of productive cough and bronchospasms, making the ivy extract adequate for the treatment of acute bronchitis and chronic obstructive pulmonary disease (including allergic bronchitis). Usual preparations are tablets/pastilles and a syrup made of dried ivy leaf extracts alone or in combination with thyme.

Clinical studies with ivy leaf

Although many studies on ivy leaf extracts deal more with chronic obstructive pulmonary disease-specific parameters, some of them reveal valuable information on the alleviation of common cold symptoms. When applied over a median duration of treatment of 12 days to 62 patients, both doctors and patients assessed the tolerability of a cough syrup with ivy and thyme as good or very good (97% of all responses). The efficacy in reducing irritating cough in consequence of common cold was also considered good or very good [109]. The results are in line with earlier publications on different types of ivy leaf preparations [110].

In one randomized double-blind, placebo-controlled study on 24 children aged 4–12 years, a daily dose of 35 mg ivy extract (3-day treatments followed by 3–5-day washout periods) resulted in clinically relevant improvement in airway resistance during the 3–4 weeks of treatment [111].

In a multicenter, prospective, post-marketing study, focusing on chronic bronchitis, 1350 male and female patients received an ivy leaf special extract. During an observational period of 4 weeks, over 90% of patients (adults and children) displayed an excellent amelioration of symptoms for cough and expectoration when treated with daily doses of 97.5–130 mg of dried ivy extract [112].

The antitussive and expectorant effects are apparently related to the saponins hederacosid C and α-hederin. They increase the mucociliary transport and the liquefaction of bronchial mucus, combined with a relaxation of bronchiolar muscles [113, 114].

Adverse and side effects

No significant adverse effects have been reported so far. According to German Commission E, suggested doses of dried herb for oral administration are between 0.002–0.005 g/day (infants up to 1 year of age) and 0.2–0.3 g/day (10–16 years) [115].

Natural product-drug interactions

No significant interactions reported.

Apitherapy/bee products (honey, propolis, pollen, royal jelly)

Honey is a traditional home remedy for colds and cough. It is very popular, alone or with hot tea, both in the eastern hemisphere (India, Pakistan, Korea, Sri Lanka) or in the western one (USA, Guyana, Puerto Rico) [86].

Honey contains enzymes, hormones, inhibins, and, dark-colored honey in particular, phenolic antioxidants. Honey may work by coating and soothing an irritated throat, but possesses in addition an antibacterial and antiviral potential, which is equally ascribed to pollen and propolis (bee glue) [116, 117].

In a randomized, partially double-blinded study, 105 children aged 2–18 years received honey, honey-flavored dextromethorphan or no treatment 30 minutes prior to bedtime. Significant differences in symptom improvement were detected between treatment groups, with honey consistently scoring the best and no treatment scoring the worst. Hence, honey may be a preferable treatment for cough and sleep difficulty associated with childhood URTIs [117, 118].

A study on therapeutic experiences with bee products among beekeepers describes positive experiences in using honey, propolis, pollen and royal jelly, which they employ for various indications. Propolis is most frequently used for treating the common cold, wounds and burns, sore throats, gingival disorders and also as a general prophylactic. It shows good antibacterial, antiviral and antifungal properties and stimulates the immune system. In addition, propolis inhibits inflammations, improves blood circulation in mucous membranes and alleviates pains and tensions. No adverse experiences were reported by the beekeepers [119].

Adverse and side effects

Honey is not recommended for infants younger than 1 year old, because of the risk of botulism.

Ayurvedic remedies for common cold

According to Ayurveda principles most of the illnesses of the respiratory system originate from a disturbance of *kapha* (phlegm). Patients with an excess of *kapha* are prone to develop common colds, flu, tonsillitis, pharyngitis, bronchitis, asthma or pneumonia. On the other side excess *vata* energy reduces *agni* (here understood as gastric fire) producing chills and shivers.

In case of colds or flu Ayurveda proposes an anti-*kapha* and anti-*ama* diet. The patients should avoid red meat, dairy products, oily, heavy or humid food. Recommended are lemon juice and preparations with ginger, holy basil, clove, cinnamon, long pepper (pippali), eye of bamboo, licorice, fennel seeds, turmeric, mint (to mention just a few).

In both ayurvedic and traditional Chinese medicine, ginger is considered the best home remedy for colds. Special appreciation is given also to long pepper (*Piper longum*), which is a good stimulant for the digestive and respiratory systems, is strongly heating, diminishes congestion and helps improving the lung function.

Ayurvedic recipes that are effective in treatment of common cold are, for example, Talisadi churna (demulcent, sedative, expectorant) or Sitopaladi churna (decongestant, expectorant). Prolonged and stubborn cough may be controlled by karkata shringi (*Rhus glabra*), bibhitaki (*Terminalia belerica*) and kalmus (*Acorus calamus*) together with honey in different preparations [120]. Also widespread is Pippali Rasayana based on long pepper and containing a multitude of herbal extracts and powders. The Chyavanprash formula helps building immunity and prevents recurrent colds.

Homeopathic remedies

Introductory remarks

In spite of the huge number of notes and articles dealing with homeopathy, it is still difficult to select a sufficient number of papers from the open literature to form an opinion on the effectiveness of this type of remedies against common cold. This stems to a large extent from the particularities of homeopathic therapy, making the interpretation of study results far from easy. For a better understanding of the data and of the encountered difficulties, some laws and principles of homeopathy have been outlined below.

- The central doctrine of homeopathy coined by S. Hahnemann and known as the law of Similia says: "Similia similibus curantur" (like shall be cured by like). A substance provoking a certain range of symptoms in a healthy person has (in a more or less diluted form) the potential to cure or alleviate the illness featuring exactly the same signs. The intake of the remedy triggers antagonistic reactions to the pathological process and mobilizes the body's own regenerative forces.

- Illness is an individual expression of imbalance and disharmony in the body. Symptoms are nothing else than reactions of the body's defense mechanisms attempting to restore order and harmony.
- An illness appears under many variations, every person may have a different array of symptoms. Before establishing a diagnosis and prescribing a remedy the homeopath will not only go through a careful case history and ask very detailed questions about type of signs, their appearance and time course but will also study the patient's personality, temperament, emotions, preferences and aversions.
- The selection of the right remedy is individualized to a high degree too. Five persons suffering apparently from the same illness may receive five different prescriptions.
- Homeopathy states that the smaller the dose, the quicker and better the curative effect of it. Not the number of molecules is important for the effect but the power of information incorporated in the carrier material. Therefore, drugs are prepared by a series of dilutions using a decimal, a centesimal or an LM (1:50000) scale. The dilutions follow a standard operational procedure (e.g., by succession). The higher the dilution, the more "potentized" the resulting mixture will be.

Homeopaths bring, among others, the following arguments in favor of their therapy:

- Allopathy treats more or less individual symptoms (e.g., inflammation or hypertension). A person is treated and not cured. On the other hand, homeopathy uses a holistic approach to re-establish the homeostatic balance of the patient, as the remedy addresses physical, mental and emotional deregulations.
- Homeopathic remedies are safe, free of side effects. They may produce in the early phase of treatment stronger symptoms, this "initial worsening" is regarded as a proof for their effectiveness and is not long lasting.
- Homeopathic remedies are relatively cheap.

The critic of homeopathy includes:

- The selection of the remedies was not based on logical, deductive thinking. Hahnemann and his followers tested substances on healthy people, registered the signs and hoped that these compounds will be effective for sick people showing similar symptoms.
- Within a group of patients, homeopaths may propose a multitude of remedies for the same illness. This is *per se* a major obstacle when assessing the results of a clinical study.

- A homeopath may change repeatedly during the course of the treatment both the potency and/or the remedy. Hence, it is very difficult to have here adequate data for a solid statistical analysis.
- There is, up to now, no proof for the allegation that information of the remedy is getting more powerful through potentiation, and may be kept and transmitted by water or sugar molecules.
- Even in the case of positive results in a study, a repetition of the study will not lead to a duplication of results. Positive outcomes after a homeopathic treatment are either based on spontaneous healing or spontaneous improving of health status and on the placebo effect.

Despite this controversy homeopathy should be mentioned here to provide a comprehensive overview about traditional and alternative methods to deal with common cold.

Evaluation of clinical trials

A good overview of the available homeopathic literature (1978–2006) in the fields of immunology and common inflammatory diseases was delivered by Bellavite et al. [121]. The authors analyzed, among others, nine trials dealing with conditions reported as acute rhinitis, common cold and flu, respiratory tract complains or ear complains, or URTIs.

Considering the test conditions, four trials were double-blind and randomized [122–125], three were non-blinded, randomized clinical trials (two of them using acetylsalicylic acid as allopathic term of comparison) [126–128], and two studies were non-randomized and used again allopathic drugs for equivalence [129, 130].

Considering the test compounds, in two trials [124, 126] patients received either a single homeopathic remedy or had to select one single out of three homeopathic medications. Four trials [122, 123, 127, 130] used commercial available fixed-mixtures of homeopathic remedies, and in the other three trials [125, 128, 129] individualized homeopathic medicine was used. The results of these studies allow following conclusions:

- The particularities of homeopathy make it very difficult to get substantial benefits when treating a large number of individuals with one single remedy at one fixed potency.
- It is easier to perform trials to prove the effectiveness of complex homeopathic medicines than trials that require individualized treatment. In two [122, 130] out of four of the performed studies with homeopathic mixtures, some slight improvements regarding symptom relief and number of asymptomatic patients at end of treatment were noticed. However, the results are not statistically significant and in toto still not convincing.

- Double-blinded, randomized clinical trials with individualized and adjusted type of homeopathic medication seem to offer some advantages when compared both against placebo as well as against allopathic medication. Better scores were obtained for mean daily symptom score and for the duration of symptoms. The data are more difficult to interpret, as randomization and blinding are rather obstacles when dealing with in-depth anamnesis and individual adjustment of remedy and potency.

The above-mentioned trials support the conclusion that homeopathic treatments seem to have rather a potential to cure than to prevent URTIs.

Bellavite et al. concluded their review by stating "we are in the situation that if we adopt the strict criteria of evidence-based medicine ...the analysis of published literature on homeopathy finds little evidence of superiority of homeopathic medicines over placebo. If we accept observational studies and equivalence studies as valuable tools of investigation, we find many proofs of effectiveness of homeopathy".

Traditional homeopathic treatments for common cold

General remarks

The list of remedies outlined below does not claim to be complete or irrefutable. It reflects, however, the agreement of many homeopaths based on their knowledge and experience. In addition, the 'recommendation' as below refers mostly to [131, 132].

In the case of the acute rhinitis, homeopathy may propose starting the treatment with an organotropic remedy. Especially in the case of a longer illness or frequent reinfections, and sometimes from the very beginning, the analysis of the person's constitutional type will precede the selection of the remedy.

The use of combination remedies is becoming more and more popular. The ready-to-use mixtures for treating common cold often contain *Aconitum*, *Bryonia*, *Echinacea*, *Eupatorium*, *Gelsemium*, and *Lachesis*.

Aconitum napellus (monkshood)

Main indications are: illnesses with a quick onset of symptoms and intense, almost unbearable pains, inflammations with fever, sunstroke, shock, cystitis, and delayed menstruation.

Controlled clinical studies for common cold are not known. Recommended in the early stages of the illness, in the case that the symptoms are intense and come on suddenly after initial strong headache (especially frontal region). Signs include a dry stuffy nose with a hot thin discharge, repetitive sneezing, a burning sore throat, a tension in the chest. A chocking, barking cough is accompanied by a bitter taste lingering in the patient's mouth.

Warning: *A. napellus* is highly toxic; therefore, extreme caution is required when selecting the potency.

Allium cepa (onion)

Main indications are: colds, allergic rhinitis, cough, and inflammations of the eyes, with watery discharge.

Controlled clinical studies for common cold are not known. Recommended for common colds with clear watery discharge that burns and/or irritates the nostrils and upper lip. The person has red, burning, watery eyes, a teasing cough and much sneezing on certain occasions (e.g., when getting up out of bed). The signs worsen in warm rooms and in the evening; the general condition improves in open air.

Arsenicum album (arsenic)

Main indications are: common cold, flu, allergic rhinitis, digestive disorders, skin rash, dysuria. The patient feels chilly, weak and restless and has pains like burning pinpricks.

Controlled clinical studies for common cold are not known. Recommended for persons with frequent colds (in the acute phase), showing a congested nose and a thin watery to white discharge that irritates nose and upper lip. Also frequent are a sore throat, throbbing headache and chest problems. Nasal congestion is not relieved by sneezing. The person feels thirsty and drinks small sips of cold fluids.

Warning: Arsenicum album is toxic and especially harmful in the case of a prolonged intake; therefore, extreme caution is required when selecting the potency.

Solanum dulcamara (bittersweet, woody nightshade)

Main indications are: respiratory tract (rhinitis, angina, bronchitis, asthma bronchiale) digestive tract (vomitus, watery-yellow diarrhea), urinary tract (cystitis, stranguria) and conjunctivitis.

Controlled clinical studies for common cold are not known. Recommended when feeling ill after getting wet and chilled, or when the cold is brought by weather changes from hot to cold. Also indicated when an already existing cold tends to aggravate. Patients needing *S. dulcamara* also tend to allergies. Frequent signs are profuse, watery discharge from nose and eyes (nasal discharge worse in warm rooms) and facial pain.

Euphrasia (*E. officinalis*, *E. stricta*, *E. rostkoviana*) (eyebright)

Main indications are: ophthalmological complaints (conjunctivitis, blepharitis, blepharospasmus, dakryorrhea), rhinitis, flu, chronic gastritis, ulcus duodeni.

Controlled clinical studies for common cold are not known. Recommended when rhinitis is accompanied by clear ophthalmological complaints. The persons show excessive ocular watery discharge with or without burning sensation. Nasal discharge especially in the morning hours without dermal or mucosal irritation. Signs tend to worsen at night and in the morning; the person avoids sunlight and bright lights (tendency to photophobia).

Gelsemium (gelsemium, yellow jessamine)

Main indications are: muscle tissue (aching, weakness), nervous system (tremor, twitching, paralysis), colds, flu, inflammations, children's illnesses. The gelsemium type of patient feels weak, lethargic, exhausted, sleepy, is trembling and has occipital headaches.

Controlled clinical studies for common cold are not known. Recommended when the illness starts in hot weather and with a gradual onset. Patients describe the sensation of a lump on one's throat and a stuffed up nose, although irritant nasal discharge is mostly present. Also frequent are otolaryngeal pains or a pressure felt in the face and nose.

Hepar sulfuris calcareum (mixture of calcium carbonate and sulfur)

Main indications are: skin, mucous membranes. Important in the treatment of purulent inflammations (suppurating abscesses, pyoderma, bronchitis, pneumonia). Indicated for persons showing increased sensitivity toward sensorial stimuli in general.

Controlled clinical studies for common cold are not known. Recommended for late stages of common cold when nasal discharge turns from watery to thick, is yellow and has an acid or foul odor; proneness to coughing fit (hacking) when exposed to cold air. Patients express strong perspiration and symptoms tend to worsen in the evening.

Mercurius solubilis (mixture with mercury oxide as main component)

Main indications are: lymphatic system, salivary glands, tonsils, mucous membranes. Can be used to cure inflammations in the buccal cavity, in the pharyngeal/laryngeal region, and to relieve some ear and eye complaints.

Controlled clinical studies for common cold are not known. Recommended when tonsils or ears may become involved, the patient shows swollen lymph nodes and complains about bad breath and a sore throat that resists treatment. Nasal discharges may be either thin, acid, burning and unpleasant smelling or thick and green-yellow.

Warning: mercury is toxic and has a strong bioaccumulation potential. Extreme caution is required when selecting the right potency (especially with kidney function impairment, gestation and lactation period, babies and toddlers).

Nux vomica (poison-nut)

Main indications are: digestive tract complains, headache, evident proneness to catch a cold. The *nux vomica* type of personality shows an enhanced irritability and nervosity, is impatient, annoyed and sensitive to sounds and lights.

Controlled clinical studies for common cold are not known. Recommended for common cold when abundant nasal discharge during the day is followed by a congested nose and a stuffy head during the night time or in open air. Also present are violent sneezing, a sore throat, harsh cough and chilliness.

Pulsatilla (*Anemone nigricans*, pasque flower)

Main indications are: psychosomatic illnesses, mucous membranes, genital organs. Appropriate remedy for children and persons with psychic instability, quick mood swings and who succumb easily to external influence.

Controlled clinical studies for common cold are not known. Recommended in cases where a congested nose prevails despite repetitive sneezing and production of thick yellow-green mucus. Symptoms tend to worsen in warm environment and when lying in bed, they get better when sitting up or in cold open air.

Short mentions of further homeopathic remedies

Barium carbonicum

This is best suited for children with a tendency to repetitive colds, status lymphaticus and slow physical and mental development. Swollen upper lip, lymph nodes, tonsils and adenoids are typical signs.

Belladona (deadly nightshade)

For sudden onset with high fever (delirium possible), flushed face, restlessness, throbbing, hammering headache (worse when moving). Bright, red and dry sore throat; sometimes a sensation like nagging tickle in the throat.

Warning: *Belladona* is highly toxic; therefore, extreme caution is required when selecting the potency.

Bryonia alba (bryony)
For colds which move to pharynx, larynx and bronchi having as main sign a spastic cough with sharp chest pain. Other symptoms may include burning eyes, a dull headache, little or no nasal discharge and diarrhea.

Carbo vegetabilis (charcoal)
Especially appropriate for treatment of colds with frequent but not so easy sneezing and congested nose. Coughing provokes difficulties in breathing and produces large quantities of thick, sticky mucus.

Eupatorium perfoliatum
Effective against fever, exhaustion, muscular and joint pains. In addition, it boosts the immune system (best in combination with *Echinacea*) and helps the self-healing processes.

Ipecacuanha (Brazilian or Para ipecac)
Congested nose during the night followed by fits of hoarse coughing with choking and vomiting in the morning.

Kali bichromicum (potassium bichromate)
Indicated for the late stages of a cold when sinusitis is also present. Congested nose; the person may experience pain at the root of the nose. Thick, stringy mucus, difficult to clear from nose and throat.

Phosphorus
Indicated for colds where the lungs may be also affected. Patients responding well to this remedy show laryngitis, hoarseness with strong tickling feeling of the vocal cords and often nosebleeds after blowing his/her nose. Unilateral headaches (above the eye) are also probable.

Warning: Phosphorus is toxic and strong irritant. Extreme caution is required when selecting the right potency.

Rhus toxicodendron (*Toxicodendron radicans*)
Colds often begin with stiffness and body aches, especially during cool damp weather or weather changes. Main signs are violent sneezing and strong nasal discharge in the morning hours, sore throat or even dysphagy, swollen dry lymph nodes and permanent thirst. The person feels extremely restless.

Medication according to Dr. Schuessler's method

Main remedies offered by Schuessler's biochemistry to treat common cold are Ferrum phosphoricum and Manganum sulfuricum; some authors mention also Natrium muriaticum [133–135]. In spite of clinical observations and reports on individual treatments, no data on clinical studies have been found in the open literature.

Ferrum phosphoricum is often taken to prevent a cold and can stop rhinitis from developing if taken right away. The typical patient feels weak, very weary, has slight fever, a flushed face or rosy cheeks and a short hard cough.

Manganum sulfuricum is a salt that has a stimulating action on the immune system and can be always recommended to prevent or treat common cold, flu or non-viral laryngitis.

Acupuncture and acupressure

Traditional Chinese acupuncture [136–139]

A main point for treatment of common cold is LI 4 (Hegu) located on the large intestine (LI) meridian. It is a source point recommended for rhinorrhea, nasal obstruction, epistaxis and pharyngitis. Provided that LI 4 is alerted during the right time window in the prodromal phase of the common cold, one may even block the further development of the illness. Using LI 4 alone at a later stage brings only smaller benefits.

One widespread option to influence an ongoing common cold is the combination LI 4 + LI 19 or LI 20 + SI 3. LI 19 (Kou Heliao) is very effective to reopen a blocked nasal passage. LI 20 (Yingxiang) regulates the nasal discharge. SI 3 (Houxi) is located on the small intestine (SI) meridian, acts in general on all mucous membranes and is helpful in case of a sore throat.

To improve breathing through the nose, Chinese acupuncture selected a triad composed of LI 20 + B 2 + PdM. B 2 (Zanzhu), located on the urinary bladder meridian, is also indicated in cases of sinusitis, pain in the supraorbital region as well as for ocular conjunctivitis and lacrimation. PdM (Point de Merveille/Yintang) a.k.a GV 24.5 (located on the governing vessel) helps in cases of rhinorrhea, headache, and increases the mucosal discharge.

Worth mentioning among other points are SJ 17 and Ren 17. SJ 17 (Yifeng), situated on the triple heater/Sanjiao meridian, is important in the treatment of rhinitis, sinusitis, otitis and tinnitus; it also improves breathing through the nose. Ren 17 (Shanzhong/Tanzhong), a point on the conception vessel, plays a role in most of thoracic complains and illnesses, clears the lungs, resolves phlegm and helps to control asthma.

Japanese style acupuncture

In one multi-center randomized-controlled test, 321 subjects were evaluated over a 2-week experimental and a 2-week follow-up period in terms of preventive and curative potential of acupuncture against common cold. The Y point at the throat was used bilaterally and four sessions were performed in total during the treatment time. The evaluation was done on the base of a common cold diary and questionnaire.

While statistically significantly fewer symptoms were reported in the questionnaire by the acupuncture group ($p=0.024$, general linear model, repeated measure), the difference between groups for the diary score was not significant. On the other hand the test detected significant inter-center and sex differences [140].

Although the test design has been subsequently modified, changing acupuncture for indirect moxibustion and elongating the treatment period to a maximum of 12 weeks, clear differences could not be reported [141].

Acupressure for common cold [142, 143]

In case of rhinitis, one should press on the point ST 3 (Juliao), located on the stomach (ST) meridian, directly below the pupil in a depression of the zygomatic bone, on a level with the lower border of the ala nasi. Pressure is applied upwards (to the eye). It is possible to continue by acupressure of LI 4, LI 20 (see above) and on G 20 (Fengchi) located on the gall bladder meridian.

Especially in the case of a cold with a dry cough and fever the points of choice should be K 27 + G 20 + LI 20 (some sources recommend to also activate GV 14. K 27 (Shufu) is situated in the depressions directly below the protrusions on the left and right side of the collar bone (sternoclavicular joint) on the kidney meridian. GV 14 (Dashui) is located in a small depression below the C 7 spinous process.

Saline nasal irrigation

This was originally a traditional Hatha-Yoga and Ayur Veda technique, called Jala-neti, pouring warm salty water (jala) into one nostril at a time and letting it to flow out through the other nostril. It is thought to cure disorders of *kapha* including headache, sinusitis, eye and ear illnesses. Traditionally, a neti pot is used; however there are nowadays a variety of more modern and convenient devices available.

The twice-a-day use of the nasal irrigation with isotonic (physiological) saline over several days can significantly contribute to the alleviation of symptoms triggered by a URTI [144, 145].

A clear improvement of the function of the ciliated epithelium is achieved through rinsing of mucous membranes of nose and sinuses.

Slightly hypertonic (hyperosmolar) saline solutions may be more effective, having in addition an anticongestive effect [146]. One may add a few drops of ethereal oils to the lukewarm saline or use a chamomile concoction for nasal irrigation.

The procedure appears to be safe and beneficial with no apparent or only very minor side effects.

Inhalation

Inhalations may be more effective than nasal irrigation because the ingredients vaporize and are optimally dispersed onto the nasal mucosa. A simple and easy to use mixture can be prepared on the base of a very hot chamomille tea by adding some drops of thyme or eucalyptus oil. Inhalation should last 10–20 minutes and be repeated two to three times per day [147, 148].

Other remedies or methods

Not mentioned are methods such as: moxibustion, use of suction cups to draw blood and relieve congestion of respiratory tract, massages and ointments with oils, alcohols, aromatic preparations or with mustard paste, teas and soups (including the famous chicken soup), gargling with warm salt (or salt/vinegar) water, procedures to stimulate the immune system such as: auto blood transfusion, aerobic exercise, hydrotherapy (like hot bath and steam, sauna, Kneipp's cure), aromatherapy, diet (refraining from some types of products). This should not be understood as a sign of nonappreciation but as a result of the limited available space or paucity of adequate data.

Acknowledgement

The author thanks Gabrielle Schmuck, Ph. D. And Mrs. Lieselotte Wolff for their great assistance with literature search and data selection.

References

1 Poolsup N, Suthhisisang C, Prathanturarug S, Asawamekin A, Chanchareon U (2004) *Andrographis paniculata* in the symptomatic treatment of uncomplicated upper respiratory tract infection: systematic review of randomized controlled trials. *J Clin Pharm Ther* 29 (1): 37–45

2 Coon J T and Ernst E (2004) *Andrographis paniculata* in the treatment of upper respiratory tract infections: a systematic review of safety and efficacy. *Planta Med* 70 (4): 293–298

3 Kigler B, Ulbricht C, Basch E, DeFranco Kirkwood C, Abrams TR, Miranda M, Kahlsa KPS, Giles M, Boon H, Woods J (2006) *Andrographis paniculata* for the treatment of upper respiratory infection: a systematic review by the Natural Standard Research Collaboration. *Explore* 2 (1): 25–29
4 Gabrielian ES, Shukarian AK, Goukasova, GI, Chandanian GL, Panosian AG, Wikman G, Wagner H (2002) A double-blind, placebo-controlled study of *Andrographis paniculata* fixed combination Kan Jang in the treatment of acute upper respiratory tract infections including sinusitis. *Phytomedicine* 9 (7): 589–597
5 Melchior J, Spasov AA, Ostrovskij OV, Bulanov AE, Wikman G (2000) Double-blind, placebo-controlled pilot and phase III study of activity of standardized *Andrographis paniculata* Herba Nees extract fixed combination (Kan Jang) in the treatment of uncomplicated upper-respiratory tract infection. *Phytomedicine* 7 (5): 341–350
6 Spasov AA, Ostrovskij OV, Chernikov MV, Wikman G (2004) Comparative controlled study of *Andrographis paniculata* fixed combination, Kan Jang and an *Echinacea* preparation as adjuvant, in the treatment of uncomplicated respiratory disease in children. *Phytother Res* 18 (1): 47–53
7 Caceres DD, Hancke JL, Burgos RA (1997) Prevention of common colds with *Andrographis paniculata* dried extract; a pilot double blind study. *Phytomedicine* 4: 101–104
8 Caceres DD, Hancke JL, Burgos RA, Sandberg F, Wikman GK (1999) Use of visual analogue scale measurements (VAS) to assess the effectiveness of standardized *Andrographis paniculata* extract SHA-10 in reducing the symptoms of common cold. A randomized double blind-placebo study. *Phytomedicine* 6: 217–223
9 Mkrtchyan A., Panosyan V, Panossian A, Wigman G, Wagner H (2005) A phase I clinical study of *Andrographis paniculata* fixed combination Kan Jang *versus* ginseng and valerian on the semen quality of healthy male subjects. *Phytomedicine* 12 (6–7): 403–409
10 KLIGLER B (2003) *Echinacea. Am Fam Physician* 67: 77–80
11 Dorn M, Knick E, Lewith G (1997) Placebo-controlled, double-blind study of *Echinaceae pallidae* radix in upper respiratory tract infections. *Complement Ther Med* 5: 40–42
12 Basch E, Ulbricht C, Basch S, Dalton S, Ernst E, Foppa I, Szapary P, Tiffany N, Orlando CW, Vora M (2005) An evidence-based systematic review of *Echinacea* (*E. angustifolia* DC, *E. pallida*, *E. purpurea*) by the Natural Standard Research Collaboration. *J Herbal Pharmacotherapy* 5(2): 57–88
13 Schapowal A (2007) Phytopharmaka bei Atemwegsinfekten in der Pädiatrie (Herbals for respiratory tract infection in paediatrics). *Z Phytother* 28 (4): 174–180
14 Barrett B, Kiefer D and Rabago D (1999) Assessing the risks and benefits of herbal medicine: an overview of scientific evidence. *Alt Therapies* 5(4): 40–49
15 Snodgrass WR (2001) Herbal products: risks and benefits of use in children. *Current Therapeutic Research* 62(10): 724–737
16 Sun LZ, Currier NL, Miller SC (1999) The American coneflower: a prophylac-

tic role involving nonspecific immunity. *J Altern Complement Medment Med* 5(5): 437–46
17 Jurkstiene V, Kondrotas AJ, Kevelaitis E (2004) Compensatory reactions of immune system and action of Purple Coneflower (*Echinacea purpurea* (L.) Moench) preparations. *Medicina (Kaunas)* 40(7): 657–62
18 Burger RA, Torres AR, Warren RP, Caldwell VD, Hughes BG (1997) *Echinacea*-induced cytokine production by human macrophages. *Int J Immunopharmacol* 19(7): 371–9
19 Luettig B, Steinmüller C, Gifford GE, Wagner H, Lohmann-Matthes ML (1989) Macrophage activation by the polysaccharide arabinogalactan isolated from plant cell cultures of *Echinacea purpurea. J Natl Cancer Inst* 81(9): 669–75
20 See DM, Broumand N, Sahl L, Tilles JG (1997) *In vitro* effects of *Echinacea* and ginseng on natural killer and antibody-dependent cell cytotoxicity in healthy subjects and chronic fatigue syndrome or acquired immunodeficiency syndrome patients *Immunopharmacology* 35(3): 229–35
21 Mishima S, Saito K, Maruyama H, Inoue M, Yamashita T, Gu Y (2004) Antioxidant and immuno-enhancing effects of *Echinacea purpurea. Biol Pharm Bull* 27(7): 1004–9
22 Sullivan AM, Laba JG, Moore JA, Lee TD (2008) *Echinacea*-induced macrophage activation. *Immunopharmacol Immunotoxicol* 30(3): 553–74
23 Schwarz E, Metzler J, Diedrich JP, Freudenstein J, Bode C, Bode JC (2002) Oral administration of freshly expressed juice of *Echinacea purpurea* herbs fail to stimulate the nonspecific immune response in healthy young men: results of a double-blind, placebo-controlled crossover study. *J Immunother* 25(5):413–20
24 Schwarz E, Parlesak A, Henneicke-von Zepelin HH, Bode JC, Bode C (2005) Effect of oral administration of freshly pressed juice of *Echinacea purpurea* on the number of various subpopulations of B- and T-lymphocytes in healthy volunteers: results of a double-blind, placebo-controlled cross-over study. *Phytomedicine* 12(9): 625–31
25 Goel V, Lovlin R, Chang C, Slama JV, Barton R, Gahler R, Bauer R, Goonewardene L, Basu TK (2005) A proprietary extract from the *Echinacea* plant (*Echinacea purpurea*) enhances systemic immune response during a common cold. *Phytother Res* 19(8): 689–94
26 Melchart D, Linde K, Workau F, Bauer R, Wagner H (1994) Immunomodulation with *Echinacea* – a systematic review of controlled clinical trials. *Phytomedicine* 1: 245–254
27 Bräunig B, Dorn M, Knick E (1992) Zur Stärkung der körpereigenen Abwehr bei grippalen Infekten durch *Echinaceae purpureae* radix (*Echinacea purpurea* radix fort the enhancement of the body's own immune defense mechanisms in influenza-like infections). *Z Phytother* 13: 7–13
28 Barrett B, Vohmann M, Calabrese C (1999) *Echinacea* for upper respiratory infections. *J Fam Pract* 48(8): 628–635
29 Giles JT, Palat CT 3rd, Chien SH, Chang ZG, Kennedy DT (2000). Evaluation of *Echinacea* for treatment of the common cold. *Pharmacotherapy* 20(6):690–7
30 Melchart D, Linde K, Fischer P, Kaesmayr J (1999) *Echinacea* for preventing

and treating the common cold. *Cochrane Database Syst Rev* (1):CD000530. pub2

31 Cohen HA, Varsano I, Kahan E, Sarrell EM, Uziel Y (2004) Effectiveness of an herbal preparation containing *Echinacea*, propolis, and vitamin C in preventing respiratory tract infections in children: a randomized, double-blind, placebo-controlled, multicenter study. *Arch Pediatr Adolesc Med* 158(3): 217–21

32 Caruso TJ, Gwaltney JM Jr (2005) Treatment of the common cold with *Echinacea*: a structured review *Clin Infect Dis* 40(6): 807–10 Epub 2005 Feb 18.

33 Taylor J, Weber W, Standish L, Quinn H, Goesling J, McGann M, Calabrese C (2003) The efficacy of *Echinacea* in treating upper respiratory tract infections in children. *JAMA* 290: 2824–30

34 Barrett B, Locken K, Maberry R, Brown R, Bobula J, Alessio D (2002) Treatment of common cold with unrefined *Echinacea*. *Ann Intern Med* 137: 1–8

35 Schoop R, Klein P, Suter A, Johnston SL (2006) *Echinacea* in the prevention of induced rhinovirus colds: a meta-analysis. *Clin Ther* 28(2): 174–83

36 Shah SA, Sander S, White CM, Rinaldi M, Coleman CI (2007) Evaluation of *Echinacea* for the prevention and treatment of the common cold: a meta-analysis. *Lancet Infect Dis* 7(7): 473–80

37 Linde K, Barrett B, Bauer R, Melchart D, Wölkart K (2008) *Echinacea* for preventing and treating the common cold (review). Cochrane Database Syst Rev. prepared by the Cochrane Collaboration. *The Cochrane Library* 4: 1–91

38 Woelkart K, Linde K, Bauer R (2008) *Echinacea* for preventing and treating the common cold. *Planta Med* 74: 633–637

39 Huntley AL, Thompson Coon J, Ernst E (2005) The safety of herbal medicinal products derived from *Echinacea* species: a systematic review. *Drug Safety* 28(5): 387–400

40 The Natural Standard Research Collaboration *Echinacea* (*Echinacea angustifolia* DC, *Echinacea pallida*, *Echinacea purpurea*) *MayoClinic.com; Drugs & Supplements; Patient Monograph*, Copyright © 2008

41 Ang-Lee MK, Moss J, Yuan C-S (2001) Herbal medicines and perioperative care. *JAMA* 286(2): 208–216

42 Blumenthal M, Busse WR, Goldberg A, Gruenwald J, Hall T, Riggins CW, Rister RS (eds) (1998) *The Complete German Commission E Monographs: Therapeutic Guide to Herbal Medicines.* Austin (TX): American Botanical Council; Boston: Integrative Medicine Communication

43 Miller LG (1998) Herbal Medicinals – Selected clinical considerations focusing on known or potential drug-herb interactions *Arch Intern Med* 158: 2200–2211

44 The University of Texas – MD Anderson Cancer Center (2008) *Echinacea* (*Echinacea angustifolia* DC, *Echinacea pallida*, *Echinacea purpurea*). *Natural Standard Monograph*, Copyright © 2008, accessed Dec. 8, 2008

45 Budzinski JW, Foster BC, Vandenhoek S, Arnason JT (2000) An *In vitro* evaluation of human cytochrome P450 3A4 inhibition by selected commercial herbal extracts and tinctures. *Phytomedicine* 7(4): 273–82

46 Gorski JC, Huang SM, Pinto A, Hamman MA, Hilligoss JK, Zaheer NA, Desai

M, Miller M, Hall SD (2004) The effect of *Echinacea* (*Echinacea purpurea* root) on cytochrome P450 activity *in vivo*. *Clin Pharmacol Ther* 75(1): 89–100

47 Freeman C, Spelman K (2008) A critical evaluation of drug interactions with *Echinacea* spp. *Mol Nutr Food Res* 52(7): 789–98

48 Hansen TS, Nilsen OG (2008) *In vitro* CYP3A4 metabolism: inhibition by *Echinacea purpurea* and choice of substrate for the evaluation of herbal inhibition. *Basic Clin Pharmacol Toxicol* 103(5): 445–9

49 Heinrich M, Modarai M, Kortenkamp A (2008) Herbal extracts used for upper respiratory tract infections: are there clinically relevant interactions with the cytochrome P450 enzyme system? *Planta Med* 74(6): 657–60

50 Medline plus, a service of the U.S. National Library of Medicine and the National Institutes of Health (update as of January 1, 2008)

51 Cordier H (2003) Verschnupftes Kind Ein Fall für "Schwarzen Holunder" (Child stuffed up with a cold. A case for black elder). *Münchner Med Wochenzeits Fortschr Med* 145 (15): 12

52 Roxas M and Jurenka J (2007) Colds and influenza: a review of diagnosis and conventional, botanical, and nutritional considerations. *Altern Med Rev* 12(1): 25–48

53 Knox Y M, Hayashi K, Suzutani T, Ogasava M, Yoshida I, Shiina R, Tsukui A, Terahara N, Azuma M (2001) Activity of anthocyanins from fruit extract of *Ribes nigrum* L. against influenza A and B viruses. *Acta Virol.* 45 (4), 209–215

54 Zakay-Rones Z, Thom E, Wollan T, Wadstein J. Randomized study of the efficacy and safety of oral elderberry extract in the treatment of influenza A and B virus infections. *J Int Med Res.* 32 (2):132–140; (2004)

55 Zakay-Rones Z, Varsano N, Zlotnik M, Manor O, Regev L, Schlesinger M, Mumcuoglu M (1995) Inhibition of several strains of influenza virus *in vitro* and reduction of symptoms by an elderberry extract (*Sambucus nigra* L) during an outbreak of influenza B Panama. *J Altern Complement Med* 1 (4): 361–369

56 Anon. (2005) Monograph *Sambucus nigra* (Elderberry). *Alternative medicine review* 10 (1): 51–55

57 Foerster-Waldl E., M. Marchetti, I. Schoell, M. Focke, C. Radauer, T. Kinaciyan, I. Nentwich, S. Jaeger, E. R. Schmid, G. Boltz-Nitulescu et al. (2003) Type I allergy to elderberry (*Sambucus nigra*) is elicited by a 33.2 kDa allergen with significant homology to ribosomal inactivating protein. *Clin Exp Allergy* 33 (12) 1703–10

58 Amagase H (2006) Clarifying the real bioactive constituents of garlic. *J Nutr* 136 (3 Suppl): 716–725

59 Ivker RS (2002) Respiratory disease – sinusitis, upper respiratory infection, otitis media. *Clinics in family practice* 4 (4): 929–946

60 Abdullah T (2000) A strategic call to utilize *Echinacea*-garlic in flu-cold seasons J *Nat Med Association* 92 (1): 48–51

61 Josling P (2001) Preventing the common cold with a garlic supplement.; a double-blind, placebo controlled study. *Adv Ther* 18(4): 189–193

62 Andrianova IV, Sobenin IA, Sereda EV, Borodina LI, Studenikin MI (2003) Effect of long-acting garlic tablets "allicor" on the incidence of acute respiratory viral infections in children. *Ther Arkh* 75 (3): 53–56

63 Shamseer L, Charrois TL, Vohra S (2006) Complementary, holistic and integrative medicine: garlic. *Pediatr Rev* 27: 77–80
64 Hiltunen R, Josling PD, James MH (2007) Preventing airborne infection with an intranasal cellulose powder formulation (Nasaleze travel). *Adv Ther* 24 (5): 1146–53
65 Pittler MH, Ernst E (2007) Clinical effectiveness of garlic (*Allium sativum*). *Mol* Nutr *Food Res* (51(11): 1382–1385
66 Anon (2008) *Herbs and Supplements – Garlic.* Copyright © 2008 EBSCO Publishing; last reviewed November 2008 by EBSCO CAM Review Board. Accessed Dec.14, 2008
67 Bielory L (2004) Complementary and alternative interventions in asthma, allergy, and immunology. *Ann Allergy Asthma Immunol* 93 (2 Suppl 1): 45–54
68 Schulz V, Hansel R, Tyler VE (1998) *Rational Phytotherapy: A Physicians' Guide to Herbal Medicine.* 3rd ed. Berlin, Germany: Springer-Verlag; 1998: 121
69 Scott GN and Elmer GW (2002) Update on natural product-drug interactions. *Am J Health Syst Pharm* 59(4): 339–47
70 Scharbert G, Kalb ML, Duris M, Marschalek C, Kozek-Langenecker SA (2007) Garlic at dietary doses does not impair platelet function. *Anesth Analg* 105(5): 1214–8
71 Hu Z, Yang X, Ho PC, Chan SY, Heng PW, Chan E, Duan W, Koh HL, Zhou S (2005) Herb-drug interactions: a literature review. *Drugs* 65(9): 1239–82
72 Macan H, Uykimpang R, Alconcel M, Takasu J, Razon R, Amagase H, Niihara Y (2006) Aged garlic extract may be safe for patients on warfarin therapy. *J Nutr* 136(3): 793–95
73 Aimbire F, Penna SC, Rodrigues M, Rodrigues KC, Lopes-Martins RA, Sertie JA (2007) Effect of hydroalcoholic extract of *Zingiber officinalis* rhizomes on LPS-induced rat airway hyperreactivity and lung inflammation. *Prostaglandins Leukot Essent Fatty Acids* 77 (3–4): 129–138
74 Ghayur MN, Gilani AH, Janssen LJ (2008) Ginger attenuates acetylcholine-induced contraction and Ca^{+} signalling in murine airway smooth muscle cells. *Can J Physiol Pharmacol* 86 (5): 264–271
75 Hong H, Yang F, Liu X-C, Yang y-Q (2006) Effect of shegan mahuang decoction on the changes of interleukin 5 and interleukin 10 in peripheral plasma of asthma guinea pigs. *Chin J Clin Rehab* 10 835): 63–65
76 Park KJ, Lee HH (2005) *In vitro* antiviral activity of aqueous extract from Korean medicinal plants against influenza virus type A. *J Microbiol Biotechnol* 15 (5): 924–929
77 Imanishi N, Andoh T, Mantani N, Sakai S, Terasawa K, Shimada Y, Sato M, Katada Y, Ueda K, Ochiai H (2006) Macrophage-mediated inhibitory effect of Zingiber officinale Rosc., a traditional Oriental herbal medicine, on the growth of influenza A/Aichi/2/68 virus. *Am J Chin Med* 34 (1): 157–169
78 Srivastava KC (1984) Aqueous extracts of onion, garlic and ginger inhibit platelet aggregation and alter arachidonic acid metabolism. *Biomed Biochim Acta (Berlin)* 43 (8/9): 335–346
79 Srivastava KC (1986) Isolation and effects of some ginger components on

platelet aggregation and eicosanoid biosynthesis. *Prostaglandins Leukot Essent Fatty Acids* 35: 183–185
80 Weidner MS, Sigwart K (2000) The safety of a ginger extract in the rat. *J Ethnopharmacol* 73: 513–520
81 Kruth P, Brossi E, Fux R (2004) Ginger-associated over anticoagulation by phenprocoumon. *Acta Pharmacother* 38: 257–260
82 Mascolo N, Jain R, Jain SC, Capasso F (1989) Ethnopharmacologic investigation of ginger. *J Ethnopharmacol* 27: 129–140
83 Bordia A, Verma SK, Srivastava KC (1997) Effect of ginger and fenugreek on blood lipids, blood sugar and platelet aggregation in patients with coronary artery disease. *Prostaglandins Leukotrienes and Essential Fatty Acids* 56 (5): 379–384
84 Mukhopadhyay M, Mukherjee A (2000) Clastogenic effect of ginger rhizome in mice. *Phytother Res* 14: 555–557
85 Erkan ML, Findik S, Tatlisoez H, Ugurlu D, Atici AG (2000) A new etiology of occupational asthma: rhizoma zingiberis. *Ondokuz Mayis Univ Tip Derg* 17(3): 184–186
86 Pfeiffer WF (2005) A multicultural approach to the patient who has common cold. *Pediatrics in review* 26(5): 170–175
87 McElhaney JE, Goel V, Toane B, Hooten J, Shan JJ (2006) Efficacy of Cold-fX in the prevention of respiratory symptoms in community-dwelling adults; a randomized double-blinded, placebo-controlled trial. *J Altern Complement Med* 12(2): 153–157
88 Predy GN, Goel V, Lovlin R, Donner A, Stitt L, Basu TK (2005) Efficacy of an extract of North American ginseng containing poly-furanosyl-pyranosyl-saccharides for preventing upper respiratory tract infections: a randomized controlled study. *Can Med Association J* 173(9): 1043–48
89 McElhaney JE, Gravenstein S, Cole SK, Davidson E, O'Neill D, Petitjean S, Rumble B, Shan JJ (2004) A placebo-controlled trial of a proprietary extract of North American ginseng (CVT-E002) to prevent acute respiratory illness in institutionalized older adults. *J Am Geriatr Soc* 52(1): 13–19
90 Scaglione F, Cattaneo G, Alessandria M, Cogo R (1996) Efficacy and safety of the standardised Ginseng extract G115 for potentiating vaccination against the influenza syndrome and protection against the common cold. *Drugs Exp Clin Res* 22(2): 65–72
91 Vuksan V, Sievenpiper JL, Koo VY, Francis T, Beljan-Zdravkovic U, Xu Z, Vidgen E (2000) American ginseng (*Panax quinquefolium* L) reduces postprandial glycemia in nondiabetic subjects and subjects with type 2 diabetes mellitus. *Arch Intern Med* 160(7): 1009–13
92 Scaglione F, Ferrara F, Dugnani S, Falchi M, Santoro G, Fraschini F (1990) Immunomodulatory effects of two extracts of *Panax ginseng* C.A. Meyer. *Drugs Exp Clin Res* 16(10):537–42
93 Wang M, Guilbert LJ, Ling L, Li J, Wu Y, Xu S, Pang P, Shan JJ (2001) Immunomodulating activity of CVT-E002, a proprietary extract from North American ginseng (*Panax quinquefolium*). *J Pharm Pharmacol* 53(11): 1515–1523
94 Wang M, Guilbert LJ, Li J, Wu Y, Pang P, Basu TK, Shan JJ (2004) A proprietary

extract from North American ginseng (*Panax quinquefolium*) enhances IL-2 and IFN-gamma productions in murine spleen cells induced by Con-A. *J Am Geriatr Soc* 52(1): 13–19

95 Yuan CS, Wei G, Dey L, Karrison T, Nahlik L, Maleckar S, Kasza K, Ang-Lee M, Moss J (2004) Brief communication: American ginseng reduces warfarin's effect in healthy patients: a randomized, controlled trial. *Ann Inten Med* 141(1): 23–7

96 Rabbani GH, Butler T, Knight J, et al. (1987) Randomized controlled trial of berberine sulfate therapy for diarrhea due to enterotoxigenic *Escherichia coli* and *Vibrio cholerae*. *J Infectious Dis* 155(5): 979–984

97 Hwang BY, Roberts SK, Chadwick LR, Wu CD, Kinghorn AD (2003) Antimicrobial constituents from goldenseal (the Rhizomes of *Hydrastis canadensis*) against selected oral pathogens *Planta Med* 69(7): 623–27

98 Anon (2000) Berberine Monograph. *Alternative Medicine Review* 5 (2): 175–177

99 Ckless K, Schlottfeldt JL, Pasqual M, Moyna P, Henriques JA, Wajner M (1995) Inhibition of *in-vitro* lymphocyte transformation by the isoquinoline alkaloid berberine *J Pharm Pharmacol* 47 (12a): 1029–31

100 Huang CG, Chu ZL, Yang ZM (1991) Effects of berberine on synthesis of platelet TXA2 and plasma PGI2 in rabbits. *Chung Kuo Yao Li Hsueh Pao* 12: 526–528

101 Hawkins EB, Ehrlich SD: Goldenseal: online review University of Maryland, Medical Center, review date: 1/24/2007

102 Bedard, M (2002) Goldenseal: high on promises, low on evidence. *Can Pharm J* 135 (9): 44–48

103 Palanisamy A, Haller C, Olson KR (2003) Photosensitivity reaction in a woman using an herbal supplement containing ginseng, goldenseal and bee pollen. *J Toxicol Clin Toxicol* 41 (6): 865–7

104 Chichon PG (2000) Herbs and the common cold. *Evidence for nurse practitioners* 31–32, August 2000

105 Mills Simon, Bone Kerry (2000) *Principles and Practice of Phytotherapy.* Philadelphia, Churchill Livingstone (cited by Hawkins and Ehrlich)

106 Yao M, Ritchie HE, Brown-Woodman PD (2005) A reproductive screening test of goldenseal. *Birth Defects Res B Dev Reprod Toxicol* 74(5): 399–404

107 Jahnke GD, Price CJ, Marr MC, Myers CB, George JD (2006) Developmental toxicity evaluation of berberine in rats and mice. *Birth Defects Res B Dev Reprod Toxicol* 77(3): 195–206

108 Sandhu RS, Prescilla RP, Simonelli TM, Edwards DJ (2003) Influence of goldenseal root on the pharmacokinetics of indinavir. *J Clin Pharmacol* 43(11): 1283–88

109 Büechi S, Voegelin R, von Eiff MM, Ramos M, Melzer J (2005) Open trial to assess aspects of safety and efficacy of a combined herbal cough syrup with ivy and thyme. *Forsch Komplemetärmed Klass Naturheilkunde* 12 (6): 328–333

110 Büechi S and Kähler D (2003) Efeu (*Hedera helix*) bei Atemwegserkrankungen. Eine offene Studie mit Efeu Pastillen (Ivy (*Hedera helix*) for respiratory tract infections. An open study with ivy pastilles). *Schweiz Zschr GanzheitsMedizin* 15, 125–128

111 Mansfeld HJ, Höhre H, Repges R, Dethlefsen U (1998) Therapie des Asthma bronchiale mit Efeublätter-Trockenextrakt (Therapy of asthma bronchiale with ivy leaf dry extract). *Münchner Med Wochenzeits Fortschr Med* 140: 26–30
112 Hecker M, Runkel F, Voelp A (2002) Treatment of chronic bronchitis with ivy special extract – multicenter post-marketing surveillance study in 1350 patients. *Forsch Komplementärmed Klass Naturheilkunde* 9 (2): 77–84
113 Anon (2004) Präparate aus der Efeupflanze lindern lästigen Husten: Molekularer Wirkmechanismus entschlüsselt (Preparations from ivy plants relieve troublesome cough: Molecular mechanism of action deciphered). *Ärztez für Naturheilverfahren* 45 (2): 84 + 86
114 De Mello FB, De Mello JRB (2006) Evaluation of antitussive/expectorant effects of two phytotherapeutic formulations existent in the Brazilian market. *Acta Farm Bonaer* 25 (1) 64–70
115 Hrastinger A, Dietz B, Bauer R, Sagraves R, Mahady G (2005) Is there clinical evidence supporting the use of botanical dietary supplements in children? *J Pediatr*. 146:311–317
116 Wagner L (2004) Die gesundheitliche Wirkung von Bienenerzeugnissen (The health effect of bee products). *Naturheilpraxis* 57(4): 533–537
117 Paul IM, Beiler J, McMonagle A, Shaffer ML, Duda L, Berlin CM Jr (2007) Effect of honey, dextromethorphan, and no treatment on nocturnal cough and sleep quality for coughing children and their parents. *Arch Pediatr Adolesc Med* 161(12): 1140–1146
118 Warren MD, Pont SJ, Barkin SL, Callahan ST, Caples L, Carroll KN, Plemmons GS, Swan RR, Cooper WO (2007) The effect of honey on nocturnal cough and sleep quality for children and their parents. *Arch Pediatr Adolesc Med* 161(12): 1149–1153
119 Hellner M, Winter D, von Georgi R, Münstedt K (2007) Apitherapy: Usage And Experience In German Beekeepers. *eCAM Advance Access* published June 30, 2007, doi:10.1093/ecam/nem052
120 Frawley D (2005) *Das große Ayurveda-Heilungsbuch – Prinzipien und Praxis* (Ayurvedic healing: a comprehensive guide, Lotus Press). Knaur MensSana
121 Bellavite P, Ortolani R, Pontarollo F, Piasere V, Benato G and Conforti A (2006) Immunology and Homeopathy. 4. Clinical Studies – Part 1. *Evid Based Complement Alternat Med* 3(3): 293–301
122 Lecoq PL (1985) L–52. Les voies thérapeuthiques des syndromes grippaux. *Cah Biothér* 87: 65–73.
123 Heilmann A (1994) A combination injection preparation as a prophylactic for flu and common colds. *Biol Ther* 13: 249–53
124 Steinsbekk A, Bentzen N, Fonnebo V, Lewith G (2005) Self treatment with one of three self selected, ultramolecular homeopathic medicines for the prevention of upper respiratory tract infections in children. A double-blind randomized placebo controlled trial. *Br J Clin Pharmacol* 59: 447–55
125 de Lange de Klerk ES, Blommers J, Kuik DJ, Bezemer PD, Feenstra L (1994) Effect of homoeopathic medicines on daily burden of symptoms in children with recurrent upper respiratory tract infections. *BMJ* 309(6965): 1329–32
126 Gassinger CA, Wunstel G, Netter P (1981) A controlled clinical trial for testing

the efficacy of the homeopathic drug *Eupatorium perfoliatum* D2 in the treatment of common cold. *Arzneimittelforschung* 31:732–6
127 Maiwald VL, Weinfurtner T, Mau J, Connert WD (1988) Treatment of common cold with a combination homeopathic preparation compared with acetylsalicylic acid. A controlled, randomized single-blind study. *Arzneimittelforschung* 38: 578–582.
128 Steinsbekk A, Fonnebo V, Lewith G, Bentzen N (2005) Homeopathic care for the prevention of upper respiratory tract infections in children: a pragmatic, randomised, controlled trial comparing individualised homeopathic care and waiting-list controls. *Complement Ther Med* 13: 231–8
129 Riley D, Fischer M, Singh B, Haidvogl M, Heger M (2001) Homeopathy and conventional medicine: an outcomes study comparing effectiveness in a primary care setting. *J Altern Complement Med* 7: 149–59
130 Rabe A, Weiser M, Klein P (2004) Effectiveness and tolerability of a homoeopathic remedy compared with conventional therapy for mild viral infections. *Int J Clin Pract* 58(9): 827–32
131 Danheisser I, Edwards P (1999) *Homöopathie – Sanfte Wege zur Gesundheit.* Könemann Verlagsgesellschaft mbH (Originalausgabe: *Homeopathy, an Illustrated Guide*, element Books Ltd., 1998)
132 *Homöopathisches Repetitorium*, Ausgabe 2007, Deutsche Homöopathie-Union Karlsruhe
133 Leibold G (2004) *Schüßler-Salze*, Oesch/Jopp Verlag, Zürich, 1. Auflage 2004
134 Anon (2008) Ferrum phosphoricum Epub, lexikon-der-schüsslersalze.de, Nr. 3 ferrum phosphoricum, accessed Dec 23, 2008
135 Rother C (2007) Efficacy and tolerance of the anthroposophical remedy Ferrum phosphoricum comp (Infludoron) for beginning and advanced common cold Epub www.anthromed.org, accessed Dec.23, 2008
136 Bischko J (1994) *Einführung in die Akupunktur* (an introduction to acupuncture) Band I, 16. Auflage, Karl F. Haug Verlag, Heidelberg
137 Bischko J (1980) *Akupunktur für mässig Fortgeschrittene* (acupuncture for moderate advanced practitioners) Band II, Textband, 2. Auflage, Karl F. Haug Verlag, Heidelberg
138 Jayasuriya A, Hühne U (1986) *Klinische Akupunktur* (clinical acupuncture) Ulrich-Hühne-Verlag, Colombo, Vertrieb: Karl F. Haug Verlag, Heidelberg, Germany
139 Wertsch, Schrecke, Küstner (1986) *Akupunkturatlas* (Acupuncture Atlas) 6. Auflage, WBV Biologisch-Medizinische Verlagsgesellschaft mbH & Co KG, Schondorf, Germany
140 Kawakita K, Shichidou T, Inoue E, Nabeta T, Kitakouji H, Aizawa S, Nishida A, Yamaguchi N, Takahashi N, Yano T, Tanzawa S (2004) Preventive and curative effects of acupuncture on the common cold: a multicentre randomized controlled trial in Japan. *Complement Ther Med* 12: 181–188
141 Kawakita K, Shichidou T, Inoue E, Nabeta T, Kitakoji H, Aizawa S, Nishida A, Yamaguchi N, Takahashi N, Sumiya E et al. (2008) Do Japanese style acupuncture and moxibustion reduce symptoms of the common cold? *Evid Based Complement Alternat Med* 5: 481–489

142 Ody, Penelope (2000) *Practical Chinese medicine.* Godsfield Press Ltd, German edition 2001 by Urania Verlag AG, Neuhausen/Switzerland
143 Hin, Dr. Kuan (1992) *Chinesische Massage und Akupressur* (Chinese massage and acupressure) 2. erweiterte Auflage 1992, Hallwag Verlag Bern und Stuttgart
144 Neumaier J (2004) Kasse propagiert Nasenspülungen – Billiges Rezept gegen Erkältungen. *MMW-Fortschritte der Medizin* Nr. 3–4, S. 16
145 Papsin B, A McTrevish (2003) Saline nasal irrigation: Its role as an adjuvant treatment. *Can Fam Physician* 49: 168–73
146 Rabago D, Pasic T, Zgierska A, Mundt M, Barrett B, Maberry R (2005) The efficacy of hypertonic saline nasal irrigation for chronic sinonasal symptoms. *Otolaryngology – Head and Neck Surgery* 133 (1): 3–8
147 Leibold G (2002) *Erkältung und Grippe. Hilfe durch bewährte Naturheilverfahren* (Common cold and flu. Help through reliable alternative therapies). Oesch Verlag Zurich (Jopp/Oesch Programm)
148 Ivker RS (2002) Respiratory disease – sinusitis, upper respiratory infection, otitis media. *Clinics in family practice* 4 (4): 929–946

Index

The BAID-Series

Birkhäuser Advances in Infectious Diseases

Infectious diseases remain a substantial drain on human well-being and economies despite the availability of modern drugs. New pathogens emerge and known pathogens change their geographical distribution and their susceptibility to the available drugs. An understanding of the structure and function of infectious disease pathogens is a major scientific challenge with important potential applications.

This new cross-disciplinary monograph series will provide up-to-date information on the latest developments in infectious disease research. The multi-authored volumes will cover basic biology and biochemistry of pathogens as well as applied medical aspects and implications for public health and policy.

The contributions are written by leading infectious disease researchers and pharmaceutical scientists with a wide range of expertise.

The envisaged readership includes academic and industrial researchers in medicine and infectious diseases as well as clinicians and others involved in diagnostics and drug development.

Available volumes:

Coronaviruses with Special Emphasis on First Insights Concerning SARS, A. Schmidt, M.H. Wolff, O. Weber (Editors), 2005

The Grand Challenge for the Future. Vaccines for Poverty-Related Diseases from Bench to Field, S.H.E. Kaufmann and P.-H. Lambert (Editors), 2005

Community-Acquired Pneumonia, N. Suttorp, T. Welte, R. Marre (Editors), 2007

Poxviruses, A. Mercer, A. Schmidt, O. Weber (Editors), 2007

Pediatric Infectious Diseases Revisited, H. Schroten, S. Wirth (Editors), 2007

Comparative Hepatitis, O. Weber, U. Protzer (Editors), 2008

Influenza Vaccines for the Future, R. Rappuoli, G. del Giudice (Editors), 2008

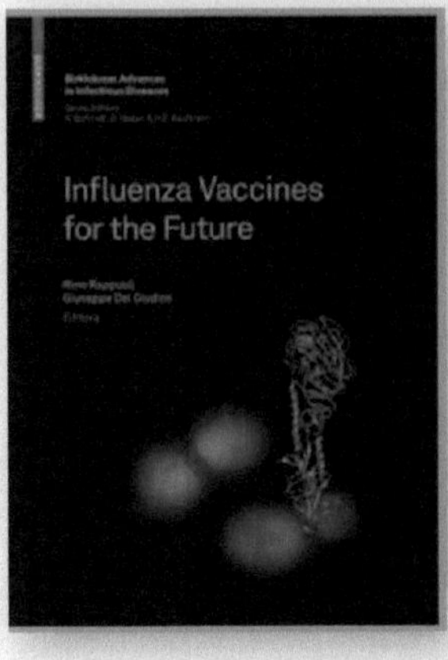

BAID – BIRKHÄUSER ADVANCES IN INFECTIOUS DISEASES

BIRKHÄUSER

Influenza Vaccines for the Future

Rappuoli, R., Del Giudice, G. (Eds),
both Novartis Vaccines, Siena, Italy

Rappuoli, R., Del Giudice, G. (Eds)
BAID
Influenca Vaccines for the Future
2008. 299 p. Hardcover.
ISBN 978-3-7643-8370-1

The threat constituted by the multiple outbreaks of avian influenza during the last few years is urgently calling for the development of new influenza vaccines. Fortunately, a quantum leap in technology has revolutionized the study of influenza and the engineering of new vaccine strains by reverse genetics. This volume provides a historical background and state-of-the-art information about the recent advances in the biology of influenza and the design of new influenza vaccines.

From the Contents:
Influenza virus: The biology of a changing virus.- Influenza vaccines have a short but illustrious history.- The epidemiology of influenza and its control.- Influenza and influenza vaccination in children.- The immune response to influenza A viruses.- Correlates of protection against influenza.- The role of animal models in influenza vaccine research.- Live attenuated influenza vaccine.- MF59: A safe and potent oil in water emulsion adjuvant for influenza vaccines, which induces enhanced protection against virus challenge.- Non-recent history of influenza pandemics, vaccines and adjuvants.- Waiting for a pandemic.- Modeling influenza pandemic and interventions.

www.birkhauser.ch

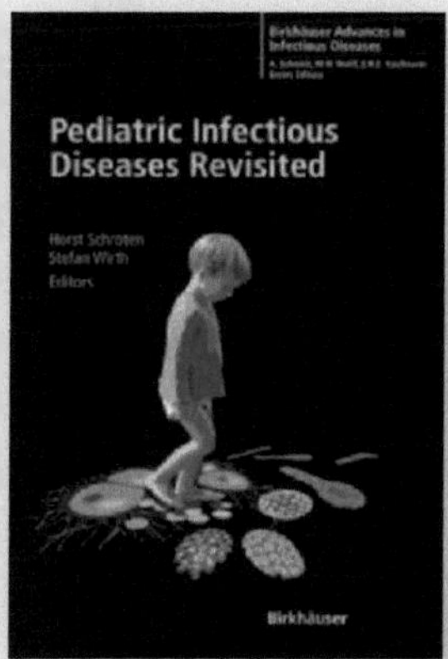

BIRKHÄUSER

BAID – BIRKHÄUSER ADVANCES IN INFECTIOUS DISEASES

Pediatric Infectious Diseases Revisited

Schroten, H., Universitätskinderklinik Düsseldorf, Germany / **Wirth, S.**, Helios Klinikum Wuppertal, Germany (Eds)

Schroten, H., Wirth, S. (Eds.)
BAID
Pediatric Infectious Diseases Revisited
2007. XIV, 503 p. 35 illus.
Hardcover
ISBN 978-3-7643-7997-1

The successful prevention of childhood diseases like diphtheria, tetanus and pertussis has made a major contribution to the improvement of public health, and vaccines and a variety of drugs are amongst the most fruitful applications of 20th-century research. Today pediatric infectious disease research is closely interconnected with other disciplines. Understanding the biology of the causative agents and the pathogenesis of disease is an essential step in achieving control and elimination of the diseases. Starting with historical, epidemiological and sociocultural issues, the volume presents clinical as well as molecular biological aspects of pediatric infectious diseases. New insights into the pathogenesis of infection are presented and an update on diagnostics, prevention and treatment of pediatric viral, fungal and bacterial diseases provided. The role of emerging new pathogens is also highlighted. The book aims at an interdisciplinary audience of clinicians and non-clinicians: pediatricians, infectious disease researchers, virologists, microbiologists, public health politicians and university libraries.

From the contents:
Global control of infectious diseases by vaccination programs.- Potential impact of rotavirus vaccination on the mortality of children in developing countries.- Controversially discussed indications for immunization.- Gonorrheal ophthalmia neonatorum: historic impact of Credé's eye prophylaxis.- Malnutrition and infection in industrialized countries.- Implications for early childhood development programs in developing countries.- ECC and childhood periodontal diseases.- Role of the blood-brain barrier and blood-CSF barrier in the pathogenesis of bacterial meningitis.- The molecular basis of paediatric malarial disease.- Kawasaki disease.- *Helicobacter pylori* infection in children.- Human metapneumovirus infection.- Avian influenza viruses: a severe threat of a pandemic in children?.- Human papillomavirus infections in children. - New treatments for hepatitis B and C.- Invasive fungal infections.- Pediatric aspects of bioterrorism.-Pediatric infectious diseases – Quo vadis 2015?

www.birkhauser.ch

MIX
Papier aus verantwortungsvollen Quellen
Paper from responsible sources
FSC® C105338

If you have any concerns about our products,
you can contact us on
ProductSafety@springernature.com

In case Publisher is established outside the EU,
the EU authorized representative is:
Springer Nature Customer Service Center GmbH
Europaplatz 3, 69115 Heidelberg, Germany

Printed by Libri Plureos GmbH
in Hamburg, Germany